T0339291

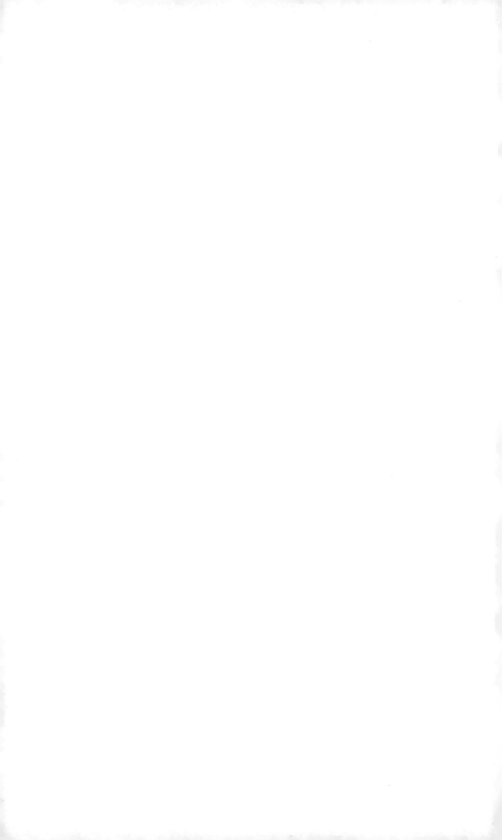

THE DIAGNOSTIC SYSTEM

JASON SCHNITTKER

THE DIAGNOSTIC SYSTEM

WHY THE CLASSIFICATION
OF PSYCHIATRIC DISORDERS
IS NECESSARY, DIFFICULT,
AND NEVER SETTLED

Columbia University Press

New York

Columbia University Press
Publishers Since 1893
New York   Chichester, West Sussex
cup.columbia.edu
Copyright © 2017 Columbia University Press
All rights reserved

Library of Congress Cataloging-in-Publication Data

Names: Schnittker, Jason, author.
Title: The diagnostic system : why the classification of psychiatric disorders is
necessary, difficult, and never settled / Jason Schnittker.
Description: New York : Columbia University Press, [2017] | Includes
bibliographical references and index.
Identifiers: LCCN 2016056249 (print) | LCCN 2017008748 (ebook) |
ISBN 9780231178068 (cloth : alk. paper) | ISBN 9780231544597 (e-book)
Subjects: LCSH: Mental illness—Diagnosis. | Psychodiagnostics.
Classification: LCC RC469 .S36 2017 (print) | LCC RC469 (ebook) |
DDC 616.89/075—dc23
LC record available at https://lccn.loc.gov/2016056249

Cover by Lisa Hamm

CONTENTS

ACKNOWLEDGMENTS

No book is the product of a single author, even a book that lists just one. My thinking on the *DSM* has changed over the years, but a number of colleagues have been especially helpful in recent years. Rob DeRubeis provided me with critical insights regarding cognitive-behavioral therapy, as well as RDoC. Owen Whooley provided me with some of his unpublished work, supplementing the great deal I had already learned from his articles in print. Robby Aronowitz has shaped my thinking on risk and much more besides. Other colleagues at Penn have been helpful, even though—or perhaps especially *because*—their interests do not center on mental illness, including Dave Grazian and Sam Preston. An especially rewarding aspect of studying mental illness is how the topic invites conversation with many different people who hold many different perspectives. I have regularly taught the Sociology of Mental Health at Penn, and, over the years, students in the class have shaped my thinking about the *DSM* in many ways. I am grateful for their input and enthusiasm. I am grateful, too, to Eric Schwartz, my editor, for his encouragement and his keen insights into what I was trying to accomplish. Finally, there is nothing nominal, contingent, or provisional about the encouragement of Julie and Claudia. Their support is beyond classification.

THE DIAGNOSTIC SYSTEM

1

THE CONTESTED ONTOLOGY
OF PSYCHIATRIC DISORDERS

The best place to start a discussion of psychiatric classification is with the people that psychiatric disorders affect directly. Consider two cases, both involving people at the boundary of formal classification. These cases are drawn from the American Psychiatric Association's most recent volume of clinical cases, designed to help mental health professionals learn more about the latest edition of the *Diagnostic and Statistical Manual*.[1] All of the cases in the volume are based on real people, though their identities have been disguised and their names changed. The cases are not necessarily typical of a disorder. Indeed, many were selected precisely to illustrate the ambiguities surrounding the manual's criteria. They are, however, illustrative, especially for those who must struggle with implementing the criteria. The first is Olaf Hendricks, a fifty-one-year-old father.[2] Olaf's daughter lives overseas, and she recently had a baby. Olaf would like to visit his grandchild, but he is severely anxious about flying. His anxiety began three years ago when the plane he was on landed during an ice storm. He has flown since that incident, but on his last complete flight he cried during landing and takeoff. Subsequent to that, when Olaf was scheduled to fly to his daughter's wedding, he ultimately refused to board the plane after arriving at the airport. His fear of flying affects more than his family life. It played a role, for instance, in his refusing to accept a promotion that would have involved significant travel. According to Olaf, his anxiety is limited to flying, though with some questioning his psychiatrist discovered that as a child Olaf feared being attacked by a wild animal. His earlier fear of animals was similar in its intensity to his current fear of flying, though it had dissipated because he now lives in a large city where encounters with wild animals are rare. According to the criteria in the *Diagnostic and Statistical Manual*, Olaf suffers from a specific situational phobia, in this case of flying. His disorder meets all the diagnostic criteria in the manual. It involves intense situational anxiety, it has caused significant distress, and it has caused significant functional impairment. In addition, Olaf also meets the diagnostic criteria for a specific phobia pertaining to animals, but, probably because he is unlikely to encounter wild animals in his current environment, that anxiety plays little obvious role in his life. The *DSM* permits this additional diagnosis, in part to allow for "significant impairment" that might be entirely unconscious; for example, Olaf might choose to live in a big city precisely to avoid wild animals. Olaf is not required to acknowledge or state this, however, for the psychiatrist to infer that it might matter.

The second case is Andrew Quinn, whose son recently died.[3] His son had suffered from depression and substance abuse and, after a struggle, died of an apparent suicide. Andrew visited his psychiatrist two weeks after his son's death, reporting that he felt life had lost its meaning. The psychiatrist continued to see him on a weekly basis in order to monitor his progress. His symptoms worsened over the next four weeks, with Andrew growing increasingly preoccupied with his son's death and ruminating over what he might have done differently. Andrew also reported the other symptoms that compose a depressive episode, including sleeplessness, fatigue, sadness, feelings of worthlessness, and a loss of self-confidence. Although these symptoms are recent and form the reason for Andrew's visit, there are other diagnostically relevant experiences in his history. Andrew had two prior episodes of depression, both occurring more than thirty years ago. According to the diagnostic criteria in the most recent *DSM*, Andrew is suffering from a major depressive episode. Although his symptoms are typical of grief and his son's death happened less than two months prior—well within the timeframe in which we might ordinarily still expect some grieving—the *DSM* emphasizes how depression that begins in grief can eventually grow "autonomous" of that experience and thus be regarded as indicative of a deeper problem.[4] Other features of Andrew's situation are relevant to discerning whether this is a case of clinical depression and not just bereavement. In particular, the risk of depression following grief is presumed to be higher for Andrew given his history of depression.

What do these two cases reveal? At one level they reveal something simple: how matters of formal diagnosis hinge on seemingly slight matters. Andrew's diagnosis hinges on what we regard as real depression and what we believe is an adequate time to grieve. Making a diagnosis also appears to depend on evidence of a preexisting risk, even if, as in Andrew's case, that risk appeared many years ago. With almost exactly the same experiences and symptoms, a person without a history of depression might be regarded as simply bereaved, not depressed, especially this soon after a son's death. Olaf's case raises similar issues. In particular, for Olaf there are two sources of anxiety, even though he is concerned about only one. In this case, too, the past is critical. The *DSM* allows for a diagnosis based on what Olaf experienced in the past. According to the *DSM*, a disorder might still be present even when it has no apparent symptoms. In this way, the *DSM* assumes authority over and above what Olaf himself recognizes or appreciates. These two cases also point to the importance of professional judgment in addition to the words and rules of a text. A reliable diagnosis requires that the psychiatrist use the *DSM* faithfully. Yet a diagnosis also requires that the psychiatrist exert a considerable amount of judgment. In Andrew's case, the psychiatrist must decide whether Andrew is really suffering from clinical depression, based on insights that probably stretch beyond the *DSM*. In particular, the psychiatrist must decide if the particular set of symptoms better describes grief or major depression, even though they are closely related. In Olaf's case, the psychiatrist must probe further to learn about Olaf's other fears, even if those fears have no obvious relationship with his current anxiety. What, though, compels a psychiatrist to use the *DSM* faithfully? And when presented with complex patients for whom a diagnosis requires reading between the lines, often based on issues that go well into a patient's past, will all psychiatrists make the same determination? Regardless of the details provided in the *DSM*, psychiatrists are still left wrangling with the meaning of its text when presented with actual patients.

This book is concerned with the ambiguities surrounding psychiatric classification, of which these examples illustrate only a few. I hope these two cases illustrate something else, too. Much of my discussion will be abstract, in the sense that I will focus on the principles guiding the creation and revision of psychiatric nomenclature. Much of my discussion, too, will pertain to aggregate-level data, including prevalence rates, correlations, and population averages. It is my hope, though, that readers will always keep in mind that these issues, in the end, are not abstract; they are personal. They are not about lists of symptoms; they apply to people who are suffering. And debates regarding the best classification systems ultimately seek to impose some sort of significance (or insignificance) over the day-to-day experiences of individuals. The ambiguity surrounding psychiatric classification is not, however, a simple or self-evident matter. It is rooted in the deep ambiguity surrounding mental illness, one that is hard to clarify with even the most scientifically credible diagnostic criteria.

THE DEEP AMBIGUITY OF MENTAL ILLNESS

Many illnesses are foreign to the experience of the average person. Epilepsy is serious for those who suffer from it, but most people will never have a seizure. Minor jolts to the head happen periodically, but a traumatic brain injury is severe and has lasting consequences. The flu is seasonal and pervasive, but there are many other diseases that will never infect the average person. Some symptoms are simply remote to our experience, even if we occasionally experience a hint of what lies just beyond the border.

Many of the core symptoms of mental illness, however, are familiar to virtually everyone. Furthermore, in the case of mental illness, differences between the sick and well can appear only a matter of degree. Most people, for example, might not regard themselves as "depressed" in any significant way, but the feeling of being sad or unmotivated is hardly unusual. In fact, such feelings are routine features of everyday life. They are characterized by a wide variety of idiomatic expressions far removed from any medical connotations, as when we say we are feeling "blue" or "downhearted." Similarly, most people might not panic in the face of something they fear, but virtually everyone can appreciate the unease of, for example, public speaking. At a minimum everyone can easily name those things they fear the most. And chances are your fears—whether of snakes, heights, or enclosed spaces—are shared by many other people. We might not even regard these experiences as symptoms at all and, instead, actively seek them out, as when people enjoy the pensive melancholy of music in a minor key.[5]

Perhaps there is a limit. Hallucinations might be regarded as the most severe kind of psychological symptom. Hearing voices when no one is around or seeing things that are not present represent especially bizarre experiences. And perhaps we can agree that such symptoms are the boundary, the point at which normal and abnormal part ways. Our commonsense view of the world allows only for externally generated auditory and visual cues. Yet even here the case is not so clear. Everyone appreciates the idea of a "delusion," and the word is used frequently. But the term is more complex than is suggested by the ease with which people deploy it. "Delusion" implies beliefs that are incorrect, and assessing when thoughts are faulty is difficult. "You're crazy" is an epithet, of course, but it is also an evaluation. It is an assessment of another person's motives, beliefs, or rationality, and the term is often used indiscriminately. Furthermore, hallucinations are not entirely uncommon, suggesting that the frequency with which something occurs provides no guidance regarding its normality. Many people can appreciate the feeling of dislocation, for example, that comes from not getting enough sleep. Indeed, some studies find that more than a third of people experience hallucinations of some kind in their lifetime, even if most of those experiences are not associated with any specific psychiatric disorder.[6] The symptoms of mental illness, then, are the "stuff of life."

Not only does the public have a reasonable sense about what the symptoms of mental illness feel like; it also has some intuitive grasp about what causes them. This, too, makes mental illness different from many other kinds of illness. The average person might have little sense about what causes epilepsy, for example, and so will seek the authority of an expert to diagnose it. Similarly, many people intuit that good and bad health "run in the family" and, thus, recognize the importance of genetic influences. Even so, people still leave the formal diagnosis of inherited conditions to professionals. For some things, like a broken bone, everyone understands the traumas that can cause it, but they still accept that the final determination of whether a bone is broken rests with an X-ray. For mental illness, the situation is quite different. The average person can easily appreciate the role of stress in feeling overwhelmed or maybe even depressed, without any sort of technological intermediary. The issue is not that such causes lack reality for being common. To the contrary, "everyday" causes gain credibility precisely because we appreciate how potent they are. The death of a loved one can produce profound sadness, one seemingly impervious to time and the support of friends. When individuals recognize themselves as suffering from depression they can almost always identify a precipitating cause and have little doubt about its significance. Science, too, has confirmed the reality of environmental causes of this sort, but the public has not waited for the insights of empirical research to draw its own conclusions.

Perhaps because the symptoms of mental illness are so common and explanations so easy to grasp, the concept of mental illness invites controversy. When everyone knows *something* about sadness—about what it feels like, about what causes it—claims of authority, even with respect to official diagnosis, can appear unnecessary or dubious. The public is quick to judge whether they think someone is "really" depressed, even as they withhold judgment about most other medical disorders. And when people are presented with so many potential causes of mental illness, the boundaries between what is or is not illness become porous. If sadness—even severe sadness—comes from living an ordinary life, how can depression ever be considered a disease? What sort of treatment could we deem absolutely necessary?

These debates are not merely matters of idle speculation. They have deep consequences. Parents struggle with whether to seek treatment for their misbehaving or underperforming children. Spouses struggle with the addictions of their partners. Policy makers struggle with how to provide health care to those who need it most. And psychiatrists struggle with crafting the most accurate diagnostic criteria. In the end, these concerns are concrete. The form of the question becomes personal: What causes my suffering? Do I have a problem, and, if so, what can I do about it? Questions of this sort are existential as much as medical. Formal diagnostic criteria are a different matter—the *DSM* provides some answers—but they have no less settled answers, and they, too, are at least partly a matter of philosophy.

CONTROVERSIES SURROUNDING FORMAL DIAGNOSTIC CRITERIA FOR PSYCHIATRIC DISORDERS

Formal diagnostic criteria for psychiatric disorders have existed for decades. They provide the "rules" for making professional diagnoses. They also provide the "catalogue" of relevant psychiatric symptoms. When applied correctly and consistently, formal diagnostic criteria are intended to produce a lingua franca for mental health professionals. They admit some experiences as symptoms but exclude others. They also provide thresholds and decision rules for adjudicating significance. *This* is what we regard as depression. *These* symptoms are significant. *This* is the point at which we say these symptoms reflect clinical depression rather than normal sadness.

Mental illnesses are real, but there is little that is settled about the classification of psychiatric disorders. This is perhaps especially so in the twenty-first century—a statement that would appear paradoxical given the advanced state of contemporary science but is not in light of the details of this science. Scientists continue to debate what psychiatric disorders are, what causes them, and even the degree to which they are significant in the lives of those who experience them. The pages of leading scientific journals are filled with new breakthroughs, but so, too, are they replete with ongoing controversies about what diagnostic criteria ought to be. Indeed, the controversies seem quickly to follow the breakthroughs. Even basic premises—ones scientists in a certain field might presumably agree upon—are contested. Discussing a study that reported a high prevalence of psychiatric disorders in the general population, for instance, Jerome Wakefield argues that the evidence for this claim, although based on popular and official formal diagnostic criteria, was premised on "invalid" measures that showed little fidelity to "true" disorders and wrongly included "normal" variation in distress.[7] Whereas most scientists who study cancer can agree on what cancer is and, given proper tests, can diagnose whether a person has it, no such consensus exists among those who study psychiatric disorders. There is perhaps a stubborn insistence on using the *DSM*, but, if anything, the science of psychiatric disorders has pushed the field further from consensus.

Even among those who can agree on what a valid measure of a psychiatric disorder is, there is controversy. At this point, for example, there is considerable evidence that genes play a role in mental illness. Studies of this sort are featured prominently in the news media, with outlets reporting, for example, the discovery of a gene for depression, a gene for alcoholism, or a gene for autism. These claims are provocative, but behind the bold headlines there remains a lot of debate. New studies routinely overturn previous ones. Even when researchers can agree generically that there are genes—if not *a* gene—for a disorder, they rarely agree on every single gene that is relevant or even on the scope of the list. Moreover, mounting evidence suggests that the genes underlying one disorder might underlie many other disorders as well. The genes for depression, for example, might be the same as the genes for anxiety. The further science progresses, the less focused genetic influences seem to be—and to some critics the more ephemeral the nature of psychiatric disorders appears. Like a mirage, a final and settled scientific understanding is continuously receding over the horizon.

Occasionally these debates assume a fervid character. Scientists argue, as they always do, but in some debates they *fight*. Even parties that would otherwise seem to be united in their efforts have drifted further apart over time. Consider, for instance, the architects of the various versions of the *DSM*. The form of the *DSM* has changed little over time, and some might regard the various revisions—especially between immediately consecutive editions—as mere updates. Yet a chairman of the taskforce behind the fourth revision of the *DSM* recently disparaged the authors of the fifth. And he did so in no uncertain terms. The title of his book reveals his standpoint: *Saving Normal: An Insider's Revolt Against Out-of-Control Psychiatric Diagnosis, "DSM-5," Big Pharma, and the Medicalization of Ordinary Life.*[8] Not only is there disagreement about the *thing* that scientists interested in mental illness should actually study, there is also, it would appear, debate and doubt about whether that thing is good to study at all.

It is tempting to regard these controversies as transitory. Some might argue that it is better to consider the *trajectory* of science, which clearly shows progress if not a solution to some longstanding problems. The argument goes something like this: Yes, there is controversy surrounding genetic influences, especially regarding the precision of their effects, but no one really doubts that genes play *some* role. And soon, because there is a natural evolution to scientific knowledge, we will have better treatments, better classifications, and a much better understanding of what causes suffering. All the current controversies derive from an unsettled understanding of what psychiatric disorders are. Eventually, though, the nature of mental illness will be revealed.

This is a popular line of thought, and it is easy to appreciate the aspirations behind it. Some aspects of the contemporary science surrounding psychiatric disorders do indeed feel revolutionary. One thing that distinguishes the present era from earlier ones, for instance, is the overwhelming optimism surrounding the explanatory power of neuroscience and the human genome. And, to be sure, research on the anatomical and molecular foundations of psychiatric disorders is promising. In the twenty-first century, scientists have an extraordinary number of new tools available to them and, thus far, have put them to good use. Science can now explore the functioning of the brain with high resolution and, in so doing, has discovered real differences between the brains of those who suffer from psychiatric disorders and those who do not.

But enthusiasts generally have something more in mind than simply good science. According to some, contemporary science has the potential eventually to eliminate the cultural baggage that still clings to the concept of psychiatric disorders. In this vein, they see the study of mental illness moving toward the clinical ideal that is already in place for other illnesses. Thomas Insel, a former director of the National Institute of Mental Health, sees a revolution underway.[9] He argues that this revolution will fundamentally transform diagnostic classification from a guessing game into an objective enterprise. Recognizing the controversies of the past but looking forward to the future, he joins with others in urging scientists to "set [their] sights higher" and aim for "precision" medicine.[10]

It is tempting, too, to regard public beliefs as evolving in much the same fashion as science. In many respects, public beliefs regarding mental illness are more sophisticated than they were in the past. Thirty years ago the representation of people with mental illness in the media was hardly flattering, and the stigma surrounding psychiatric disorders was strong. Many of the public's beliefs betrayed a level of ignorance that is hard to imagine today. In 1972, Thomas Eagleton withdrew as George McGovern's vice presidential running mate over concerns regarding his earlier treatment for depression. Today, having received treatment for a psychiatric disorder is perhaps less concerning. Indeed, if taking psychiatric medications was summarily disqualifying, there would be far fewer capable politicians and professionals. In addition, public-opinion data reveal a more attuned and responsive culture. Whereas the public was once ill informed, it is now knowledgeable. The public is increasingly adopting the biomedical model of mental illness, for instance, accepting the idea that psychiatric disorders have biological causes. Furthermore, the idea that people are personally responsible for mental illness has receded. For example, the public is less likely to attribute alcohol abuse to personal character or weakness, accepting it, at least in part, as a disease. In short, the argument goes, science and culture can and will evolve together, together fomenting a medical approach. Whatever misconceptions the public had in the past, they are merely reflections of an imperfect understanding, which can be remedied with education.

THE FRAMEWORK OF THE DIAGNOSTIC SYSTEM

In this book, I ask us to take a step back. Let me be clear about what I mean. I will not ask us to ignore fifty years of progress. In fact, this book will discuss the contemporary science of psychiatric disorders in some detail and with approval. Nor will this book ask us to entertain the possibility that a much earlier era was, in some sense, a more tolerant one. Michel Foucault famously questioned whether the modern approach to psychiatric disorders was superior to the premodern one, wondering, in particular, whether regarding a psychiatric disorder as an illness was truly better than regarding it as, say, a product of divine intervention or as simply an unremarkable expression of the natural order.[11] Nor is this book another critique of the *DSM*, at least not in a narrow sense. To be sure, I will review the controversies surrounding the *DSM* up to its latest iteration, but I do so not to argue that one side of a debate is superior to another but rather to illustrate how the *form* of the controversies surrounding the *DSM* has remained consistent over time. In addition, I also hope to show how some debates regarding the best classifications rest more on differences in first principles than on differences in empirical matters. In this way, this book will focus on the social, cultural, and scientific conditions that have set the stage for prolonged controversy, whether in earlier eras, in the present one, or, in all likelihood, in future eras as well. Another way to put this is to say this book adopts a more *meta* approach to the issue of classification, casting a wide eye on the many different parties and interests involved.

This book seeks to answer three related questions: why the classification of psychiatric disorders is so difficult, why it is necessary to classify in the first place, and what problems (and solutions) follow from the kinds of classifications we create. Answering these questions requires a capacious and multidimensional approach, which this book advances in a couple ways. For one, it explores definitions of mental illness from the standpoint of different stakeholders. It looks at what diagnostic criteria are and how they were developed, focusing naturally on the *DSM*. It also explores how *clinicians* think about psychiatric disorders. It then explores how *scientists* think about mental illness. At the same time, though, this book takes seriously what the *public* thinks about mental illness. Indeed, this book takes as its starting point that these different standpoints—from the lay to the expert, the impressionistic to the scientific, and the general to the specific—cannot be entirely segregated. The science of psychiatric disorders, for example, proceeds from how clinicians define disorders. And controversies surrounding how the public understands mental illness have corollaries in debates surrounding how scientists conceptualize mental illness. Mental illness sits within a remarkably large public sphere, and partly for that reason, it resists any sort of consensus.

At the same time, this book focuses on what different groups *do* with diagnoses. It focuses on the production of the *DSM* and the rules it contains, but, perhaps more importantly, it focuses on the *reception* of the *DSM*. Much has been made about how the *DSM* is useful, but answering the question of useful *for whom* and *for what reasons* makes the pragmatic aspects of the *DSM* more complicated and also makes appeals to crafting useful diagnostic criteria less compelling. This focus on how the *DSM* is received by different groups also helps us think about the various critiques of the *DSM*. Rather than assume the significance of formal diagnostic criteria a priori —that is, assume that the *DSM* is hegemonic in its influence across many domains—this book is concerned with how diagnoses are used and what significance or insignificance different groups attribute to them. Much of the debate surrounding the *DSM* naturally focuses on how it has been produced and the principles that have guided it. These controversies are ongoing, and there is no doubt they are significant. Controversies inhere to the text itself—what sentences and paragraphs are revised, what disorders are added, and what disorders are dropped—and for good reason. The *DSM* is regarded as the bible of modern psychiatry, and, befitting the analogy, many regard its criteria as sacrosanct. But a study of the Bible is not the same thing as a study of the church, the clergy, or the laity. This book focuses on the afterlife of the *DSM* and, in effect, the many different forms of apostasy. It explores the social, clinical, and scientific consequences of the *DSM* critically and in detail, providing a ledger of sorts. It examines, for example, how clinicians actually use the *DSM* in their daily practice. It also explores what patients do when they receive a diagnosis (and, before that, how they decide whether to seek a diagnosis in the first place). We can study what psychiatric disorders truly are, and we can debate what they ought to be, but it is important not to overlook the actual consequences of formal diagnostic criteria as they are written. In this book, I will try to provide a more complete ledger of these consequences, both positive and negative, and in so doing I hope to address whether our fears regarding the *DSM* (not to mention our hopes) are realized or not.

THE STRUCTURE OF THE CHAPTERS

The structure of the book will play an important role in the development of my argument. The book starts in the next chapter by exploring the origins of the *DSM*, focusing in particular on its third revision. It will also consider the most recent revision, the fifth (with periodic mention of the others), but it focuses on the third because that revision set the form for the revisions that followed. In chapter 3, I will explore the descriptive science of psychiatric disorders as those disorders are defined in the *DSM*, followed in chapter 4 by the various proposals regarding how best to revise the *DSM* further in light of what that descriptive science revealed. This sequence implies a certain circularity between classification and science, and these chapters will elaborate on their imperfect and recursive interface in some detail. As a way of thinking about this problem, most of my discussion will focus on the principles, goals, and intentions of a classification system like the *DSM*.

Then I dig deeper. In chapters 5 through 8, I will turn to the reception of the *DSM*: not what diagnoses are in description or intent but how they operate in actuality and practice. In this regard, I will begin with a natural starting point, discussing how mental health professionals use the *DSM*. There is no doubt that clinicians are interested in providing accurate diagnoses and that patients, too, are interested in learning exactly what is wrong with them. The *DSM* is critical to this task and so helps satisfy patients and clinicians alike. Yet mental health professionals do not use the *DSM* with perfect fidelity. The relationship between the use of mental health services and whether patients actually meet the formal diagnostic criteria for a psychiatric disorder is quite weak. Furthermore, clinicians tend to depart from formal diagnostic criteria in predictable ways, premised on a prototype they have in mind and not necessarily the sort of prototype detailed in the *DSM*. In this way, the *DSM* is not a binding document when it comes to clinical practice, although it is, nonetheless, a powerful one.

I turn in chapter 6 to how the public uses the *DSM* as well as to how it uses psychiatric concepts more generally. In this vein, I will discuss public beliefs about mental illness. I will also discuss how the public comes to regard diagnoses—which are essentially only names—as explanations. The *work* of a diagnosis—the meaning it harbors and the light it sheds—is significant for the public. Diagnoses illuminate experiences, and they help create new identities for individuals. But there is a potential shadow falling behind the light. Some observers, for example, fear that formal diagnostic criteria can artificially create the disorders they are merely meant to describe. They worry, for instance, about false epidemics, the problem of false positives, and diagnostic creep. Furthermore, some fear the *DSM* has created an overly therapeutic culture, one intolerant of individual differences and that incorrectly regards social problems as medical ones. Although most sociologists no longer regard labels as the central cause of mental illness, labels do play a role in how mental illness is experienced. For instance, clinical diagnoses of autism have increased precipitously over time. Has the "true" prevalence of autism increased as well? The use of antidepressants has, likewise, increased much more than the prevalence of depression would seem to have increased. How are we to regard these facts? Have the diagnostic criteria for mental illness somehow been unleashed into the larger culture, encouraging the encoding of normal suffering as full-blown illness? Can the profession of psychiatry no longer contain its diagnostic authority? It is important to be precise in our discussion of these issues. This book will entertain the possibility of labeling, as well as related issues such as looping, but it will do so in light of empirical evidence. The public certainly *uses* psychiatric diagnoses—in fact, the language of formal psychiatric nomenclature is suffused throughout popular culture, and the ascendance of psychiatric thinking can be linked directly to the publication of the *DSM*—but it is not clear that the public is unequivocally enthusiastic about diagnoses or that it embraces the *DSM* without qualification.

Chapter 7 explores how scientists use the *DSM*. Although earlier and later chapters explore this issue as well, chapter 7 focuses on how scientists have approached the dilemma stemming from both using the *DSM* as a requisite tool for their research and recognizing its many limitations. This chapter, then, provides a more focused account of the use and misuse of the *DSM* in scientific settings, rather than a report of the findings of science, as discussed in chapter 3.

In chapter 8, I move to the broadest possible level—I explore how cultures use psychiatric diagnoses. Any discussion of culture is, of course, related to a discussion of the public—a culture is, after all, made up of people—but I intend to show how cultures operate with their own prerogatives and interests, many of which are independent of the mission of the *DSM*. Scientists frequently talk about how the *DSM* "reifies" diagnostic criteria, creating disorders that appear real in a formal sense but for which the underlying foundation is weak. Institutions perform a lot of the work of reification, and it is important to understand how they do so. More generally, though, diagnoses serve a variety of functions for a culture. They demarcate who is responsible for addressing certain behaviors. They shape how distress is expressed and determine which are regarded as the most credible symptoms of a disorder. They also, in some instances, serve as a conduit for the expression of power. In chapter 8 I explore the consequences of the *DSM* for how cultures think about and write about suffering.

The next two chapters turn to the contemporary science of psychiatric classification, discussing, in this case, something more than descriptive science: I discuss what science has to say regarding what psychiatric disorders might actually be. Chapter 9 provides a broad overview of the natural and social-scientific evidence regarding psychiatric classification, and chapter 10 discusses why searching for more "valid" psychiatric classifications is so difficult and why the issue of validity is unlikely to be resolved using even the best empirical and scientific tools. Chapter 11 ends with a synthetic overview of the contradictions of the diagnostic system. It also provides principles for thinking about the next revision of the *DSM*.

Proceeding step by step across these different aspects of psychiatric classification is useful for illustrating a number of things. For one, it illustrates the sharp discontinuity between what we intend psychiatric diagnoses to accomplish and what they actually do. Furthermore, it illustrates where the controversies surrounding the *DSM* come from and, ultimately, why they are unlikely to be resolved any time soon. I regard the actors described in these chapters as composing an ecology of diagnosis, in reference also to how these actors interact (or not) with one another.[12] The controversies surrounding psychiatric disorders reflect, I will argue, the contradictions and tensions embedded in this ecology and the inability of any single classification system to resolve all of these tensions simultaneously. I will also argue that this ecology explains why a focus on a single sector is incomplete. For instance, a focus on the science of psychiatric disorders will not necessarily produce insights that lend themselves to better revisions of the *DSM*, especially insofar as different actors have very different views about what a "valid" diagnosis looks like. Validity, unfortunately, is not given in nature, revealed once and for all when we discover the right tools. On the flip side, the criteria provided in the *DSM* are used by clinicians but do not always provide diagnoses that are appropriate for science. Controversies flow from other points of intersection as well. People rely on psychiatric diagnoses to make sense of their experiences, but formal diagnoses do not always serve this purpose well. Despite the promise of a more objective view of mental illness, for instance, scientific progress is not producing a uniformly more tolerant public. A genetic approach to psychiatric disorders serves science well, but the public sometimes becomes *less* tolerant when it regards mental illness as deeply rooted in biology.

My emphasis on the ecology of diagnostic classification has other implications. Although many have critiqued the power of the *DSM*, referring to its "tyrannical" aspects (if still couching it as a benevolent tyrant), I intend to show that the *DSM* is nestled in a system of checks and balances that transmute and blunt its influence.[13] The *DSM* is fundamentally useful, even if it is not perfectly valid relative to the biological entities we can now identify. This implies a good deal of flexibility and uncertainty in classification. But the fact that clinicians, scientists, and the public use diagnostic classifications in their own particular ways and to their own ends is not in itself a problem. Indeed, it ought to alleviate some of the pressure the authors of the *DSM*—or even the scientists who try to help them craft better criteria—feel to derive the best possible classification over all possible considerations. Furthermore, there is incommensurability embedded in how clinicians, scientists, and the public use psychiatric diagnoses. It is difficult to envision a time when science might serve as the ultimate arbiter of these differences and resolve all the contradictions in a way that satisfies everyone.

An emphasis on the ecological setting of diagnoses also highlights the importance of *judgment*, something that has perhaps been elided in recent years. Despite the optimism surrounding genes and neuroscience, the contemporary science of psychiatric disorders does not provide unambiguous insights regarding the nature of psychiatric disorders. Nor does it absolve scientists and clinicians of the difficult task of making decisions about what psychiatric disorders are. Decisions of this sort involve many considerations. They involve values, competing interests, and public interest. They also involve *choices*. We might regard science as the unassailable authority on what psychiatric disorders are, but it is difficult or impossible to split scientific evidence from all the other issues that psychiatric disorders intersect with. It is difficult, for instance, to impose objective criteria over symptoms that are, in their essence, *subjective.* It is also difficult to produce accurate diagnostic criteria when validity can be evaluated in numerous ways. Some recent controversies reflect an implicit acknowledgment of this tension even as scientists have seemingly sought to obviate it. For instance, the recently proposed Research Domain Criteria (RDoC), emerging from the National Institute of Mental Health, is explicit in attempting to cleave the science of psychiatric disorders—that is, attempts to understand "real" disorders based on biological and neurological evidence—from the normative aspects of psychiatric disorders—that is, discussions of values or debates regarding what is or is not "normal." The RDoC also attempts to minimize some of the cultural aspects of the *DSM*, including, especially, its dependence on subjectively reported symptoms. In particular, the RDoC attempts to circumvent reliance on verbal reports, such as "I feel depressed," by using neuroanatomical traces of that emotion instead. But such efforts raise larger questions about what we as a society are prepared to regard as the most authoritative signals of experience. Prioritizing the signals of the brain over the reports of a person involves complex tradeoffs.

There is a reason the title of this book refers to the diagnostic *system*. As I am sure the reader has already discerned, the title is a double entendre: When most people think of a diagnostic system in the context of mental illness, they almost certainly think of the *DSM*. But in using the title, I am hoping for an additional connotation: By diagnostic system I am referring to how the entire diagnostic enterprise, including but not limited to the *DSM*, is situated in a complex social and cultural ecology. A system, too, implies some sort of organization or persistence, even when haphazard in appearance.

Some other terms are useful to define up front, in part because their definitions get to the heart of the matter. A *diagnosis* refers not only to the formal diagnostic criteria that define a psychiatric disorder but also to the application of those criteria to a person. The word is a noun, but it can be converted to a verb. A person receives a diagnosis, and a clinician diagnoses a disorder. Other terms refer to psychiatric classification per se and not to its application.[14] Ultimately I am interested in describing *classification*, that is, the procedures used for constructing categories of psychiatric disorder. A *classification system* provides a framework for organizing different entities.[15] A *taxonomy* is a more precise term. It refers to the *theory* that guides classification, allowing entities to be arranged according to deeper features of similarity. It refers, then, to the logic of a classification system or to the abstract principles that guide it. The term *nosology* is the clinical equivalent of the more general concept of a taxonomy. It refers to the classification of diseases in particular, rather than the many other entities that can be organized under a taxonomy, such as species. It turns out, though, that even seemingly clear taxonomies, like those for species, struggle with some of the same issues as the *DSM*.

Defining these terms foreshadows some of the distinctions that will later emerge as important. The next chapter, for example, describes the *DSM* as a classification system. It discusses the *DSM*'s underlying philosophy and principles. Yet I want to be clear that even as a classificatory *system* the *DSM* is far from a formal *taxonomy*. The theory underlying the *DSM* is generally quite superficial, even though the principles guiding it were well thought out and well intentioned. The next chapter also describes the process by which the *DSM* has been written and revised. Here, too, the lesson is less one of gradual improvement than of ongoing renegotiation among interested parties. Although the manual is now more than thirty years old, a review of the *DSM-III* is the best place to start a discussion of the contested ontology of psychiatric disorders.

2

WHAT DIAGNOSES ARE

DSM-III and the Form of Contemporary
Psychiatric Diagnoses

Although it is difficult to determine what mental illness is in nature, it is not at all difficult to define mental illness operationally. In the United States, psychiatric diagnoses are based on the *Diagnostic and Statistical Manual of Mental Disorders*.[1] The *DSM* is currently in its fifth edition, which I will discuss in more detail later. Perhaps the most important revision in the history of the manual, however, was *DSM-III*, which set the form—if not the content—that subsequent revisions have adhered to. The publication of *DSM-III* was a watershed moment in the history of psychiatry, and the manual still represents the strongest statement regarding what psychiatric disorders are.

In its essence, the *DSM* is little more than a catalogue of symptoms. The manual is overlaid with decision rules regarding the number of symptoms that constitute a disorder. Furthermore, disorders are organized along axes of similarity. The *DSM* also provides a general definition of mental disorder, designed to set the theme of the criteria. Yet the essence of the *DSM* is its assorted specific diagnostic criteria, which can be appreciated on their own. The *DSM* contains a wide variety of disorders and, naturally, contains an even wider variety of symptoms. Indeed, its editions have grown in size with each consecutive revision. The first contained 128 diagnoses. The second contained 193. Both editions were well under two hundred pages and, in fact, the second edition was shorter than the first, consisting of many pages consisting only of numerical codes denoting otherwise undescribed disorders. These editions of the *DSM* received little attention apart from professionals, and even for them, the manual was regarded as little more than a reference. With the third edition, however, the number of diagnoses jumped to 228, and the manual spread to 494 pages.[2] The upward trend has continued since. *DSM-III-R* was regarded as only a slight revision of *DSM-III* (hence it lacks promotion to a new roman numeral), but it, too, introduced many new disorders. It contained 353 diagnoses spread over 567 pages. Seven years later, *DSM-IV* contained 383 diagnoses over a remarkable 886 pages (which was followed by a text revision, referred to as *DSM-IV-TR*). *DSM-5* was published in 2013 and contained 541 diagnoses over 947 pages.

The *DSM* is routinely referred to as the "bible" of psychiatry. Yet for a document of such material heft and apostolic significance, it is constructed using a relatively small number of principles. Before discussing these principles, it is important to appreciate the deeper historical and scientific context in which *DSM-III* was written. *DSM-III* was crafted to solve a number of practical problems and should, in the first instance, be appreciated for how well it solved them. Although I will return to the fear and ambiguity surrounding the *DSM*, from at least one important standpoint, *DSM-III* was a clear and unambiguous success.

A BRIEF HISTORY OF *DSM-III*

The guiding principles behind *DSM-III* did not emerge in a vacuum. In fact, they reflected a very long history, a lot of professional circumspection, and a broader cultural context that pushed the revision process further along its path. For all the attention psychiatric disorders receive in the twenty-first century, the need to name and categorize disorders is quite old. Indeed, even the idea that classification should fundamentally be used to meet certain administrative ends is old. In the middle of the nineteenth century, for instance, the U.S. census recorded "the idiotic and insane" as a single class, doing so in order to enumerate those who might be dependent on the state.[3] This category was later revised in order to count only the "insane" (the "idiotic" were counted in another way), and, later still, the insane category was split into more fine-grained groups. Although among the people working on the census there was support for splitting the category further, there was little consensus about what the appropriate subgroups ought to be. The initial pass included disorders that are similar to those used today, including mania, melancholia, dementia, and epilepsy, but that hardly included the full variety that would materialize in the twentieth century.

The modern *DSM* reflects the same instinct to categorize and avoid crude groupings, but it pushes in an even more granular direction. *DSM-III* is especially emblematic in this regard. *DSM-III*, published in 1980, represented a significant departure from *DSM-I* and *DSM-II*, published in 1952 and 1968 respectively. Much of the dissatisfaction surrounding these initial editions reflected something similar to what earlier eras saw in the category of "insane." The category was regarded as crude and as poorly matched to the specificity required of the modern and sophisticated clinical enterprise. The initial versions of the *DSM*, likewise, did not provide explicit diagnostic criteria, even if they provided lots of names for specific disorders, leaving the clinician responsible for defining the disorder. In *DSM-II*, for instance, manic-depressive illness (a precursor to bipolar disorder) was described in terms of "severe mood swings and a tendency to remission and recurrence," with additional short descriptions provided for three different subtypes.[4] At the time, clinicians perhaps had a strong intuition about what manic-depressive illness looked like, whether through training or experience, but a detailed description was plainly not provided in the *DSM*. Similarly, the main symptoms of involutional melancholia (a precursor to what is now termed a major depressive episode) were listed simply as "worry, anxiety, agitation, and severe insomnia."[5] In this case, the description of melancholia is richer than manic-depressive illness—it at least described four symptoms—but it still provides little in the way of specific criteria. In total, all major affective disorders—a category essentially synonymous with what is now referred to as mood disorders—were described in about two pages.[6]

This cursory discussion might appear odd or even careless, especially to contemporary audiences. With all the current debate regarding, for example, whether someone is *truly* depressed, or whether depression is a *real* disorder, or how many different *types* of depression there are, how could the primary professional organization for psychiatry provide its practitioners with such limited guidance? How could they be so seemingly unable—or perhaps unwilling—to describe a disorder's core features? The answer reflected more than the profession's faith in the acumen of its practitioners. Indeed, at the time there was little consensus regarding the characteristics of psychiatric disorders. Opinions varied even about whether diagnosis per se was important. Early editions of the *DSM* reflected this uncertainty and indifference. In being so opaque, the *DSM*, in effect, permitted and even encouraged a variety of perspectives and definitions. It allowed clinicians to infer what a patient suffered from. Moreover, the profession felt little imperative to fix the *DSM*'s criteria or settle on one perspective or another. Among professionals, the act of diagnosis was not especially fraught or worrisome.[7] Their primary concern was, instead, providing patients with treatment and appreciating the idiopathic aspects of psychiatric disorder. Among clinicians there was little interest in discerning a disorder's typical features, lest they disregard the patient in front of them. What was typical was regarded as uninteresting, often for good reason. At the time many mental health professionals worked in hospital settings, where the patients they treated suffered from "obvious" psychiatric problems, or at least disorders that plainly required long-term in-patient care. Taken to an extreme, the art of diagnosis was regarded as little more than a superficial act of applying a convenient label to a plainly troubled person. If there was a tendency to classify at all, it was more consistent with "splitting" diagnoses into finer units, rather than "clumping" disorders into larger bins. Even in more conventional office-based settings, which were becoming more prominent as a site of treatment, diagnosis was superficial. It was dispensed with quickly, and, in the end, the diagnosis was regarded as little more than vaguely descriptive, often made for purposes of satisfying some outside audience rather than anything internal. In short, the *case*—the patient, his or her symptoms, history, and challenges—was more important than the disorder.

The emphasis on the idiopathic aspects of disorder also reflected the dominance of psychoanalysis in outpatient settings. As a system for explaining the origins of mental illness, psychoanalysis also spoke to how disorders manifested. Among its precepts was that the same underlying conflict could produce symptoms spanning many types of disorder, some symptoms related, for example, to depression, others to anxiety, and still others to impulsive behavior. In this context, the role of the analyst was to uncover and treat the underlying *conflict*, rooted in, for example, family upbringing, rather than focus on the mere surface features. Symptom-based diagnosis per se was not terribly informative. A diagnosis alone could not reveal the conflict, and it might very well mislead the analyst, insofar as rendering a single diagnosis mitigated against a more synthetic approach. In this respect, the root was seen as far more important than the branch.

At the time, the relevance of psychoanalysis to diagnostic practice was mostly latent, but it became very apparent in light of the discipline's sharp resistance to *DSM-III*. Many psychoanalysts saw *DSM-III* not merely as too focused on the issue of diagnosis—a concern shared by clinicians of other orientations as well—but as wholly antagonistic to the psychodynamic approach. After the publication of *DSM-III*, Charles Brenner, a prominent American psychoanalyst, questioned in particular the diagnostic criteria for depression, citing the role of childhood conflicts in producing a variety of unpleasant emotions, only some of which were related to depression.[8] To him, *DSM-III* was misleading and unproductive. A diagnosis of depression might suggest something about a patient's defenses, he argued, but it did not actually reveal anything about the underlying problem and, thus, the real disorder. In the end, Brenner recommended dropping depression-related diagnostic terms altogether, and his feelings were likely shared by many other analysts.[9]

DSM-I was certainly more amenable to his tastes. *DSM-I*, published in 1952, included an especially expansive understanding of mental illness, with only weakly delimited borders. Most of the disorders were listed in short prose-based descriptions. To the extent that they included symptoms, they often referred to concepts that were part of psychoanalysis, such as reactions to psychosocial forms of stress.[10] Disorders that were not an obvious product of brain dysfunction were classified as "psychogenic" in origin, divided into those that were, for example, psychotic or psychoneurotic.[11] Yet even these categories were quite porous. Symptoms shared a concatenated flavor: Through a chain of influences, symptoms from different disorders were described as related to one another. Depression, for instance, was characterized as one of several psychological defense mechanisms experienced in light of anxiety.[12] In the end, *DSM-I* is perhaps more appropriately regarded as a brief statement about psychodynamic causes than as a diagnostic instrument per se.

Even those clinicians not wed to a psychodynamic approach saw little value in sharpening the *DSM*. The legacy of World War II loomed large over both *DSM-I* and *DSM-II*.[13] The psychological experiences of returning soldiers had subtly shifted the focus of psychiatry in ways that mitigated against diagnosis, even if those experiences also rendered some psychiatric disorders more real. The experiences of veterans suggested several things: that even "normal" individuals—those, for example, drafted into the conflict with no preexisting problems—could succumb to mental illness given sufficient trauma; that the symptoms of mental illness had psychological roots reflecting the individual's inability to adapt to his environment; that symptoms contained an underlying meaning, especially with respect to flashbacks; and that mental illness existed on a continuum of severity, with some soldiers experiencing only mild anxiety and others experiencing full-blown psychosis. The nature of combat-based trauma in particular also shifted diagnosis to the background and etiology to the foreground. When the focus is on variation in severity among at-risk people, diagnosis is secondary to treatment. Indeed, insofar as clinicians had gradations in mind, they considered earlier intervention—even before symptoms were present—as a good strategy for forestalling a slide into madness. This approach is not unlike how we regard intervening at "prehypertension" as a strategy to prevent full-blown hypertension: The end diagnosis is important, to be sure, but the insistence on prepositions betrays support for a continuum. At the same time, if symptoms are interpreted in light of a unique trauma, the symptoms are secondary: They can point to the underlying and far more significant problem. Under these conditions there might be little need to judge whether a veteran is truly experiencing "shell shock," for example, when their flashbacks alone suggest a problem that can be treated.

This situation reflects specific historical influences, but things changed. As the dominance of psychoanalysis faded, new concerns emerged. And, in this context, the limitations of *DSM-I* and *DSM-II* became clear. In the

1960s and 1970s, psychiatry was increasingly criticized for its lack of reliability, an abrupt shift from an earlier era that focused on variation in how disorders were manifest. Reliability is the idea that the same patient, if he has a real disorder, should receive the same diagnosis regardless of the clinician he sees. By the same token, a person who does not have a disorder should not be diagnosed with a disorder, regardless of the clinician who evaluates him. Reliability is consistency. A focus on unreliability might seem like an unusually specific critique to level at the *DSM*, especially in light of the more or less untroubled acceptance of *DSM-I* and *II*. Yet the issue of reliability is in fact closely related to concerns about the reality of mental illness. Over time it was becoming increasingly clear that psychiatric disorders might not be as real as they once seemed and that clinicians might not have the fine-grained expertise the public once presumed. Several studies made the case in especially vivid ways.

In a now famous study, David Rosenhan unveiled a remarkable and troubling instability in psychiatric diagnosis.[14] His research design was simple. He sent eight confederates to twelve different psychiatric hospitals. The confederates did not suffer from any psychiatric disorder but were instructed during the intake interview to complain of hearing voices. This insured a credible admission to the facility, but after being admitted the "pseudopatients" (as Rosenhan referred to them) were instructed to stop simulating any symptoms. All other biographical details of the pseudopatients were drawn from real life, though Rosenhan used pseudonyms to protect their identities (for good reason, as it turned out). The hospital staff was not informed about the presence of the pseudopatients or the nature of Rosenhan's study.

Assuming a reliable definition of what a psychiatric disorder is, or at least a strong prototype firmly in the minds of experienced professionals, the hospital staff should have been able to detect the presence of the pseudopatients just as easily as they should have been able to detect "real" patients. Even if *DSM-II* did not provide especially detailed diagnostic criteria, the nature of psychiatric disorder should have been sufficiently well understood to allow hospital staff to identify imposters. The pseudopatients were, after all, "sane," apart from their fabricated initial reports of auditory hallucinations.

And despite these limited initial symptoms—which are, to be clear, troubling in themselves—the clinicians should have been able to update their impressions enough to recognize the deception (or, barring that, at least to regard the once sick patients as cured). Yet not one of the pseudopatients was detected. To be sure, the pseudopatients were eventually discharged, but the average stay was more than two weeks, and all but one of the pseudopatients was discharged with a diagnosis of schizophrenia in remission. They were not diagnosed as cured and certainly not as an inappropriate initial admission. Their status as patients was never questioned—except occasionally by other patients. Put differently, the label "schizophrenic," for all intents and purposes, stuck. It was virtually impossible to eliminate.

In defense of the profession of psychiatry, it could be argued that the hospital staff operated with the reasonable presumption that everyone under their care suffered from *something*, even if it wasn't immediately apparent in their behavior. Hospitals, after all, treat the sick, not the well. And the pseudopatients were in fact admitted with a diagnosis of schizophrenia, which cannot be cured overnight and involves some ebb and flow in day-to-day symptoms. In a second study, however, Rosenhan flipped the design: He informed another hospital, one that was aware of his initial findings, that he had placed one or more pseudopatients in their care, and he asked if they could identify the patients. In fact, however, Rosenhan had placed no pseudopatients in the hospital. In this case, the task of the clinicians was more focused than it was in the earlier study: In effect, the clinicians were only asked to identify the sane rather than treat the sick. Yet here, too, clinicians did poorly. Of the 193 patients the hospital assessed during the window of Rosenhan's study, the staff reported—and with great confidence—that forty-one were pseudopatients, just over one in five patients. Rosenhan delivered his results with a flourish. He published his study in *Science*—perhaps the most prestigious journal in all the sciences, social and natural—with a title that revealed its essence: "On Being Sane in Insane Places."

This study represents a particularly vivid demonstration of the unreliability of psychiatric diagnoses, and Rosenhan was not reluctant to amplify its implications. Yet there was equally damaging evidence—albeit perhaps less *dramatic* evidence—coming from other studies as well. Indeed, there was reasonably compelling evidence published well before Rosenhan's work, including a study appearing in the late 1940s in a psychiatry journal.[15] This study explored agreement among three clinicians regarding thirty-five cases. Here, too, agreement was very weak. In about 46 percent of cases, clinicians could at least agree on a major *category* of disorder, but only in about 20 percent of cases could they agree on a specific diagnosis. Other studies pointed to cultural differences and, in so doing, revealed the importance of idiosyncratic prototypes over any stable understanding of mental illness. One particularly influential study along these lines found that when presented with vignettes depicting exactly the same symptoms of psychosis, American psychiatrists preferred a diagnosis of schizophrenia whereas British psychiatrists preferred a diagnosis of manic-depressive psychosis.[16] One interpretation of this finding is that culture exerts an unusual degree of influence, even over disorders that are so severe we might ordinarily regard them as transcultural. Another interpretation, though, is simply that diagnosis is a sloppy enterprise governed by local habits. This study, too, sent shudders throughout the profession of psychiatry. Evidence was mounting that something was missing at the core.

These studies were not published in a vacuum. Their influence and reception was abetted by a growing antiauthoritarian streak in American culture. Armed with clear evidence for unreliability among professional psychiatrists, critics required only a small step to impugn the entire enterprise of psychiatry. In the early 1960s, Thomas Szasz—perhaps the strongest antipsychiatry critic—took the next step and declared mental illness a "myth."[17] In an attempt to strip psychiatry of any credibility, especially any it had assumed simply from being affiliated with traditional medicine, Szasz contrasted physical disorders with mental disorders. Physical disorders, he argued, were real, often rooted in anatomical dysfunctions that could be identified. He conceded that mental disorders *could* exist in the same way, but only to the extent that they, too, were rooted in identifiable lesions or malfunctions of the brain. Without such evidence, Szasz argued, mental illness was merely an analogy in search of a reality. To Szasz, psychiatry sought to validate mental disorders by appropriating the form of physical disorders, but mental disorders had none of the actual content. Much of his argument was premised on the seemingly fluid nature of psychiatric classification, merged with an emphasis on biology as the ultimate arbiter of true illness. In this regard, he was not unlike many contemporary critics of the *DSM*, as I will discuss later. Yet Szasz added a much stronger focus on social control as the underlying motive of psychiatry—on this he truly was different. For him, diagnoses served authority figures more than patients. *Labeling*—the preferred term among critics, as it connotes the artificiality of diagnosis—occurred when professionals sought to exert some control over nonconformists who could not be designated as deviant through some other means, such as a criminal conviction. What we cannot describe as "bad," he argues, can be recast as "mad," to much the same effect. Although Szasz's ideas perhaps look extreme in retrospect—and his work is no longer a cornerstone of discussion—they haven't disappeared altogether. Modern critics of the *DSM* still emphasize the fundamental difference between mental illness and ordinary physical illness, and, indeed, the emphasis on biological forms of validity is the foundation for much of contemporary science's ongoing critique of the *DSM*.

Later, Thomas Scheff articulated a very similar argument, albeit one less committed to the idea that mental illness was a wholesale fabrication.[18] For Scheff, the symptoms of mental illness represented violations of "residual" rules, not quite against any laws or revealing an obvious physical disorder, but nonetheless symptoms that society was interested in treating and thereby controlling in some fashion. For both Scheff and Szasz, the underlying concern was partly one of unreliability. And, in this regard, their concerns were not so different from that of mental health professionals at the time. Psychiatrists, too, were bothered by the growing evidence of unreliability. Yet Scheff and Szasz differed from the mental health establishment in emphasizing how powerful institutions emerged to fill the breach left by weak diagnostic criteria. Despite the problems with unreliability, psychiatrists remained confident in their ability to treat patients, while in light of the same facts Scheff and Szasz saw only a morass of judgment and control. In the 1960s, these arguments were perhaps especially well received. In the presence of very flexible diagnostic criteria, seemingly ineffective treatments, and growing social unrest, it was easy to appreciate how an institution like psychiatry could be deployed as one arm of a much larger social-control enterprise.

Other aspects of the debate surrounding formal diagnostic criteria resonated as well. In the 1970s, gay rights advocates lobbied for the removal of homosexuality from *DSM-II*. In that edition of the manual, homosexuality was categorized as one of several "sexual deviations," a category designed for those "whose sexual interests are directed primarily toward objects other than people of the opposite sex, toward sexual acts not usually associated with coitus, or toward coitus performed under bizarre circumstances as in necrophilia, pedophilia, sexual sadism, and fetishism."[19] There were many concerns regarding the inclusion of homosexuality at all and especially within this diagnostic category, but among the most critical issues was the alignment of homosexuality with necrophilia and pedophilia. The American Psychiatric Association responded to these concerns, and they did so independent of other changes to the *DSM*. They voted to remove homosexuality from the manual in 1973, well in advance of the more wholesale revisions that would come with *DSM-III*. Furthermore, they did so at a time when homophobia was not altogether uncommon. Gay marriage is legal today and has been met with considerable public support, but at the time it is hard to imagine even 10 percent of Americans supporting gay marriage (or even regarding such a thing as conceivable). This is all to the American Psychiatric Association's credit, but for many critics the apparent progressivity of the association's decision betrayed something more damning: The mere existence of a diagnosis of this sort made the political dimensions of psychiatry clear. With homosexuality as a disorder—or, more generally, the diagnostic criteria's regular invocation of the term "bizarre" and its focus on coitus as the standard of sexuality—the *DSM* could hardly be regarded as above the fray, as beyond moral concerns, or as purely medical. The existence of homosexuality as a diagnosis opened up the possibility of seeing other diagnoses, too, as reflections of judgment about problems rather than objective statements about disorders. In fact, though, the integration of science in the *DSM* has never been straightforward.

PSYCHIATRY, SCIENCE, AND MEDICINE

Many of the controversies regarding diagnostic criteria would seem to be easy to address. Old diagnoses can be removed. More specific diagnostic criteria can be crafted. Vaguely described symptoms can be clarified. Moralizing can be clipped. Latent assumptions can be addressed once they are brought to light. Yet in the 1970s psychiatry faced other challenges that were not so readily remediated. For one, the status of psychiatry as a division of medicine was unstable. The foundations of a strong clinical science rest on its practitioners' ability to deliver effective treatments, not just render accurate diagnoses. Scientists studying psychiatric disorders hardly dismissed mental illness as a "myth," but they nonetheless recognized that they were standing on a weak classification system for the purposes of evaluating treatments. Clinical trials, for instance, rely on identifying a homogenous pool of subjects in order to test the effectiveness of pharmaceuticals for specific disorders. When testing a drug for the treatment of heart disease, for example, it is best to identify a group of people suffering from a typical case of heart disease and ideally *only* a case of heart disease. Otherwise it would be unclear what exactly the medication was treating (or not), and, in the end, drugs are approved for specific indications. But if the definition of major depression is poorly established, it is difficult to design a study that can meet the requirements of demonstrating specific effectiveness. The pool of study participants the scientist has identified as suffering from "depression," for example, might be suffering from a variety of other ill-defined disorders as well (or no disorder at all). A historical example of a clinical trial is useful for purposes of illustration. Two studies published in 1965 and 1966 tested the effectiveness of diazepam, one of the popular psychiatric medications in the treatment of anxiety (known by its brand name, Valium), relative to another pharmaceutical. In both studies, the description of the participants was a single sentence, describing, in one case, patients suffering from "anxiety states" and, in the other case, in a slightly more specific and differentiating fashion, patients "with symptoms predominantly those of anxiety and in whom an underlying depressive illness had been excluded."[20] In practice, researchers eventually recognized this problem with sample identification to the point that they coordinated with one another regarding a solution. They developed definitions and protocols to ensure some degree of homogeneity in what they were calling "depression." Yet these definitions were not derived from the *DSM* (or any other single authoritative document), and the availability of shared criteria of this sort varied from disorder to disorder. Shared criteria were certainly not available for all the disorders contained in the *DSM*.

In the end, the research enterprise remained highly idiosyncratic, and the science surrounding psychiatric disorders floundered. Results of one study could not be easily compared with another. A study could be promising but not easily reproduced in another setting. The literature, such as it was, did not develop in a cumulative fashion, and treatments, when found effective, were developed in a mostly ad hoc and occasionally entirely accidental fashion. Other parties were taking note of these problems. Throughout the 1960s and into the early 1970s the number of research grants awarded by the National Institute of Mental Health—ordinarily the primary source of funding for basic science regarding mental illness—declined by 17 percent.[21] In addition, the grants themselves grew smaller and, thus, less ambitious. The dollar amount of grant support, adjusted for inflation, declined by about 5 percent per year during this time period.

For similar reasons, psychiatry's interface with medicine was deteriorating. Psychiatry is a specialty within medicine, but its fit has never been seamless. Modern medicine relies on the notion of disease specificity. Disease specificity refers to the idea that diseases have their own ontology, which can be separated from the characteristics of the patient experiencing the disease. Cancer, for instance, is represented by malignant cells situated at a site. Because of its ontology, cancer has an identity apart from the patient. Even if two cancers share the same symptoms, the underlying pathology defines each illness uniquely. The prototype of a specific disease is, of course, infectious disease, for which the disease is known only when the pathogen is identified. Beyond involving specific pathologies, specific diseases imply specific etiologies, prognoses, and treatments. The idea of specificity allows for a more seamless integration between science and clinical medicine: Modern medicine works best when its targets are narrow. The most high-tech medicine, such as proton therapy, is regarded as cutting edge precisely because it is directed. Similarly, the best diagnostic tools are regarded as frontline because they allow the clinician to see pathologies they could not envision otherwise. Indeed, the entire enterprise of modern clinical medicine would not be possible without first accepting the idea of disease specificity. Physicians could not be well trained were it not for the fact that knowledge about disease can be thought of as typical and, therefore, as separate from the individual experiencing it.[22] When physicians learn the tools of their trade, they do so in terms of studying the pathology, course, and treatment of diseases.

DSM-I and *II* did not cohere well with the idea of specificity. For one, the *DSM* provided little in the way of an explicit classificatory scheme. To be sure, the *DSM* provided diagnostic labels and corresponding numerical codes, but it provided little in the way of actual descriptions of those disorders. The *DSM* was further out of sync because of its underlying model of disorder. At the time, the dominant mode of treatment for mental illness was psychotherapy. When properly applied, psychotherapy can be valuable, but its practitioners were increasingly viewed as *different* from standard physicians. Diagnosis was not terribly important in psychotherapy, but in clinical medicine it remained the cornerstone of treatment. The fluid application of psychiatric diagnoses was not limited to psychotherapists. Prior to the early twentieth century, much of the treatment of psychiatric disorders occurred in psychiatric hospitals, wherein diagnosis was seen as less important than maintaining order.[23] Further complicating matters was the inability of psychiatrists to link diagnosis to other aspects of care, including prognosis. Although the prognosis of many forms of cancer, for example, was reasonably well characterized, the prognosis of many psychiatric disorders was understood only in the most general terms. About all a psychiatrist could say was that a disorder was chronic. These limitations in knowledge complicated the patient-clinician relationship in ways that were not as apparent in the standard doctor-patient encounter. When seeking treatment for a psychiatric disorder, patients could not receive the same kind of information from a psychiatrist that they could from a physician about most other diseases. In a more prosaic way, clinicians were also having a difficult time communicating their craft to those who were paying the bills.

THE *DSM* AND HEALTH INSURANCE

For all the critical focus on psychiatry and psychiatrists, the *DSM* was, in fact, making a lot of people uncomfortable. Into the 1970s, psychotherapists were providing much of the care for mental illness, but the range of their responsibilities stretched beyond what many regarded as mental illness. They were providing care for an array of problems, many of which were thought of as beyond the remit of medicine, from treating troubled marriages to addressing thwarted careers. Addressing personal problems in a professional fashion is a worthwhile endeavor, but it invites controversy when it is conceived in terms of *medicine.* The skepticism was perhaps greatest among those paying for such medical services. And the number of people paying for those services was suddenly much larger than it was before. During the 1960s, health insurance companies began handling psychotherapy as a partially reimbursable expense. This was true of private insurers, who might be expected to provide a range of policies covering more or fewer procedures, but it was also true of public insurers including Medicaid, which began in 1965. For this reason, psychotherapy was increasingly coming under the scrutiny of state and federal governments.[24] Other government-sponsored social welfare programs, such as Supplemental Security Income, were involved with mental health issues as well. The widespread closure of psychiatric hospitals starting in the 1950s meant that more patients were seeking treatment in other settings, including community mental health centers. With growing treatment-unit expenses applied to ever more patients, insurers began to demand more accountability from providers. In the end, their skepticism was quite broad. They wondered, in the first instance, about the diseases they were paying to treat. It hardly escaped their attention that mental health was defined in a more opaque fashion than, say, diabetes. At the same time, they had little actuarial ability to forecast future expenditures, something that is critical for budgeting. They understood their anticipated expenses only in the broadest possible strokes. Insurers anticipated that treatment for psychiatric disorders would probably become more expensive over time, but they had little guidance in anticipating the number of people who might seek treatment. If entirely new diagnoses could be created easily, seemingly with little more than a stroke of the pen, the number of potential patients might grow well beyond the sort of slow and predictable growth insurers could ordinarily anticipate with respect to, for example, heart disease in an aging population. From a financial perspective, skepticism regarding psychiatric disorders is easy, especially when the manual of psychiatric disorders is as superficial in its appearance as was *DSM-II*. It is notable, though, that this skepticism continues today, with spending for mental health care being subject to more utilization review than physical health care, suggesting insurers remain reluctant to pay for anything and everything a mental health professional might prescribe.[25]

In addition to concerns about what they were paying for, insurers had concerns about *whom* they were paying.[26] Psychiatrists have been around for a long time. Psychiatry was a specialty within medicine as early as the 1920s.[27] Its practitioners were (and still are) trained in medical schools, and they practiced, at the time, mostly in psychiatric hospitals. But with the emergence of psychotherapy as the dominant mode of treatment, the field of mental health treatment was open to more competitors who were able to practice in a wider variety of sites. Some psychologists, for instance, could reasonably claim to have the qualifications and competencies necessary to perform psychotherapy.[28] In addition, social workers could claim to have at least some of the same skills and could certainly claim much of the same clientele. Social workers also vastly outnumbered both psychiatrists and psychologists.[29] Insofar as the common tool among all these professionals was some version of psychotherapy, broadly understood, the pool of potential providers and clients was large and diverse. Faced with this issue, insurers were in a bind. They could choose not to reimburse for certain services or for certain providers, but any such decision would require justification on the basis of what they regarded as real mental disorders and/or worthwhile treatments. Insurers could not expect to make such claims without a fight, even if there were strong budgetary forces compelling them to do so.

THE GUIDING PRINCIPLES OF *DSM-III*

It is in this context that the American Psychiatric Association (APA) set out to write *DSM-III*. The authors of *DSM-III* were well aware of all of these issues. Indeed, they had been dealing with them for years and had successfully negotiated the case of homosexuality recently. It is worth describing the revision process in detail in order to illustrate how the APA sought to quell some of the anxiety festering among its ranks, not to mention the pressures mounting from the outside. It is also worth reviewing the *human* dimensions of the process, if only because little of the writing of *DSM-III* was entirely impersonal. *DSM-III* is not a reflection of purely scientific matters or of univocal objectivity. The *DSM-III* was written by committee, with the presence of a strong leader who was surrounded by many allies. The first step of the process was appointing a chair. Robert Spitzer, a psychiatrist at Columbia University, was chosen for the role. Spitzer was a natural choice to lead the task force, which was effectively the steering committee for the operation. He was a natural for several reasons. He had worked on *DSM-II*, he had spent much of his academic career studying issues regarding the standardization of diagnosis, and he was well aware of the forces producing unreliability in diagnoses. He had also played a leading role in the removal of homosexuality from the *DSM*, demonstrating a good deal of leadership. The committee that Spitzer assembled tilted heavily toward medically oriented researchers, especially those interested in diagnosis, which was certainly not something every psychiatrist at the time focused on.[30] The committee consisted primarily of highly reputable scientists familiar with the research literature, but they also shared personal connections. Many had previously worked with Spitzer. By one count, ten of the nineteen task force members were drawn from the group of researchers Spitzer had been working with already.[31] At least in this regard, the committee was already in agreement on some important matters.

Given the many challenges facing psychiatry, it is difficult to imagine a revision that would satisfy everyone. Furthermore, it is difficult to imagine how a single *text* could solve problems that were partly institutional. The committee set to the task, however, and they were guided by a few principles. These included a focus on symptom-based diagnosis, an emphasis on categorical diagnoses, the development of specific diagnostic criteria, and the maintenance of a neutral stance regarding the causes of psychiatric disorders. Altogether these principles provided a remarkably clean solution to some of the challenges the committee faced. They were also adopted very early in the process, with essentially no controversy or even discussion among task force members.[32] As fine as these principles were—they can be articulated in a straightforward manner—they were enormously consequential. And once they were in place, the task of crafting better diagnostic criteria proceeded apace (and they continue to inform the subsequent revisions of the *DSM*). The principles are worth elaborating in detail because they will set many of the parameters of my later discussion.

SYMPTOM-BASED DIAGNOSIS

The *DSM* is based on symptoms, but it assumes that symptoms are significant because they provide clues regarding the underlying disorder. In absence of strong information about the underlying cause of mental illness, surface features provide the best indicators of the presence and nature of a disorder. The *DSM*, then, is roughly premised on the framework depicted in figure 2.1.

The figure presents major depression as an example, although the same framework applies to virtually all the disorders contained in the *DSM*. The key is the relationship between the symptoms and the disorder. The nine symptoms of depression, depicted in the square boxes, are what we observe and what the patient experiences. They are part, then, of the phenomenology of psychiatric disorders; they are what is present in the patient. But we are trying to diagnose whether the person has major depression, which is depicted in the large circle. Major depression itself cannot be observed directly, and so the symptoms are taken as the best signs of its presence. This

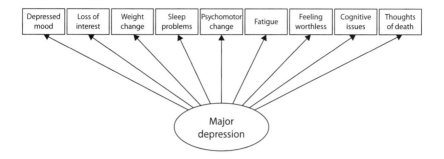

FIGURE 2.1 Major depression as represented by its symptoms.

framework has another implication, one that is perhaps less appreciated in the scientific literature but that stems naturally from a symptom-based focus. In this framework the symptoms are seen as resulting from the underlying disorder, a connection represented by the arrows pointing from the disorder to the symptom. These arrows represent causal relationships. Although the symptoms of depression can occur on their own—one can, of course, feel sad without suffering from major depression—when they occur together and simultaneously, they are regarded as having been caused by the entity that is major depression.

This framework represents the modern approach to psychiatric disorders, but it has a long intellectual lineage. Its most important forebear was Emil Kraepelin, a late nineteenth-century psychiatrist. Kraepelin believed that psychiatric disorders had unique symptom patterns, which, he insisted, must be carefully observed in order to distinguish different kinds of disorders. His ideas were controversial at the time but are remarkably uncontroversial today, as they fit neatly with the idea of disease specificity. Certainly those on the *DSM-III* task force found his ideas compelling, perhaps owing to how well his ideas advanced the goals of their project. Kraepelin's approach requires no inference regarding the underlying causes of a disorder—it fit squarely with the idea of being neutral regarding the underlying causes. A disorder might be neurological, chemical, or genetic, but diagnosing the disorder and rendering an accurate diagnosis, according to Kraepelin, required only close observation of its specific symptoms. Although it was not wed to the goal of uncovering causes, Kraepelin's approach was still scientific in the sense that it demanded detailed and methodical observation.[33]

A related emphasis was on *polythetic* criteria. The *DSM* is guided by the idea that psychiatric disorders can be identified by their symptoms, but there was no presumption that every case of a given disorder will present itself in exactly the same way. Diagnostic criteria are polythetic when there are symptoms common to a disorder but where there are few or no symptoms essential for a diagnosis. The same disorder can be realized with different combinations from a finite set of symptoms. In *DSM-IV*, for example, post–traumatic stress disorder (PTSD) is characterized by portfolios of different kinds of symptoms, each with its own diagnostic threshold, such as experiencing at least one of five reexperiencing-related symptoms (reexperiencing the original trauma), three of seven avoidance-related symptoms, and two of five hyperarousal symptoms.[34] With these symptoms and thresholds, along with rules regarding qualifying traumas, there are nearly eighty thousand potential profiles of PTSD.[35] There are even more possibilities in *DSM-5*, which sought even greater sensitivity to variation in how PTSD manifests. Indeed, in *DSM-5* there are over a half-million ways to have the disorder. In *DSM-III*, the use of polythetic criteria was partly a reflection of what the task force presumed to be the nature of psychiatric disorders: It recognized that psychiatric disorders were complex phenotypes that might appear messy from the standpoint of standard categorization systems.[36] But the use of polythetic criteria was also a compromise: Critics of most specific *DSM* criteria have argued that such criteria fail to capture adequately the variety of ways in which disorders are expressed. The use of polythetic criteria allowed for this variation while keeping its range within a tolerable limit for purposes of promoting reliability. Though the combinatorics grow complex from even small numbers, the *DSM*'s diagnostic criteria do provide a finite list of symptoms. In addition, the use of polythetic criteria spoke to the task force's ecumenical approach to latent causes. It allowed for a potentially broad understanding of the epidemiology of psychiatric disorders. Many psychiatric disorders are characterized by both emotional and more somatic symptoms. And the *DSM*'s criteria generally do not emphasize one sort of symptom over the other, at least for these two types of symptoms. The criteria for a major depressive disorder, for instance, require one of two primary symptoms—depressed mood or loss of interest or pleasure—but thereafter contain a list of nine symptoms, each of which is diagnostically equivalent. Somatic symptoms, thus, will not naturally assume more significance than affective symptoms. A similar approach was adopted for other disorders.

Though important, the symptom-based focus of *DSM-III* should not be overemphasized. The authors of *DSM-III* favored descriptions that richly detailed the symptoms, to be sure, but they were guided by a general idea about what mental disorders were. In fact, they took tentative steps toward defining the general concept of "mental disorder." Their definition was broad and hardly amounted to a *theory* of mental disorder—as critics continue to point out—but it was influential nonetheless. In their definition, mental disorder was characterized by a "clinically significant behavioral or psychological syndrome or pattern."[37] Furthermore, symptoms were regarded as painful in and of themselves or were regarded as significant because they led to impairment in one or more areas of functioning.[38] Finally, the authors assumed that mental disorders were chronic and involved some "behavioral, psychological, or biological dysfunction" and, thus, were not merely situational.[39] Symptoms, though, hinted at the underlying pathology. A group of symptoms might be observed at only one point in a person's life, and maybe only during a narrow window of time, but even this brief period was presumed to reveal the initial emergence of a long-term dysfunction. In these ways, the authors of *DSM-III* explicitly sought to distance themselves from a value-based definition of disorder, stating that a disorder involved *dysfunction*, that it was not based only on *deviance* from social norms, and that it was a *chronic* problem, not unlike more traditional physical illnesses.

Other aspects of *DSM-III*'s organization were designed to alert clinicians to the principal characteristics of psychiatric disorder. *DSM-III* employed a multiaxial organizational structure, with five axes. The first three represented the official diagnostic system: Axis I described conventional clinical disorders; Axis II focused on personality disorders; and Axis III focused on physical disorders that were related to mental disorders and, thereby, were diagnostically relevant. The remaining two axes were designed to alert clinicians to aspects of the case that were relevant to treatment but were regarded as optional for purposes of diagnosis. In this vein, Axis IV focused on psychosocial stressors. Axis V, meanwhile, focused on mental *health* as a tool for indexing the depth of mental *illness*. Text within the axis asked clinicians to consider, for instance, the highest level of functioning the individual had achieved in the last year. Although the disorders presented in Axis I remain *DSM-III*'s most enduring contribution, the multiaxial system itself was designed to insure an ecumenical evaluation of each case, and this, too, remains an important legacy of the manual. By including some symptoms that were not formally part of a mental disorder but were related to it, the *DSM* ostensively clarifies the concept of disorder. This is a useful expository strategy: When a definition of mental disorder is hard to articulate in a general way, it might be easier to do through comparison. By seeing the "well," we can evaluate the "sick." By the same token, even when clinicians focus on Axis I disorders, the inclusion of Axis II disorders admits the influence of enduring and basic features of the personality. All this is far from a clear formal definition of mental disorder or certainly from a framework for thinking about causes, but it nonetheless provides a sketch of mental disorder's characteristic features with a user of the manual in mind.

CATEGORICAL DISORDERS

The *DSM* employs categorical definitions of disorder. In a categorical framework, a disorder is either present or absent. Further subtypes of severity are possible, including whether a disorder is mild, moderate, or severe, but a disorder is only regarded as present when an individual has a sufficient number of symptoms to exceed a diagnostic threshold. If she has too few symptoms, she does not have the disorder. And if she has the disorder, further gradations of disorder are collapsed. If a disorder requires five of nine symptoms, for instance, someone with five symptoms receives the same diagnoses as someone with nine. The categorical approach can be considered in contrast with a spectrum-based approach, wherein the severity of a dimension varies across a range or continuum, with no emphasis on where on that spectrum a disorder might be present or not. A categorical approach does not imply that depression never exists in lower degrees. It implies only that milder forms of depression are not to be regarded as major depression.

In addition, the *DSM* assumes discrete diagnoses. Although more than one disorder can certainly be present at the same time, disorders in the *DSM* are generally regarded as diagnostically distinct. Meeting the clinical criteria for a major depressive episode means someone suffers from depression, while meeting the clinical criteria for a generalized anxiety disorder means someone suffers from anxiety. If someone suffers from both disorders simultaneously, the *DSM* assumes that each of these disorders is present on its own. One disorder does not supersede another as the primary diagnosis. And the presence of both disorders does not indicate the possibility of a new third disorder. There are exceptions. In some instances, the *DSM* provides rules regarding when to rule out other disorders or to determine when one disorder should take precedence over another. In addition, the *DSM* has more subtle features that imply that some pairings of disorders are more divisible than others. Some disorders, for example, are placed within categories of resemblance. One category of disorders pertains to disorders usually diagnosed in early life; another pertains to mood disorders. This type of organization is consequential in the sense that individuals who experience one mood disorder, for example, are at a considerably higher risk of experiencing another mood disorder. The organization of the *DSM* thereby acknowledges some limits to differentiation. Yet the *DSM* does not reflect an especially deep understanding of how disorders are connected, and, in general, there is little discussion of relationships among disorders.

This emphasis on independent diagnoses represents a significant change over previous editions of the *DSM*. *DSM-I* emphasized rendering only one psychiatric diagnosis per patient, even though it provided little guidance for doing so. It stated that conditions that were "first in the chain of etiology" should be designated as the primary cause and, further, that a primary condition should be recorded as the diagnosis, while a secondary condition should be recorded as a "manifestation" of the more general process.[40] The task of determining primacy, however, requires considerable inference on the part of the clinician. *DSM-II* permitted multiple diagnoses in a more thoroughgoing way, but it was clearly ambivalent about allowing this. *DSM-II* acknowledged, for instance, that individuals could have more than one disorder and, further, that one disorder could cause another.[41] In this vein, it provided the specific example of alcoholism beginning as "a symptomatic expression of another disorder."[42] Yet it demurred that comorbidity per se should only be recorded when appropriate. It encouraged clinicians to "not lose sight of the rule of parsimony" and, to this end, asked them to rank the disorders, using their judgment to assign the more serious or underlying disorder as the first.[43] In a few instances, *DSM-II* created guidelines that prevented the recording of comorbidity. *DSM-III*, by contrast, assumed discrete diagnosis more directly and provided a structure that more readily allowed for comorbidity.[44] *DSM-III* explicitly stated that multiple diagnoses were possible, even within the same class of disorders.[45] One reason for permitting comorbidity in this fashion was to absolve clinicians of the responsibility of assigning one disorder as the primary one, something that proved a challenge.[46] This, too, can be seen as another way of moving clinical authority from the clinician to the *DSM*—in effect, *DSM-III* no longer asked clinicians to do those things it regarded as difficult—although the revision was made with practical purposes in mind.

SPECIFICITY OVER SENSITIVITY

When attempting to define mental illness, it is possible to construct criteria that are *sensitive* and those that are *specific*. A sensitive set of criteria for major depression, for instance, would correctly diagnose every case of depression in a population, though it might also incorrectly include some cases that do not involve depression. A specific set of criteria, meanwhile, would be correct in each of its diagnoses of depression, though might overlook some cases. In an ideal world, it would be possible to have criteria that maximize both sensitivity and specificity. In that case, the *DSM* would produce no false positives (no one without a disorder would be incorrectly classified as having a disorder), and therefore would be perfectly specific, but would also produce no false negatives (no one with a disorder would be incorrectly classified as not having a disorder), and therefore be perfectly sensitive. In practice, though, balancing the two is difficult, and their intersection is the site of many ongoing controversies. Critics charge, for example, that the *DSM*'s diagnostic criteria produce an unreasonably high prevalence of psychiatric disorders, a point I return to later. In their mind, then, the problem with the *DSM* is one of false positives: too much sensitivity. But it is important to emphasize here that the authors of *DSM-III* favored specificity over sensitivity. They sought more specific and detailed diagnostic criteria in order to avoid false positives, not to encourage them. In their words, they favored a "narrow" definition of disorder (one that might even miss a few cases) to a broad definition (one that risked including too many).[47]

They did so partly under the assumption that mental disorders were rare. When a disorder is rare, the consequences of a change in sensitivity are much greater than the same change in specificity. Moving too far toward specificity might result in overlooking a few cases of psychiatric disorder, but if psychiatric disorders are uncommon to begin with, it is less numerically consequential to miss a few cases among the, say, 5 percent of people who have a disorder than mistakenly to identify disorder among the 95 percent of people who do not have one. In fact, however, the true prevalence of psychiatric disorders was not well established at the time. The authors of *DSM-III* were, thus, basing the balance of their decision to favor specificity on an assumption. The assumption of a low prevalence was, nonetheless, reasonable. If relatively few people are confined to psychiatric hospitals, for instance, it is reasonable to assume that the most severe disorders, at least, are rare.

The focus on specificity was ultimately a conceptual choice. *DSM-III* emphasized specificity primarily to improve reliability.[48] Reliability was a goal in and of itself, but Spitzer also emphasized the importance of "raising the credibility of psychiatry as a profession" by providing clinicians with better tools.[49] If clinicians were able to make similar determinations about the definition of a disorder, there would be less concern about capricious evaluations and, thus, less impugning of the motives of psychiatry. The profession would be more cohesive in orientation and in practice. Yet the emphasis on specificity had to be balanced by other concerns, including clinical utility. Clinicians are, of course, concerned about the reputation of their profession, but as practitioners they might prefer sensitivity, given the risks of not providing treatment when it proves necessary. Sensitivity is especially important when clients come to their office looking for a diagnosis: Most people who decide to talk to a professional have already decided they have some kind of problem. With this in mind, the task force again reached a compromise: They favored specificity at the level of the *diagnosis* but sensitivity at the level of the *manual*.[50] The criteria for each individual disorder would be highly specific, but by including many disorders across the entire manual, the task force insured adequate coverage and, thereby, adequate sensitivity. Furthermore, the task force adopted a strategy of inclusiveness within boundaries: They sought to create very few disorders entirely outside of existing categories but to allow for a variety of new disorders within any existing category. Indeed, within this constraint, the task force welcomed all proposals. According to Spitzer, the task force was willing to consider any new disorder so long as it was relevant to clinicians, and they were willing to do so even if there was very little scientific data regarding the disorder. There was no presumption that all the disorders included in the *DSM* would be equally prevalent. Their thinking was in terms of representation: By including a variety of different manifestations of disorder, virtually all clinically relevant presentations would be represented in the *DSM* in some fashion. As we will see later, the same strategy was also used, to a remarkable degree, by the authors of *DSM-5*.

The strategy of inclusiveness had another dimension, which was perhaps even more consequential. *DSM-III* introduced a category that would permit the diagnosis of disorders that were not otherwise included in the manual but closely resembled disorders that were. The name for this category has changed over time, as have the guidelines for its use, but *DSM-III* set the basic idea in motion. *DSM-III* outlined a variety of "atypical" disorders. These disorders inhered around a certain class of disorder but failed to reflect a single disorder described therein. The label of "atypical" was to be used when "enough information is available to indicate the class of disorder that is present" but when "further specification is not possible," in part because "the clinical features of the disorder do not meet the criteria for any other categories."[51] With *DSM-III-R*, the language changed, but the idea remained the same. The "atypical" category was changed to disorders "not otherwise specified" (NOS). *DSM-III-R* further clarified that the NOS designation was to be regarded as a "residual" category, but it also acknowledged that disorders designated as NOS could, in some instances, be more prevalent than the disorders actually specified within the class.[52] Recognizing the lingering ambiguity surrounding the NOS designation, *DSM-IV* further elaborated on how it was to be used. It noted four conditions in which the use of NOS was appropriate: first, when the symptoms were consistent with disorders in a class but as a whole did not meet the diagnostic criteria; second, when the symptoms did not conform to a *DSM-IV* classification but still caused clinically significant distress or impairment; third, when it was unclear whether the disorder was caused by another medical condition; and fourth, when there was insufficient opportunity to collect more information about the patient.[53] Although there was no presumption that the earliest "atypical" designation would be used rarely, the *DSM-III* task force assumed that the ordinary criteria contained in the *DSM* would adequately capture most disorders. The atypical category was, thus, introduced in a spirit of tempered modesty, even if, as I will discuss, it has bedeviled the manual ever since.

THEORY NEUTRALITY

A key idea in the construction of *DSM-III* was theory neutrality. Theory neutrality has several dimensions, but it essentially represents an attempt to separate a formal understanding of what psychiatric disorders are from knowledge about what causes them. This is consistent with the rest of medicine in the sense that heart disease, for example, can be diagnosed without information about how much the individual exercises, the quality of his diet, or whether his parents suffered from heart disease. Earlier editions of the *DSM* frequently blended information about symptoms and causes, and they did so in light of the prevailing scientific and professional views of a disorder's causes. *DSM-I*, for instance, frequently referred to internal conflicts, as when, for example, it specified that in a conversion reaction, the symptoms were "symbolic of the underlying mental conflict."[54] By the same token, adjustment-related problems in children were thought to reflect either the immediate situation or some "internal emotional conflict."[55] *DSM-I* also made regular reference to unconscious processes[56] and repression,[57] concepts popular at the time but less important today. *DSM-II* continued with many of the same themes.[58] Neuroses, for instance, were defined according to how such disorders were thought to develop. Anxiety, for instance, "is the chief characteristic of the neuroses. It may be felt and expressed directly, or it may be controlled unconsciously and automatically by conversion, displacement, and various other psychological mechanisms."[59]

The *DSM-III* task force made an explicit effort to avoid concepts of this type and, indeed, to avoid discussion of any causes at all. First, it did so in order to avoid creating a manual that would become outdated as soon as new treatment models were developed or old ones were discarded. The looming failure of Freudian psychodynamics was clearly on their minds, not to mention problems regarding the interface between psychotherapists and traditional medicine, but more generally the task force sought to avoid *any* theories that might look naïve or speculative in retrospect.[60] Second, the task force feared the clinical utility of the *DSM* would be compromised if the manual adhered to a specific etiological theory, especially when there were many different kinds of professionals involved with treating mental illness. According to Millon, the task force sought to be accommodating in order to "alienate the smallest number of clinicians."[61]

THE FEIGHNER CRITERIA

It is easy to devise principles for revising the *DSM*, and all of the above all well motivated, but the committee still faced the difficult task of writing the actual diagnostic criteria. Fortunately, a critical resource was already available to them, at least for some disorders. In 1972 the *Archives of General Psychiatry* published a set of operational definitions for fifteen psychiatric disorders, definitions that came to be known as the "Feighner Criteria," in reference to the lead author of the study.[62] Feigner and his collaborators developed the criteria based on prior published research as well as on impressions based on their own clinical work. Their motivation for devising these criteria was based, in part, on the same issues motivating the *DSM-III* task force: Scientists were struggling with operationalizing the diagnostic criteria in *DSM-II*, just as clinicians were struggling with providing reliable diagnoses. For the task force, the Feighner criteria were a natural source of inspiration. They were well articulated and well known: The *Archives* article was the most highly cited article in psychiatry at the time. Nevertheless, the criteria were less scientific than their provenance and popularity might suggest. In fact, the Feighner criteria followed a long chain of guesswork, more or less. When an author of an early progenitor of the Feighner criteria was asked why the criteria for depression stipulated six out of ten symptoms, he reported only that "it sounded about right."[63] Furthermore, the Feighner criteria were not intended for clinical use. They were intended for use by researchers, for research purposes. Although this might seem like a fine difference in emphasis, it is a real one: Clinicians and researchers have their own set of interests and prerogatives, a point I return to later. Yet clinical applications of the Feighner criteria were certainly easy to envision. The *DSM-III* task force immediately recognized these applications and debated only how to use the criteria best, not whether to use them at all. Some proposals expressed reluctance to go too far in the direction of the Feighner criteria. An early proposal, for example, was to use the Feighner criteria merely as a supplement to a more narrative-based set of criteria, similar to *DSM-II*.[64] Another was to develop two sets of criteria, one for researchers, very similar to the Feighner criteria, and one for clinicians. In the end, however, a single Feighner-like set of criteria was adapted for use across *DSM-III*.

THE *DSM-III* CRITERIA

Perhaps the best way to illustrate the *DSM-III* criteria is by example. Below is the diagnostic criteria for a major depressive episode. It is drawn from *DSM-III*. Subsequent editions followed a very similar form but differ in some important details, especially, in fact, in the case of a major depressive episode, which I will discuss in detail later on. For now, focusing on *DSM-III* provides a way of foreshadowing the remarkable consistency of the *DSM*. Each disorder in the *DSM* usually contains an organized sequence of information, starting with essential features, followed by associated features, followed by other assorted aspects of the disorder, if those aspects are sufficiently well established, including age of onset, complications, associated impairments, and differential diagnosis. For purposes of illustration, some subclassification criteria are omitted in this example.

DIAGNOSTIC CRITERIA FOR A MAJOR DEPRESSIVE EPISODE

A. Dysphoric mood or loss of interest or pleasure in all or almost all usual activities and pastimes. The dysphoric mood is characterized by symptoms such as the following: depressed, sad, blue, hopeless, low, down in the dumps, irritable. The mood disturbance must be prominent and relatively persistent, but not necessarily the most dominant symptom, and does not include momentary shifts from one dysphoric mood to another dysphoric mood, e.g., anxiety to depression to anger, such as are seen in states of acute psychotic turmoil. (For children under six, dysphoric mood may have to be inferred from a persistently sad facial expression.)

B. At least four of the following symptoms have each been present nearly every day for a period of at least two weeks (in children under six, at least three of the first four):

(1) poor appetite or significant weight loss (when not dieting) or increased appetite or significant weight gain (in children under six, consider failure to make expected weight gains)

(2) insomnia or hypersomnia

(3) psychomotor agitation or retardation (but not merely subjective feelings of restlessness or being slowed down) (in children under six, hypoactivity)

(4) loss of interest or pleasure in usual activities, or decrease in sexual drive not limited to a period when delusional or hallucinating (in children under six, signs of apathy)

(5) loss of energy; fatigue

(6) feelings of worthlessness, self-reproach, or excessive or inappropriate guilt (either may be delusional)

(7) complaints or evidence of diminished ability to think or concentrate, such as slowed thinking, or indecisiveness not associated with marked loosening of associations or incoherence

(8) recurrent thoughts of death, suicidal ideation, wishes to be dead, or suicide attempt

C. Neither of the following dominate the clinical picture when an affective syndrome (i.e., criteria A and B above) is not present, that is, before it developed or after it has remitted:

(1) preoccupation with mood-incongruent delusions or hallucinations

(2) bizarre behavior

D. Not superimposed on either Schizophrenia, Schizophreniform Disorder, or a Paranoid Disorder

E. Not due to any Organic Mental Disorder or Uncomplicated Bereavement

The diagnostic criteria for a major depressive episode provide a good context for thinking how the principles of the task force were implemented. The criteria also contain a caveat that will later emerge as important. Section E describes what is referred to as the bereavement exclusion. Another section of *DSM-III* clarifies what is meant by this exclusion and notes that normal bereavement rarely persists after the first two or three months. In this exclusion, *DSM-III*, in effect, assumes that the death of a loved one can produce symptoms consistent with that of a major depressive episode, but precisely because the cause of these symptoms is common and the outcome "normal," the episode should not be regarded as a disorder (unless it is "complicated"). In principle, the *DSM-III* task force could have expanded exclusions of this sort to other life events and to other disorders. Their reasoning regarding the death of a loved one could easily be applied, for instance, to the loss of a job or a divorce. The task force, however, chose not to extend the exclusion, perhaps because of the complications it might introduce. As noted earlier, the task force explicitly sought theory neutrality; that is, they sought diagnostic criteria that would be independent of any consideration of the causes of mental disorder. Though it nominally involves a cause, the bereavement exclusion is not a violation of theory neutrality, at least not an unambiguous one. For one, the idea that the environment can cause psychiatric disorders—including the social environment and, therefore, the death of a loved one—is consistent with virtually any model of psychiatric disorder. It was not *only*, for instance, part of the psychoanalytic tradition. Moreover, the idea of allowing for an exclusion could be seen as consistent with the very definition of mental disorder provided in *DSM-III*, which noted in the introduction that "there is an inference that there is . . . a dysfunction, and that the disturbance is not only in the relationship between the individual and society."[65] The bereavement exclusion was seen as relevant to this inference, though the task force apparently felt sufficiently ambivalent about including it that they did not apply it to other disorders. The complication, then, pertained to what "tools" the task force was willing to provide readers to help in the difficult task of inferring dysfunction. In this regard, the task force appeared only willing to go so far.

Other complications were perhaps more subtle but no less consequential. And they, too, reflected the difficulty of sticking to all the principles simultaneously and across all disorders. In the name of specificity, the symptoms contained in the criteria are well described. And many of the symptoms can be interpreted in a plain fashion. Weight loss and weight gain can be measured, for instance, and in *DSM-III-R* the amount of weight change was further specified as 5 percent rather than just "significant," as it was described in *DSM-III*. Similarly, sleeping more or less than usual can be evaluated relative to a person's previous patterns. Other symptoms, however, presuppose some understanding of what those symptoms describe and, thus, involve some *theory*, however crude.[66] Understanding the concept of a delusion, for instance, requires some understanding of what a delusion is. Similarly, the diagnostic criteria for identity disorders frequently refer to concepts like a "coherent" or "independent" identity.[67] All of these concepts require considerable insight. A complete and adequate definition is, in fact, difficult to articulate. One definition of a delusion, for instance, is a fixed idea, especially about the self, that departs significantly from reality. But such a definition presupposes a clear understanding of the "reality" of a person. Furthermore, even a reasonably well articulated definition of a delusion contains an eye-of-the-beholder quality. Virtually everyone suffers from at least some kind of "delusion," regarding, for example, their competence, their attractiveness, or their prospects. Furthermore, many beliefs pertain to what *could be* and not what *is* and, therefore, do not involve veracity at all. It is hard to regard optimism, for example, as a disorder, just as hopelessness can sometimes be misguided. And, of course, it is hard to disprove the existence of conspiracies, which resist falsification. Similarly, a "coherent identity" requires an understanding of what an identity is, and it presupposes coherence as an ideal. In order to use the *DSM*'s diagnostic criteria, then, the clinician is required to have some insight into a concept and to render some judgment. The *DSM-III* was written to be as clear as possible. It was also written to be almost entirely sufficient for the task of diagnosis. Yet some of its ideas are difficult to describe using common-sense language, and clinicians must employ knowledge gathered from other sources in order to use the *DSM*.[68]

THE SUCCESS OF *DSM-III*

Despite these problems, *DSM-III* succeeded in providing an *operational* definition of mental disorder. In the end, *DSM-III* was *useful* for certain practical interests, starting with those of mental health professionals. In this vein, perhaps the most important concern of the *DSM-III* task force was improving reliability, and there is evidence that *DSM-III* indeed worked in this regard. In psychiatry, a key test of reliability is a field trial, wherein multiple clinicians are asked to evaluate the same patients using a shared set of criteria. In 1979, Spitzer and colleagues published the results of such a trial, albeit using a draft version of the *DSM-III* criteria and not the final version.[69] In the study, clinicians were asked to participate in at least two evaluations, along with another clinician evaluating the same case. The clinicians were instructed to use the preliminary *DSM-III* criteria and not older versions of the *DSM* they might be familiar with. Within a pair, both clinicians had the same information about a case, including records and letters of referral. Clinicians also either shared an evaluation interview or did their evaluations separately but as close in time as possible. The most often used measure of agreement between these evaluations—or what is referred to as inter-rated reliability—is the kappa statistic, for which a 1 represents perfect agreement and a 0 represents agreement no better than chance (as in, for example, both parties flipping a coin). By convention, a .7 or higher is regarded as "good" agreement. Although a field trial represents a different approach to the issue of reliability than the more casual approach provided in Rosenhan's study, the overall goal is much the same. Both approaches are interested in uncovering evidence for the ability of clinicians to render the same diagnosis for the same case. Unlike the Rosenhan study, though, the DSM-III field trials revealed some agreement. The average kappa was .74. There was, however, variation between disorders, suggesting more or less success. For some disorders, such as paranoid disorders, the kappa reached 1, whereas for others it was much lower. The kappa also varied by the conditions of the exam. The level of agreement dropped somewhat, for example, when the interviews were not conducted jointly, as expected, but in general the decline was not great. Even for more eye-of-the-beholder disorders, like the major affective disorders, the level of agreement was high. The kappa statistic is not without controversy, and what is considered "good" or "bad" might be debatable, but it seems DSM-III did provide an apparent improvement over its earlier editions. Kappa statistics from field trials based on earlier diagnostic criteria were considerably lower.[70] Previous studies found kappas as low as .32 for personality disorders, .41 and less for affective disorders, and .57 for schizophrenia.[71]

DSM-III solidified the profession of psychiatry in other ways as well. As Buchanan notes: "If you can define it, you can own it."[72] For this reason, DSM-III further elevated the authority of psychiatry over the domain of behavioral problems. To be sure, the DSM is not a secret document (nor a prohibitively expensive one), and the American Psychiatric Association can do little to prevent the DSM's criteria from being used by other parties. Indeed, with sufficiently clear diagnostic criteria virtually anyone can render diagnoses that will resemble those provided by a professional. Nevertheless,

DSM-III consolidated the influence and standing of psychiatry. Among other things, it elevated the importance of diagnosis as a clinical activity. As a result, clinicians who were not interested in diagnosis suddenly found themselves out of step with where professional psychiatry was heading. Not surprisingly, psychotherapy was perhaps the first to suffer. *DSM-III*, with its classifications and standardization, was met with resistance by practitioners of psychotherapy, whose training model bristled at rules. Yet the success of *DSM-III* insured psychotherapists' resistance was a minority position or at least made their differences from mainstream psychiatry clear.[73] *DSM-III* also paved the way for a more specific understanding of mental illness. Although in a formal way the principle of theory neutrality dictated an agnostic stance regarding causes, whether social, psychological, or biological, the *form* of *DSM-III* lent itself to understanding mental illness as rooted in some underlying pathology. Later researchers would seek to uncover some of the biological origins of this form, while others pursued a more cognitive-behavioral approach, but both groups of researchers now proceeded from the premise that mental illness was categorical in nature.

DSM-III was also hailed as a victory for research.[74] In particular, it was thought finally to cleave the science of psychiatric disorders from ideology and politics, indeed, to allow the real science finally to begin.[75] With formal diagnostic criteria in hand, researchers quickly developed a variety of structured instruments that could assess psychiatric disorders in nonprofessional survey interviews (or what researchers refer to as "lay" interviews). The research enterprise benefitted from not requiring a professional assessment of each of their research subjects. These instruments were further revised when the next revision, *DSM-III-R*, was published in 1987. Spitzer himself developed one of the most popular such instruments, the Structured Clinical Interview (or SCID).[76] Beyond the development of new measurement tools, research funding from the National Institute of Mental Health increased. The NIMH recognized how *DSM-III* in effect cleared much of the scientific clutter that had previously concerned them. For the first time, researchers could study disorders that were heretofore not explicitly codified. Researchers could also rest assured that when studying cases of depression, for example, they were, in fact, studying more or less the same thing as other researchers studying depression, regardless of where the study took place or who participated.

In all these ways, *DSM-III* was an enormous success. In fact, it was probably more of a success than its authors anticipated. *DSM-I* and *II* were largely technical documents used by a limited number of professionals. *DSM-III* was written for the same audience, but it sold like a popular novel. In the first six months, *DSM-III* sold more copies than both previous editions combined, and it was purchased by laymen and professionals alike.[77] It generated over 9 million dollars in revenue for the APA.[78] And it was eventually translated into more than twenty languages, furthering its global reach.[79]

Certainly the long-term success of *DSM-III* was not something its authors could have anticipated in the short term. Venomous criticism of *DSM-III* appeared almost immediately.[80] Criticism pertained as much to the authors' *intent* as to what was actually in the manual. Some critics charged, for instance, that *DSM-III* was an attempt to gain exclusive control over mental health services and to impose a strict medical model over treatment.[81] Other critics went even further, focusing on the large number of disorders contained in *DSM-III* and charging its authors with an attempt to medicalize everyday problems. These criticisms continue today, although in a perhaps even more piqued form, given the ever-growing number of disorders contained in the *DSM*. If critics had a problem then, they surely have a problem now.

As an initial way of understanding these criticisms, it is important to distinguish *DSM-III*'s pragmatic intentions from its ontological accuracy. There is no doubt that *DSM-III* was a *practical* success, but it left many issues unresolved. In particular, *DSM-III* left the question of *validity* open. The authors of *DSM-III* fully understood the distinction between reliability and validity. They realized that reaching some agreement about appropriate diagnostic criteria might foster reliability but would not insure validity.[82] In this way, they emphasized reliability and mostly set aside the issue of validity, seemingly comfortable in doing so. Yet they also blended the two in ways that frustrated critics. The authors of *DSM-III* saw reliability as a bridge to validity, even if they did not always say so directly. Spitzer has since clarified his thinking about the issue, albeit in a way that simply circles back to the issue of reliability and utility. According to Spitzer, a diagnosis is valid "to the extent that the defining features of the disorder provide useful information not contained in the definition of a disorder," noting that this information can pertain to etiology, family aggregation, risk factors, typical course, and so on.[83] He further clarified that previous editions of the *DSM* failed to be valid because they did not help in the management or treatment of disorder. And he states directly that science "cannot wait for a fully validated diagnostic system."[84] His understanding of validity, then, was fundamentally pragmatic.

With the publication of *DSM-III*, Spitzer and others envisioned a newly empowered science of psychiatric disorders. What, however, were the actual consequences of *DSM-III*? The next chapter discusses research that stemmed from *DSM-III* and its subsequent revisions. To a remarkable degree, agreement regarding formal psychiatric nomenclature solved one problem but introduced many more. Once the problem of reliability had been addressed, researchers were in a position to question the validity of psychiatric disorders using better evidence—and, indeed, evidence that could not be provided before the development of specific criteria. Yet the ensuing scientific controversies further fanned the flames of controversy, laying bare all the complexities of validity. In addition, *DSM-III* shifted the locus of expertise. Whereas previous versions of the *DSM* implicitly valorized the expertise of clinicians, *DSM-III* elevated the contributions of researchers.[85] The post-*DSM-III* era is one of an increasingly active scientific enterprise. It is also one of surprising insights that have reverberated back to the question of when and why, exactly, does the *DSM* fail and succeed.

3

DSM-III AND THE DESCRIPTIVE SCIENCE
OF PSYCHIATRIC DISORDERS

Before *DSM-III*, a remarkable number of facts about psychiatric disorders were hidden from view. Scientists could study psychiatric disorders, to be sure, but only in a disorganized way. Other parties struggled for the same reason. Clinicians could talk about the need for psychiatric treatment among their clients, but they ultimately had little information about the scope of mental illness nationally. In fact, before *DSM-III* it was virtually impossible to estimate the number of Americans who suffered from a psychiatric disorder. Counting requires a firm sense of what, exactly, you're counting. If clinicians routinely disagreed over how to diagnose even a single case, there was little chance they could agree on how to count all the cases in a community.

The publication of new and improved diagnostic criteria provided an opportunity. Using criteria that were specific, clear, and written in (mostly) plain language, researchers could use standardized survey instruments, administered in community samples, to estimate the number of people who met the diagnostic criteria for a psychiatric disorder. Furthermore, they could do so without the aid of clinicians. Well-articulated symptoms could be easily translated into survey questions, the answers to which could then be coded by scientists rather than psychiatrists.

Up to this point, research on the prevalence of psychiatric disorders had been inconclusive. Studies were inadequate either from the standpoint of how they assessed psychiatric disorders or the range of the populations they targeted. A large number of studies, for instance, explored nonspecific psychological distress, measured with various questions about the amount of depression, anxiety, sadness, alcohol consumption, and so on an individual had experienced recently. Questions of this sort were often summed together to create an index of overall distress, involving a range of potential scores and not just the presence or absence of a disorder. So measured, the distress was "nonspecific" in the sense that it need not involve any particular psychiatric disorder, and, in any case, the measures used by scientists did not provide the information necessary for discerning whether an actual psychiatric disorder was present. Studies of nonspecific distress also failed in one important aspect of quantification: They did not provide *counts*. They only provided averages. Measures of nonspecific distress say nothing about the number of Americans suffering from a psychiatric disorder. They only report on the average level of distress. And, in this sense, they fail to cohere with any obvious clinical benchmark. Yet when it comes to assessing suffering, many people want to know whether an experience is *normal*, not simply whether it is high or low, and they especially want to know how many people suffer from *abnormal* levels of distress and, therefore, might be considered ill.

Other studies addressed this issue better but were limited in their design. They focused, for instance, on the number receiving psychological services. The number receiving services is not the same thing as the number needing services, although scientists assumed the two groups were similar, perhaps for good reason. Other studies were more ambitious in their scope but were still limited. They explored community-based populations, but they did so within a limited geography. The Midtown Manhattan Study, for instance, explored the prevalence and correlates of psychiatric disorders among about 1,600 persons living in a section of New York City.[1] The study was influential and important. It was regarded as objective at a time when many other studies were seen as impressionistic. Yet few researchers regarded the study's classification of psychiatric disorders as adequate or saw its prevalence estimates as representative of the United States generally.

Existing studies were unsatisfying for other reasons as well. The need for more accurate estimates of prevalence was growing, especially among policy makers. In 1978, President Carter commissioned a report on mental health. The report focused on improving psychiatric services and highlighted the inadequacies of the present system. In doing so, however, the report also brought some scientific issues to the fore, including the need for estimating the prevalence of psychiatric disorders in a more credible fashion.[2] Calling for broad reform of psychiatric services is good, but with little understanding of how many people actually suffered from psychiatric disorders, it was impossible to know whether the existing mental health system was adequate or whom it might be missing. Nor was it possible to anticipate the amount a better system might cost, assuming a better system would treat those not yet reached by the current system.

With the goal of providing more useful information, researchers took the *DSM-III* criteria and crafted appropriate survey questions. The goal was to capture the manual's symptoms and decision rules in a prose-based instrument that could then be administered by lay interviewers. When using such instruments, the question is not how many have received a psychiatric diagnosis from a professional, or how many have sought formal treatment of some kind, but rather how many people have met the clinical criteria for a psychiatric diagnosis by *DSM* standards at some point in their life, regardless of whether they actually received a diagnosis or treatment. In this sense, scientists were pursuing what is referred to as the *true* prevalence of psychiatric disorders rather than the *clinical* prevalence. And, in pursuit of this, scientists used what are known as highly structured diagnostic instruments administered by lay interviewers, wherein the "structured" part refers to how tightly the survey instrument hews to the *DSM* and forces the interviewer, by virtue of a script, to ask all the relevant questions. Though the *DSM* is a good guide, transposing the symptoms and decision rules contained in the *DSM* into survey questions is more difficult than it might sound. Survey instruments must first adjust to revisions in the *DSM* itself, meaning estimates based on *DSM-III-R* will employ different diagnostic criteria *and* different survey instruments than those based on *DSM-III*. One major survey initiative used what was referred to as the Diagnostic Interview Schedule, whereas a later survey used the Composite International Diagnostic Interview (which too has again been revised). Although the researchers behind all of these instruments seek fidelity to the *DSM*, the prevalence estimates they produce are sensitive simply to how questions are asked, let alone to changes in the *DSM*'s diagnostic criteria.[3] The Composite

International Diagnostic Interview remains the cornerstone of contemporary epidemiological research, though its structure has changed over time in ways that make it difficult to compare even with immediately prior versions. In any case, these instruments provided researchers with an opportunity to see how the new *DSM* criteria actually worked.

The first large-scale study to estimate prevalence in this fashion was the Epidemiological Catchment Area Study (ECA), conducted in the early 1980s.[4] As the first of its kind, the ECA was enormously influential, but it still carried some of the same limitations as earlier studies. Perhaps the most significant was its limited geographic scope. The survey was conducted in five cities: New Haven, Connecticut; Baltimore, Maryland; Durham, North Carolina; St. Louis, Missouri; and Los Angeles, California. The survey stretched beyond these sites to some degree. The Durham site included four rural counties as well as the city, and the St. Louis site included some suburban and rural areas too. Furthermore, surveys conducted in sites can be weighted to approximate more closely the characteristics of the United States as a whole. But such techniques are imperfect, and scientists had lingering doubts about how representative the sites in the ECA sampling frame were or could be. At a minimum, the five cities were unusual in ways that prompted concern. All five, for example, had large university-based hospitals, suggesting a more robust mental health treatment sector than was probably available to the average American.

A subsequent study set out to address these limitations (and a few others). The National Comorbidity Survey (NCS) was conducted in the early 1990s, using the then-current criteria published in *DSM-III-R*.[5] The NCS was a significant improvement, especially in terms of representing the U.S. population. The study was large and broad. It contained over eight thousand respondents between the ages of fifteen and fifty-four and was collected in over 174 counties in thirty-four states. In addition, the NCS made a special effort to sample students living in group housing, the largest group of people not living in standard households and, thus, a key group to target when seeking a truly representative household sample.

The NCS still had some limitations. Efforts to estimate the true prevalence of psychiatric disorders are limited by the very conditions they seek to study (apart from whether we think the *DSM* is correct or not). The NCS, for instance, was a *household* survey. It included a wide array of dwellings, but, still, a large number of people suffering from psychiatric disorders are homeless or living in institutions. When researchers refer to "community" surveys, they are usually not, in fact, referring to *everyone* who resides in a region. In addition, researchers cannot *force* anyone to participate in a survey. They require affirmative agreement from participants. Those with psychiatric disorders tend to refuse participation in surveys at higher rates, producing a healthier sample of respondents than would be available if scientists were able to include everyone in their study. Complicating matters further, even perfect participation in a survey does not guarantee accurate data. Those with psychiatric disorders tend to suffer in ways that complicate how they respond to survey questions. Many psychiatric disorders involve, for example, cognitive impairment, and, in particular, those who suffer from psychiatric disorders are more likely to misremember the past. The converse is also true. Happy adults are often glad to forget, for example, the depression they experienced in their teens. Estimating the true lifetime prevalence of psychiatric disorders places some demands on the memories of respondents, especially those who might be suffering from a disorder or suffered from one in the past. More generally, surveys are unable to explore all the disorders cataloged in the *DSM*. For simple practical reasons—no one is willing to participate in a survey that could last most of the day—researchers must decide what disorders in the *DSM* to include in a survey instrument.[6] Researchers often choose a set they assume represents the most common disorders, but, even so, many important disorders are not assessed at all. For these reasons, estimates of the true overall and lifetime prevalence of psychiatric disorders—even from the very best community studies and the most thoughtful scientists—are prone to being *conservative*. Not all disorders are open to study, not all people suffering from a psychiatric disorder find their way into a sample, and not every participant can faithfully report the suffering they once experienced or are experiencing now.

These factors make the results of the NCS even more surprising.[7] Table 3.1 presents two types of prevalence.[8] *Lifetime prevalence* refers to the percentage of the sample who ever experienced a disorder. Because the sample represents

TABLE 3.1 PREVALENCE OF PSYCHIATRIC DISORDERS IN THE UNITED STATES, NATIONAL COMORBIDITY SURVEY

	LIFETIME PREVALENCE	TWELVE-MONTH PREVALENCE
ANXIETY DISORDERS		
Panic Disorder	3.5	2.3
Agoraphobia	5.3	2.8
Social Phobia	13.3	7.9
Simple Phobia	11.3	8.8
Generalized Anxiety	5.1	3.1
Post-traumatic Stress	7.6	3.9
Any Anxiety Disorder	28.7	19.3
MOOD DISORDERS		
Major Depressive Episode	17.1	10.3
Manic Episode	1.6	1.3
Dysthymia	6.4	2.5
Any Mood Disorder	19.3	11.3
SUBSTANCE DISORDERS		
Alcohol Abuse	9.4	2.5
Alcohol Dependence	14.1	7.2
Drug Abuse	4.4	.8
Drug Dependence	7.5	2.8
Any Substance Disorder	26.6	11.3
OTHER DISORDERS		
Antisocial Personality	2.8	—
Nonaffective Psychosis	.5	.3
Any Disorder	49.7	30.9

Source: Adapted from Ronald C. Kessler et al., "Lifetime and Twelve-Month Prevalence of DSM-III-R Psychiatric Disorders in the United States: Results from the National Comorbidity Survey," *Archives of General Psychiatry* 51, no. 1 (1994): 8–19.

people between the ages of fifteen and fifty-four, "lifetime" is limited. It means up until this point in the person's life. In this sense, the lifetime prevalence of psychiatric disorders is a misnomer. All else being equal, fifteen-year-olds should have a lower lifetime prevalence than fifty-four-year-olds, if only because they have had fewer years of life. Furthermore, a fifty-four-year-old still might experience a disorder at some point in their remaining lifespan. In fact, these issues present only a small problem, given that most psychiatric disorders have an early onset. If someone has not suffered a psychiatric disorder by the age of fifty-four, the chance they will at some point in the future is small. These issues do, however, introduce some confusion over terminology. *Twelve-month prevalence* or *current prevalence* is more straightforward. It refers to the percentage of the sample that experienced a disorder at some point in their lives and also reported an episode of the disorder during the preceding twelve months. Twelve-month disorders are considered "active" or "current." The relationship between the lifetime and twelve-month prevalence is informative. If we assume that at least some disorders go away, the twelve-month prevalence should always be lower than the lifetime prevalence. If disorders are perfectly chronic, the two numbers will be identical. No lifetime disorder is ever not also a current disorder.

The most remarkable finding of the NCS was the seemingly high prevalence. All told, the NCS discovered that nearly half (49.7 percent) of all Americans reported a lifetime history of at least one *DSM-III-R* disorder. Furthermore, just over 30 percent reported experiencing a disorder during the last twelve months. Of the specific disorders included in the study, the most common was a major depressive episode, with a lifetime prevalence of 17.1 percent and a twelve-month prevalence of 10.3 percent. The most prevalent *category* of disorders, however, was anxiety disorders, with an estimated 28.7 percent of Americans suffering from at least one anxiety disorder at some point in their life. This prevalence is followed closely by addictive disorders, especially alcohol dependence, from which 7.2 percent of Americans currently suffer.

The NCS revealed other important dimensions of mental illness. Note that the sum of the prevalence of all the individual disorders far exceeds the prevalence of those reporting any disorder. This implies that many people

TABLE 3.2 COMORBIDITY OF PSYCHIATRIC DISORDERS IN
THE UNITED STATES, NATIONAL COMORBIDITY SURVEY

NUMBER OF LIFETIME DISORDERS	PERCENT OF PEOPLE	PERCENT OF LIFETIME DISORDERS
0	52.0	
1	21.0	20.6
2	13.0	25.5
3+	14.0	53.9

Source: Adapted from Ronald C. Kessler et al., "Lifetime and Twelve-Month Prevalence of DSM-III-R Psychiatric Disorders in the United States: Results from the National Comorbidity Survey," *Archives of General Psychiatry* 51, no. 1 (1994): 8–19.

suffer from multiple disorders simultaneously; this is termed *comorbidity*. Although comorbidity is a critical feature of mental illness, it does not have a straightforward interpretation. Table 3.2 presents two quantities that shed at least some additional light. The first is the percentage who suffered from different numbers of disorders simultaneously. In the NCS, about 52 percent experienced no lifetime disorder, as already noted, but of the remainder, only 21 percent experienced a single or "pure" disorder. Twenty-seven percent experienced two or more disorders, and about 14 percent experienced three or more. If we shift the unit of analysis to *disorders* rather than *people*—that is, if we use as our base the number of psychiatric disorders in the population rather than the number of people suffering from psychiatric disorders—the significance of comorbidity is clearer. The second column indicates that only about 21 percent of lifetime disorders were pure disorders, while 79 percent occurred in tandem with at least one other disorder. Putting these two calculations together reveals the final crucial fact about comorbidity: About 54 percent of all disorders were present in the 14 percent of people who suffer from three or more disorders. Most of the disorders in the United States were, then, comorbid disorders. Comorbidity is a complex phenomenon, and I will elaborate on its meaning and significance shortly. Some implications, however, are immediately clear. The burden of psychiatric disorders in the United States appears concentrated in a relatively small group of people who suffer from several disorders simultaneously. Furthermore, the idea of discrete and independent disorders is more concept than reality. Psychiatric disorders tend to spill over the boundaries set in the *DSM.*

Further exploration the NCS data found that virtually all psychiatric disorders were positively correlated with one another. Put differently, if you have one psychiatric disorder, your risk of having another is very high. This implies a general risk for mental illness, broadly understood, but some disorders are more strongly related to one another than are others, perhaps implying a shared etiology.[9] Major depressive episodes, for example, tend to co-occur with generalized anxiety disorders. In addition, alcohol and drug abuse are positively related to each other, as one might expect if people abuse substances generally rather than just one substance in particular. By the same token, those who strongly fear one thing, such as social encounters, tend to have other fears as well. For this reason, anxiety disorders are strongly correlated with one another. Certain *sets* of disorders also tend to be related, albeit for more abstract reasons. At the broadest level, two general types of disorders can be identified: externalizing disorders, such as substance abuse and conduct disorders, and internalizing disorders, such as depression and anxiety. These categories reflect the symptoms they characterize. In externalizing disorders the symptoms are directed outward, whereas in internalizing disorders they are directed inward. Those who suffer internally, then, tend to experience a variety of internally directed symptoms and disorders, whereas those who suffer externally experience a variety of other-directed symptoms and disorders. In these ways, the NCS almost immediately revealed information useful for questions of taxonomy. It was suggesting, for instance, more synthetic ways to organize a taxonomy such as the *DSM,* even though those dimensions were not yet part of the *DSM*'s organizational structure.

Another inference that could be drawn across these two tables—and one that skeptics of the *DSM* immediately reached for—is that prevalence is not the same thing as severity. A large number of Americans might suffer from a psychiatric disorder at some point in their lives, as the NCS appeared to be saying, but merely meeting the diagnostic threshold for a disorder does not indicate much about the *severity* of that disorder. To some critics, this possibility makes the otherwise suspicious findings of the NCS more reasonable. If comorbid disorders are more severe than pure disorders, for example, then the prevalence of "real" disorders is considerably less than what the NCS was reporting overall. Furthermore, if the lifetime prevalence of psychiatric disorders is always higher than the twelve-month prevalence, many disorders would seem to be short-lived, and that, too, might be something to consider when interpreting prevalence. In the same vein, it is possible that a seemingly high prevalence might reflect a large number of people just meeting the diagnostic threshold for a disorder but progressing no higher. If so, the high prevalence in the NCS might simply reflect having drawn too low of a diagnostic threshold and, thus, of capturing too many mild and fleeting problems.

Subsequent research further explored the issue of severity, and while it shed additional light for interpreting the data, it hardly clarified matters for purposes of classification. Table 3.3 presents the severity of twelve-month disorders.[10] The table presents data from a later replication of the NCS, conducted in the early 2000s, although the prevalence of psychiatric disorders changed very little between the initial NCS and its replication, suggesting comparability at least for those disorders measured in both surveys.[11] In the replication, severity was assessed by evaluating the consequences of symptoms, not just their presence or absence. Indications of a "serious" disorder, for example, included a suicide attempt, work-related disability, and violent behavior. Based on these indicators, the severity of individual disorders was divided into three categories: serious, moderate, and mild. Those suspicious of the NCS's high prevalence initially assumed that many disorders were mild, and, indeed, the later data suggested that many were. Overall, only 22 percent of disorders were serious, and 40 percent were mild. Yet complications lurked just below the surface. The distribution of severity varied by disorder, though not in the way we might anticipate. As I will discuss shortly, a good deal of debate has centered on the meaning and significance of depression in particular. If feeling sad, for example, is regarded as an unremarkable fact of life, as many critics contend, and the *DSM* draws the threshold of depression too low, one would expect that many instances of major

TABLE 3.3 SEVERITY OF PSYCHIATRIC DISORDERS, NATIONAL COMORBIDITY SURVEY REPLICATION

	PERCENT SERIOUS	PERCENT MODERATE	PERCENT MILD
ANXIETY DISORDERS			
Panic Disorder	44.8	29.5	25.7
Agoraphobia	40.6	30.7	28.7
Specific Phobia	21.9	30.0	48.1
Social Phobia	29.9	38.8	31.3
Generalized Anxiety	32.3	44.6	23.1
Post-traumatic Stress	36.6	33.1	30.2
Obsessive-Compulsive	50.6	34.8	14.6
Separation Anxiety	43.3	24.8	31.9
Any Anxiety Disorder	22.8	33.7	43.5
MOOD DISORDERS			
Major Depressive Disorders	30.4	50.1	19.5
Dysthymia	49.7	32.1	18.2
Bipolar I and II	82.9	17.1	0
Any Mood Disorder	45.0	40.0	15.0
IMPULSE CONTROL DISORDERS			
Oppositional Defiant	49.6	40.3	10.1
Conduct Disorder	40.5	31.6	28.0
Attention-Deficit/Hyperactivity	41.3	35.2	23.5
Intermittent Explosive	23.8	74.4	1.7
Any Impulse Control Disorder	32.9	52.4	14.7
SUBSTANCE DISORDERS			
Alcohol Abuse	28.9	39.7	31.5
Alcohol Dependence	34.3	65.7	0
Drug Abuse	36.6	30.4	33.0
Drug Dependence	56.5	43.5	0
Any Substance Disorder	29.6	37.1	33.4
TOTAL TWELVE-MONTH DISORDERS			
One	9.6	31.2	59.2
Two	25.5	46.4	28.2
Three or More	49.9	43.1	7.0

Source: Adapted from Ronald C. Kessler et al., "Prevalence, Severity, and Comorbidity of Twelve-Month DSM-IV Disorders in the National Comorbidity Survey Replication," *Archives of General Psychiatry* 62, no. 6 (2005): 617–27.

depression are, in fact, quite mild and inconsequential. This was not the case, however. On the contrary, as a class of disorder, mood disorders were the most severe, with 45 percent of mood disorders regarded as serious. Moreover, some mood disorders were especially—and almost always—severe. A remarkable 83 percent of bipolar disorders, for example, were categorized as serious. By contrast, only 30 percent of substance disorders were serious, and the vast majority of cases of alcohol abuse were mild or moderate, despite the many problems caused by alcohol use in the United States.

In interpreting these patterns, it is still important to emphasize the discontinuity between the *prevalence* of disorders and the *severity* of disorders. Those suspicious of the high prevalence were largely correct in one important respect: Prevalence does not, in fact, reveal much about severity and can be quite misleading. As a class of disorders, for example, anxiety disorders are the most prevalent, but they are also the least severe. The single most severe disorder, bipolar disorder, has a prevalence of less than 3 percent, whereas the single most prevalent disorder, a specific phobia, has the highest percentage of mild cases. A focus on severity rather than prevalence reinforces the importance of comorbidity as a potentially better indicator of the real depth of disorder. In particular, mild cases of disorder are especially common among those who suffer from only one disorder. Of those with a pure disorder, for example, 59.2 percent are mild, and only 9.6 percent are serious. Among those with three or more disorders, though, 49.9 percent are serious. In isolation, then, the most common disorders tend to be mild disorders, but when disorders occur together, they tend to be severe.

The issue of severity is also related to treatment, though, again, in ways that complicate a clean interpretation. Table 3.4 presents the frequency of using mental health services.[12] The table presents findings both from the initial version of the NCS and its later replication, corresponding to the time period 1990 to 1992 and 2001 to 2003, respectively. This feature of the initial survey and its replication allows us to explore changes over a decade, although some important facts have remained the same. In both the NCS and its replication, *most* cases of psychiatric disorder receive no treatment at all, regardless of severity. Among those with serious disorders, for instance, only 24.3 percent received treatment in 1992. Although this increased to 40.5 percent

TABLE 3.4 TREATMENT OF TWELVE-MONTH PSYCHIATRIC
DISORDERS IN TWO TIME PERIODS

	1990–1992	2001–2003
ANY TREATMENT		
Any Disorder	20.3	32.9
Serious Disorder	24.3	40.5
No Disorder	8.8	14.5
TREATMENT IN PSYCHIATRY SECTOR		
Any Disorder	4.8	10.5
Serious Disorder	7.3	14.4
No Disorder	1.4	2.9
TREATMENT IN GENERAL MEDICAL SECTOR		
Any Disorder	6.8	17.3
Serious Disorder	8.2	22.1
No Disorder	2.6	6.8

Source: Adapted from Ronald C. Kessler et al., "Prevalence, Severity, and Comorbidity of
Twelve-Month DSM-IV Disorders in the National Comorbidity Survey Replication," *Archives
of General Psychiatry* 62, no. 6 (2005): 617–27.

in 2003, the percentage is still short of half. This low percentage is even more
remarkable given that the category of "any" services is very broad. It includes
things such as complementary and alternative medicine as well as human services. If we limit the focus to specialty care or to the general medical sector—
sectors that generally provide the best care for those suffering from a serious
psychiatric disorder—the percentage who received treatment is very low.
Only 14.4 percent of serious cases, for instance, received specialty care, and
only 22.1 percent received care in general medical settings.

On the flip side, a surprising number of people who suffered from *no*
discernable disorder received treatment. Among those with no disorder,
14.5 percent received some kind of treatment, including 6.8 percent in general medicine settings and 2.9 percent from specialists. To be sure, there is
a positive relationship between severity and the likelihood of receiving

treatment: As severity increases, the percentage receiving treatment increases as well. Yet the relationship between severity and treatment was no stronger in 2003 than it was in 1992. The percentage receiving treatment has gone up for *both* those with no disorder and those with a serious disorder. In short, the health care system does not appear to be especially discerning with respect to issues of severity and no more so when it has more treatments at its disposal.

Other NCS findings were equally surprising. In much of psychiatry, the origins of mental illness are thought to reside in *contemporaneous* experiences. Life events trigger depression, for example, and chronic stress makes depression worse. People are distressed by what is happening currently in their lives. To be sure, the psychodynamic approach focuses on childhood conflicts, but even in that framework the assumption is that childhood conflicts produce disorders in adults *when adult defense mechanisms fail.* In a less theoretically guided way, the various diagnostic exclusions contained in the *DSM* reflect a similar emphasis on current experience. Many exclusions, for example, focus on circumstances common in the lives of adults, such as bereavement and physical illness. The NCS revealed that this focus on current experience might be misguided: The NCS discovered that most disorders have a much earlier onset, well before the time when death and illness are common. Disorders apparent in adulthood reflect the recurrence of disorders that first emerged in childhood more than they are the emergence of entirely new disorders. In particular, studies estimated the median age of onset, corresponding to the age at which 50 percent of cases have emerged.[13] In general, the median age of onset for psychiatric disorders is quite low. For some disorders, this is true virtually by design. Impulse-control disorders, for instance, are defined in ways that emphasize early onset and, consistent with this diagnostic structure, the median age of onset for such disorders is very young, around eleven. But most other disorders show the same pattern, even when the criteria would appear to allow for more variation. The median age of onset for anxiety disorders, for example, is also eleven. Substance abuse disorders have a slightly higher age of onset, but the median age is still quite young, at twenty. Mood disorders have the most advanced median age of onset, at thirty, but the most severe mood disorder, bipolar disorder, has a median onset of twenty-five. Among those people who experience any disorder, half are affected by the age of fourteen. Furthermore, the range of ages for first onset is quite restricted. Although the interquartile range—corresponding to the age range in which 75 percent of cases will emerge—is twenty-five years for mood disorders (about a third of the average life expectancy), it shrinks to nine years for substance abuse. Psychiatric disorders, in short, begin quite early in life, and for many disorders there is a relatively brief period of vulnerability, after which the risk of initial onset declines precipitously. Once individuals have "aged out" of the most risky age groups, then, their chance of developing a disorder in later life is quite small, regardless of the stresses that might be unique to later life.

Another way to think about age patterns is in terms of cohorts. This, too, sheds light on issues relevant to classification as much as epidemiology. Social scientists frequently separate what they refer to as age, period, and cohort effects. In the case of psychiatric disorders, an age effect represents the relationship between aging and the onset of a disorder. The risk can be arrayed over ages, so that it starts low, begins to increase in childhood and early adolescence, and then subsides with older age. In an age effect, the pattern reflects something about aging itself. It happens regardless of the time period. People grow older, and their risk for developing a psychiatric disorder changes as well. A cohort effect, by contrast, pertains to an effect related to the period in which someone was born. Cohort has a natural relationship with age, of course. Those born in 1950, for instance, will be fifty years old in the year 2000, so those in a birth cohort will resemble one another if for no other reason than that they share the same age. A cohort effect, however, posits something different: It posits that cohort groups have a distinct risk for psychiatric disorders apart from the age they share. For instance, coming of age during the Great Depression might shape mental health years later, increasing the risk for an entire group born around that time (or coming of age around that time) relative to those born before or after. A period effect, meanwhile, pertains to influences apparent at any one time and affecting those across the age spectrum. All adults, for example, might be more anxious following the attacks of September 11, and so we would characterize the event as forming a period effect. Given how they are logically related to one another, age, period, and cohort effects are difficult to distinguish. Nonetheless, the replication of the NCS found evidence suggesting distinct cohort patterns, including a higher prevalence of disorders among more recent cohorts.[14] The largest cohort effect of this type was for drug use disorders, followed by mood disorders. In particular, among cohorts who passed through their adolescence during the 1970s, drug use and depression were high relative to cohorts born earlier or later.

Taken altogether, the NCS presents a striking picture of psychiatric disorders in the United States. Despite the intuition that psychiatric disorders are rare, and despite explicit efforts to craft *DSM* criteria in ways that favor specificity over sensitivity, the true lifetime prevalence of psychiatric disorders was seemingly very high. To be sure, many of these disorders were mild, and some were self-limiting. Yet, irrespective of these caveats, the high prevalence was alarming to many scientists. Other studies soon deepened the alarm. In the early twenty-first century, researchers began to expand upon the basic design of the NCS. If such a survey could be conducted in the United States, why couldn't it be replicated in other countries? And if the prevalence of psychiatric disorders was so high in the United States, why wouldn't it be even higher in more "stressful" countries, especially in countries without all the medical resources of the United States? The World Mental Health Project began in earnest at the turn of the century.

PSYCHIATRIC DISORDERS AROUND THE GLOBE

If before the NCS the picture regarding psychiatric disorders in the United States was muddled, the global picture was even more complicated. In international settings, there were very few standardized survey instruments at all, and comparisons between countries were virtually impossible. There was no diagnostic system as clear as the *DSM*, although the International Classification of Disease did help and was regularly revised. Complicating matters even more, though, was the presumed significance of language and culture. For these reasons alone, comparisons between countries seemed especially daunting. What, if anything, for example, was the equivalent of feeling "blue" in Japan? Did other countries talk about fear the same way we do in the United States? In 1998, the World Health Organization established the World Mental Health Survey Consortium in order to address these issues and to derive credible estimates of the true prevalence of psychiatric disorders on a more global scale. In effect, the WHO sought to replicate the success of the NCS in a coordinated international endeavor. The WHO was not naïve about the scope of the challenge. In an attempt to impose basic standardization, they began by using the same diagnostic criteria, drawn from *DSM-IV*, across nations in a common survey instrument. Major depression, for instance, must be at least *measured* the same way in all countries, even if we assume depression might be a different thing in Japan than in the United States. But the WHO also went a step further. They conducted field trials to see if international respondents could understand survey questions in more or less the same way as U.S. respondents. They also compared what diagnostic information their survey instruments provided relative to what clinicians might determine about the same case.[15] By 2004 the consortium had completed diagnostic surveys in fourteen countries. The countries were diverse. Six were classified as "less developed" by the World Bank; the others were classified as developed. Although the U.S. sample was the largest, each country provided a sample that was sufficiently large to be regarded as representative.

Once again, the results were surprising, deepening even more the problems of those concerned with taxonomy.[16] The results were perhaps especially surprising for those who assumed the United States was in any way typical. Table 3.5 presents the twelve-month prevalence of psychiatric disorders by country and the percentage of disorders that are considered serious. The U.S. percentages repeat what I have discussed already, although with somewhat updated figures. In the United States, just over 26 percent have suffered from a psychiatric disorder over the previous twelve months. What is remarkable, though, is how much higher the prevalence in the United States is relative to any other country or region. In Shanghai, for instance, the twelve-month prevalence was 4.3 percent. The nearest competitor to the United States was Ukraine, where the twelve-month prevalence was

TABLE 3.5 PREVALENCE OF TWELVE-MONTH PSYCHIATRIC DISORDERS,
WORLD MENTAL HEALTH

	ANY DISORDER	ANY SERIOUS DISORDER	ANXIETY DISORDER	MOOD DISORDER	IMPULSE-CONTROL DISORDER	SUBSTANCE DISORDER
United States	26.4	7.7	18.2	9.6	6.8	3.8
Columbia	17.8	5.2	10.0	6.8	3.9	2.8
Mexico	12.2	3.7	6.8	4.8	1.3	2.5
Belgium	12.0	2.4	6.9	6.2	1.0	1.2
France	18.4	2.7	12.0	8.5	1.4	.7
Germany	9.1	1.2	6.2	3.6	.3	1.1
Italy	8.2	1.0	5.8	3.8	.3	.1
Netherlands	14.9	2.3	8.8	6.9	1.3	3.0
Spain	9.2	1.0	5.9	4.9	.5	.3
Ukraine	20.5	4.8	7.1	9.1	3.2	6.4
Lebanon	16.9	4.6	11.2	6.6	1.7	1.3
Nigeria	4.7	.4	3.3	.8	0	.8
Japan	8.8	1.5	5.3	3.1	1.0	1.7
Beijing	9.1	.9	3.2	2.5	2.6	2.6
Shanghai	4.3	1.1	2.4	1.7	.7	.5

Source: Adapted from the WHO World Mental Health Survey Consortium, "Prevalence, Severity, and Unmet Need for Treatment of Mental Disorders in the World Health Organization World Mental Health Surveys," *Journal of the American Medical Association* 291, no. 21 (2004): 2581–90.

20.5 percent. Even more fine-grained comparisons reveal the United States as exceptional. Within each of the four disorder categories, the United States had the highest prevalence, with the exception of substance disorders, where Ukraine reported a prevalence of 6.4 percent compared to 3.8 percent in the United States.

To be sure, there are some patterns that are consistent across countries, but these consistencies only make the inconsistencies more difficult to interpret. For instance, in all but one country (Ukraine), anxiety disorders were the most common type of disorder. Mood disorders were the next most common, except in Nigeria and Beijing, where substance disorders were nearly as prevalent. In general, though, countries with a high prevalence were high across a variety of different disorders, while countries with a low prevalence were low across the board. No country, then, was uniquely depressed or uniquely anxious or uniquely prone to alcoholism. Countries were simply high or low in how much psychiatric distress they experienced, and this distress was expressed in a variety of ways.

One interpretation of this pattern is that in low-prevalence countries, people might be setting an especially high bar for reporting most symptoms. In Nigeria, for instance, it is possible that only those with the most severe disorders report any symptoms at all—most people, in effect, hold back—whereas in the United States people report even the most low-level symptoms. Under these conditions, even mild symptoms would be reported as potentially indicating major depression. This interpretation is fundamentally *cultural*—it relies on ideas about how residents of a country think and behave—but it has at least one testable implication. If true, the relationship between the prevalence of psychiatric disorders and the severity of psychiatric disorders would be negative: Countries with a higher prevalence should have a lower overall severity because its residents are reporting symptoms that are of little consequence. This was not the case, however. Indeed, the relationship was positive, not negative: The proportion of serious cases decreased as the prevalence decreased. In Nigeria, for instance, only 4.7 percent suffered from a psychiatric disorder at all, and less than 9 percent of those disorders could be considered serious.

Another interpretation of these patterns is simply that the diagnostic threshold for disorders varies between countries. Assuming people report symptoms accurately and completely, it is still possible that the threshold for, say, depression varies between countries, making the differences more apparent than real. The problem, then, is with accurate classification and, in an attempt to impose standardization, the *DSM*-derived survey instrument will be blind to these differences.[17] This idea, too, has at least one testable implication. If true, there would be less cross-national variation in the basic symptoms of depression (e.g., feeling depressed or losing interest in things) than in the prevalence of a major depressive episode per se. In other words, most people might experience sadness, regardless of where they live, but the link between reporting sadness and reporting major depression should vary by country. Studies show, however, that there is enormous cross-national variation even in the basic symptoms of depression. Table 3.6 shows the

TABLE 3.6 PREVALENCE OF LIFETIME MAJOR DEPRESSIVE
EPISODE, WORLD MENTAL HEALTH

	LIFETIME PREVALENCE	ANY LIFETIME SCREENING SYMPTOMS
United States	19.2	62.0
Columbia	13.3	58.6
Mexico	8.0	40.6
Belgium	14.1	49.4
France	21.0	65.0
Germany	9.9	43.1
Italy	9.9	44.9
Netherlands	17.9	53.2
Spain	10.6	37.7
Ukraine	14.6	82.4
Lebanon	10.9	57.7
Japan	6.6	29.9
China	6.5	54.6

Source: Adapted from Ronald C. Kessler and Evelyn J. Bromet, "The Epidemiology of Depression Across Cultures," *Annual Review of Public Health* 34, no. 1 (2013): 119–38.

percentage in each country who reported the symptoms necessary but not sufficient for a diagnosis, referred to as lifetime "screening" symptoms.[18] In particular, these numbers correspond to the percentage who reported ever having a time lasting several days when they were sad, depressed, or lost all interest in their usual activities. Overall, the global prevalence of these symptoms was quite high, which is not surprising, assuming that around the globe distress is a normal fact of life. More surprising, though, was the variation. Reports of sadness appear to correspond closely with reports of major depression. In places where major depression is common, milder forms of sadness are common as well. Lots of people suffer from major depression in the United States, but short of that, lots of people report several days of feeling sad as well. This suggests that between-country differences in the prevalence of major depression are not an artifact of a poor fit between the *DSM*'s diagnostic criteria and how distress is expressed in those countries. To be sure, the criteria might work *better* in some countries than in others,[19] but even in low-prevalence countries the criteria appear to work reasonably well.[20] It remains unclear why depression is so much more common in the United States, though the possibilities include relative deprivation or social and psychological isolation. In any case, we should not dismiss the World Mental Health numbers as merely reflecting "worried well" Americans feeling sad while living in a land of plenty. Their sadness appears, at a minimum, real.

Since its initial foray, the World Mental Health initiative has expanded into more countries, providing additional information. Most of the new information confirms what was established in the first round of data collection, but some additional patterns have come into focus. Across an expanded range of countries, for instance, the lifetime prevalence of major depression was shown to be somewhat higher in high-income countries (14.6 percent) than in low-income countries (11.1 percent). In addition, the ratio of twelve-month disorders to lifetime disorders—an indicator of how chronic a disorder is—tends to be lower in high-income countries, suggesting less persistent disorders in high-prevalence countries. This, then, is consistent with the idea that high-income countries experience more fleeting disorders, if not fewer of them. But the overall conclusion is that cross-national differences in the basic prevalence of psychiatric disorders are *real*. They do not reflect how people respond to surveys, at least not in any obvious way. Furthermore, psychiatric disorders tend to have real consequences, whatever else we might think about the diagnostic threshold. Even in places where psychiatric disorders are common, those experiencing disorders report significant disability. People who suffer from depression, for example, tend to be less productive and motivated, regardless of how prevalent the disorder is in their country. For this reason, depression in the United States, for instance, is just as disabling as depression in China. In addition, there is little evidence that in places where psychiatric disorders are common the use of services is entirely unrelated to a patient's actual need for services. Worldwide, the bulk of treatment for psychiatric disorders goes to those who, in fact, meet the diagnostic criteria for a psychiatric disorder. Indeed, if anything, this pattern is slightly more pronounced in high-income countries, suggesting greater sensitivity on the part of those health care systems to issues of severity.[21]

In an attempt to shed more light on the issue of culture, recent studies have focused on depression.[22] Depression is a strategic choice. It has many diverse symptoms and is among the most common of psychiatric disorders. If culture matters, there might be a number of characteristic patterns between countries. For instance, some symptoms of depression might be especially prominent in certain countries. In addition, some symptoms might be especially disabling. It is also possible that some symptoms might be more central to the experience of depression in some countries than others. If losing interest in things, for example, is especially important in the United States, it is possible that most people who suffer from that particular symptom will go on to suffer from a major depressive episode as well, whereas in other countries the symptom is experienced independent of a disorder. By the same token, more somatic symptoms, such as fatigue, might be especially important in non-Western countries, where emotional symptoms are more stigmatized. World Mental Health data indicate, however, that none of these ideas is entirely correct. There is no symptom that is especially important in one country but not in another. Even the relationship between individual symptoms and disability tends to be consistent across countries. In short, there is some cross-national stability in how depression is manifest, even if depression appears much more frequently in some countries than others.

Other studies have further fanned the flames of controversy. As high as the true prevalence of psychiatric disorders appears to be, there are reasons to suspect that even the best studies, like the NCS, underestimate it, perhaps severely. Recall that the NCS is a *cross-sectional* study. It was conducted at a single point in time (although it was replicated a decade later) and asked respondents to reflect on their life up to that point. Lifetime prevalence is, thus, estimated retrospectively: It pertains only to respondents' lives up to the time they were interviewed. Although there was no presumption that individuals could accurately recall everything they experienced, researchers did assume that people could recall those times when they suffered from a psychiatric disorder. This assumption was a logical extension of their vision of what a psychiatric disorder is and, indeed, of the vision of psychiatric disorders as codified in the *DSM*. If major depression, for example, is qualitatively *different* from ordinary sadness, individuals should be able to remember distinctly when they suffered from it, even if they forget normal bad days. Some recent studies, however, have questioned this assumption. One study explored what the lifetime prevalence of psychiatric disorders might look like if disorders were examined *prospectively*, that is, by following people over time and thereby evaluating whether they ever experienced a psychiatric disorder in their lifetime based on a string of current reports rather than on retrospective ones.[23] To be sure, the researchers were unable to follow people for their entire lives, but they did follow them from youth to age thirty-two, a time span in which most psychiatric disorders that will ever appear are likely first to appear. Their study was based in New Zealand, but presumably it has relevance to the United States, given that the prevalence of psychiatric disorders in the two countries is similar. The researchers found that the estimated lifetime prevalence of psychiatric disorders differed a great deal between a prospective and retrospective approach. Assessed prospectively, the estimated lifetime prevalence of any disorder was approximately *double* that of a retrospective assessment. The lifetime prevalence of anxiety disorders, for example, was nearly 50 percent, and the lifetime prevalence of depression was just over 40 percent. This implies that the NCS estimates—as high as they are—are probably far too low. It also implies something about the nature of psychiatric disorder, perhaps an even more unsettling implication. One interpretation of this finding is that individuals tend to forget episodes of psychiatric disorder, even when those episodes are regarded as significant by *DSM* standards. Indeed, research finds that episodes of disorder are forgotten even when those episodes are plainly severe and have seemingly memorable consequences. One study, for example, found that people often failed to recall episodes of depression even when those episodes resulted in hospitalization.[24] Another interpretation, though, is that retrospective surveys fail simply because people have a difficult time recalling events of a short duration, even if those events are consequential. Respondents might forget psychiatric disorders that were experienced only once or were experienced only over a few weeks, much like they might forget they once had food poisoning. Regardless of the interpretation, prospective studies have at least one implication of clear significance: They suggest most people in high-prevalence countries will experience a psychiatric disorder at some point in their lifetime.

INTERPRETING THE PREVALENCE
OF PSYCHIATRIC DISORDERS

In uncovering so many points of contention, all of these studies provide a kind of Rorschach test. It is instructive to dwell on how these studies have been interpreted as a way to understand not only the nature of the controversy but also the first principles that continue to inform debates about the proper classification of psychiatric disorders. For many critics, the results of the NCS and related efforts boil down to a single issue: The estimated prevalence of psychiatric disorders is implausibly high. How could it be, they ask, that half of all Americans suffer from a psychiatric disorder at some point in their lifetime? Many critics were quick to answer that the *DSM* itself must be fatally flawed. There is simply no way the prevalence of psychiatric disorders is so high, that comorbidity is so broad, and that the influence of culture is so deep. The *DSM* must, the reasoning goes, admit too many false positives, draw too many distinctions, and allow for too many external influences. In this vein, Allen Frances, among others, returned to the definition of mental disorder provided in the *DSM* as the principal way to understand why the NCS estimates were so high.[25]

In the next chapter, I will review the various proposed alternatives to the *DSM*'s diagnostic criteria. In some cases, these proposals reflect a response to the emerging science surrounding the *DSM*, including studies based on the NCS. In other cases, however, they reflect longstanding concerns that existed well before science began to produce credible research on the topic. For the moment, though, it is worth reflecting on the idea of *implausibility*. To say that something is "implausible" is to state more than just a strong opinion. It is to claim something about the parameters of truth. But where, exactly, was critics' insistence that the prevalence was "too high" coming from? What benchmark were they using? Judgments regarding plausibility are based on a reasonable standard, or a standard that most people will find compelling. Yet precisely because the NCS was among the first studies to estimate the true prevalence of psychiatric disorders, a good deal was, in fact, *unknown*. The expectations of critics were not coming from a clear scientific understanding, although, to be sure, their expectations were coming from somewhere and not from a place of total ignorance. Perhaps clinicians developed intuitions based on their caseloads. Researchers, too, had some sense about the number of people being *treated* for psychiatric disorders, if not yet the true prevalence of psychiatric disorders in the general population. In addition, a few abstract ideas could be applied to the issue of prevalence. One might assume, for instance, that psychiatric disorders are rare because we regard them as diseases. Clinical medicine is premised on a normal-pathological distinction wherein homeostasis favors health rather than disease. From this, one might infer that psychiatric disorders, too, should be uncommon, especially if they cause lots of problems for those who suffer from them. Yet none of these ideas constitutes a definitive theory or provides incontrovertible evidence regarding the prevalence of psychiatric disorders. Furthermore, none of these ideas is so compelling as to warrant clinging to it in the face of data that contradict it.

To be sure, some scientists were not alarmed by the findings of the NCS. Indeed, they argued that as a reaction to empirical findings surprise might betray a kind of prejudice. Ronald Kessler, the scientist behind the NCS, has offered this interpretation in interviews, focusing in particular on how mental illness tends to be evaluated relative to physical illness.[26] If, for example, we argued that most Americans will experience the flu at some point in their lives, no one would be surprised. And no one would conclude that the flu was not "real" in light of the fact that most people will experience it. The point of this analogy is not to trivialize psychiatric disorders by aligning it with a common seasonal infection. Depression, for instance, is one of the most disabling medical conditions in the world, as Kessler himself has made perfectly clear. The point of the analogy is rather to show how the interpretation of prevalence depends on how one regards the course and typical significance of a disease. The intuition behind how mental illness is regarded, which in turn informs how prevalence is interpreted, seems to be that mental illness ought to be rare and chronic. The same logic is not applied, however, to physical illness, where people can readily appreciate that even severe illnesses can be common and transitory. Why, then, do we apply a different and fundamentally more restrictive logic to psychiatric disorders? Still, a critic might insist that psychiatric disorders *are* different from other diseases and that it is appropriate to apply a different standard to them. One could believe, for instance, that psychiatric disorders must be chronic in order to be a disease and, therefore, that psychiatric disorders differ from the flu in a critical way. One could believe also that psychiatric disorders must be serious in order to qualify as a disease—otherwise they would be something else. Some of the proposed revisions to the *DSM* that I will discuss shortly are based precisely on these ideas. These ideas, though, betray a model for psychiatric disorders and not necessarily a fact about how they exist in nature. They reflect a premise about what psychiatric disorders are. And these ideas are not, in fact, consistent with the model we employ for most other medical conditions. Like psychiatric disorders, many other physical illnesses are self-limiting and mild, but we consider them illnesses regardless of that fact. Furthermore, for some diseases we recognize that a mild condition can become a severe one, appreciating, then, that the disease is a disease irrespective of its current severity. (Also, for the record, the flu does kill a large number of people every year.) A different but still reasonable interpretation of the high prevalence of psychiatric disorders is that it reveals only that psychiatric disorders are like other medical conditions. Much like it is normal occasionally to have an infection the immune system will eliminate, it might be normal to suffer periodically from a psychiatric disorder that gets better on its own.

Among the most important consequences of the NCS was to lay bare the assumptions researchers were harboring about psychiatric disorders. The NCS certainly gave scientists something to talk about. And, in the end, critics of the NCS were not criticizing the data, the analysis, or the researchers who collected it so much as the very concept of a psychiatric disorder as codified in the *DSM*. The NCS allowed critics to sharpen their attack on formal diagnostic criteria and to offer proposals for criteria that might better achieve one or another specific aim. In addition, with data in hand, critics could start to estimate what the prevalence of psychiatric disorders might look like if the *DSM* employed different diagnostic criteria. Over time, however, the science of psychiatric disorders has not evolved in lockstep with debates about what psychiatric disorders ought to be. The next chapter explores the imperfect intersection between science and taxometric issues, a theme that will recur throughout the remainder of the book.

4

RETHINKING THE *DSM*

The principles behind *DSM-III* led to a revolution in psychiatric classification, but the manual's publication was only the beginning of a much longer debate. In improving the situation with respect to diagnostic reliability, *DSM-III* fanned the flames with respect to diagnostic validity. It was not long before people began to rethink the *DSM* and propose alternatives. In fact, some critics were people involved with *DSM-III*'s creation, including Spitzer himself. Many of the proposed alternatives were designed with specific goals in mind. Among the most important was that any revised diagnostic criteria ought to yield a much lower prevalence of disorders in the population. This goal is relatively easy to achieve. Simply raising the diagnostic threshold by a symptom or two is usually enough. But some proposals were more ambitious in their intent and underlying philosophy. In addition to providing what their authors regarded as more reasonable estimates of prevalence, their authors envisioned revised criteria that would yield more valid diagnoses as well.

It is useful to review the full variety of proposals, which encompass a broad range and reflect an abundance of perspectives. At one extreme are proposals that essentially surrender on the question of validity. One version of this idea was articulated by Allen Francis, the architect of *DSM-IV*, in the context of addressing the fallout over *DSM-5*. Francis conceded that there was likely no way to articulate a thoroughly satisfying definition of mental disorder, even if there were ways to create useful diagnostic criteria. He went further, though, in arguing that *in reality* there might be no way to define the concept of mental disorder. In this, Francis revealed a surprising degree of deference to a longstanding strain in critical psychiatry, including themes reviewed earlier in this book.[1] Yet he was articulating something far less radical: He was only asking the authors of the *DSM* not to make the perfect the enemy of the good. He was advocating, in essence, for a conservative refinement of a document he regarded as deeply flawed. At the other extreme, however, are authors who believe that nothing short of a complete overhaul of the *DSM* is required. For them, the *DSM* is off the mark, and a more radical approach is necessary, especially because something better is now available. The conservative approach, though, is the best place to start, including its many variations and shadings.

THE CONSERVATIVE APPROACH

The conservative approach asserts that the *DSM* criteria are correct in their form but wrong in their details.[2] In particular, the approach emphasizes that some mechanical features of the form, such as the diagnostic threshold, are responsible for producing false positives. The approach further emphasizes that empirical evidence, not just judgment, can be leveraged to draw more appropriate cut points, though all within the existing parameters of the *DSM*.

With this in mind, there are various ways in which the diagnostic criteria can be improved. A good starting point is to focus on those things that cut across criteria, especially what is meant by "clinically significant impairment." *DSM-III* addressed this concept in some detail, but the definition of what constitutes "significant" has evolved over subsequent editions. *DSM-III* included a general statement specifying that the symptoms of psychiatric disorders must be either painful in themselves or cause "impairment in one or more areas of functioning," thereby eliminating symptoms that were seemingly of little consequence for daily life.[3] A similar statement appeared in *DSM-IV* but provided more detail. In *DSM-IV*, mental disorder was conceptualized as a "clinically significant behavioral or psychological syndrome or pattern that occurs in an individual and that is associated with present distress (e.g., a painful symptom) or disability (i.e., impairment in one or more important areas of functioning) or with a significantly increased risk of suffering death, pain, disability, or an important loss of freedom."[4] Definitions of this sort are intended as a metastructure. Although they hardly amount to a philosophy, these statements orient clinicians to the issue of severity before they even begin to apply the diagnostic criteria to specific disorders.

Naturally some proposals start here. They seek to set a higher threshold for impairment or to define more explicitly the most relevant dimensions of functioning, within the broad sweep of death, pain, disability, and limitation.[5] Proposals of this sort are conservative in the sense that they only seek to expand what is already in place, but they often yield very different outcomes. As a demonstration of what happens when a higher threshold of clinical significance is used, Narrow and colleagues reestimated the prevalence of psychiatric disorders using what they referred to as "enhanced" criteria.[6] They did so within an existing survey instrument, the NCS, and, therefore, using much of what is already contained in the *DSM*. This also allowed them to compare with previous estimates without using an entirely different dataset. They employed two ways of revising the definition of clinical significance. The first pertained to help seeking. Symptoms were counted as significant if respondents answered affirmatively to either of the following questions: Have you ever told a doctor, mental health specialist, or other professional about your symptoms, or have you ever taken medication more than once because of symptoms? The second question pertained to disability. Symptoms were regarded as significant if respondents answered affirmatively to the question: Did your symptoms ever interfere with your life or activities a lot? In this case, "a lot" was the critical element. Respondents could report a full range of interference, from "none" to "a lot," but "a lot" imposed a higher level of interference relative to someone who reported merely that a condition "sometimes" interfered with activities.

Not surprisingly, using the enhanced criteria did, indeed, produce a lower estimated prevalence of psychiatric disorders. The twelve-month prevalence of any disorder declined by about a third, from 30.2 percent to 20.6 percent. And some specific disorders fell even more. The prevalence of social phobia, for instance, dropped by half, implying that most cases of social phobia are not terribly disabling or concerning. The prevalence of other disorders, meanwhile, did not change at all, including bipolar disorder, post–traumatic stress disorder, and nonaffective psychosis. This implies these disorders tend to be severe regardless of how severity is assessed. Those who propose revisions of this sort are surely aware of the simplicity of their suggestions: They are only asking to set the bar a bit higher. Yet they regard this simplicity as the essence of the problem: For them the *DSM* criteria admit far too many weak symptoms and inconsequential disorders, and so raising the bar, although superficial, can improve the *DSM*'s accuracy. In their words—in reference to James Carville's famous statement about the role of the economy in the 1992 presidential election—it's "the 'disorder threshold,' stupid."[7]

Still, raising a threshold in this fashion is largely a mechanical solution. Although doing so might yield a lower prevalence, a higher threshold does not improve the validity of diagnostic criteria on any deep conceptual grounds. There is not a particularly robust philosophy behind the idea. Another way to achieve the same goal would simply be to address a *different* threshold: to increase the number of *symptoms* required for a diagnosis, moving the criteria for a major depressive episode, say, from five to seven symptoms and leaving the definition of clinical significance unchanged. A focus on clinical significance at least has the benefit of shifting the focus to *disability* as a criterion for assessing validity. And if one regards mental illness as a medical problem only when it causes significant suffering, disability is, indeed, critical. Yet as other researchers have pointed out, some revisions premised on enhancements of one sort or another present a tautology.[8] One element of Narrow and colleagues' enhanced criteria, for example, blends the identification of a disorder with the receipt of treatment: One of their criteria for assessing severity is simply whether the person thought the condition was serious enough to warrant treatment. No other medical condition requires the patient to seek treatment in order to be seen as suffering from a disease. Those who refuse renal dialysis are not suddenly cured of kidney failure. To be sure, Narrow's enhanced criteria contain *two* inclusive dimensions, not one. Using their criteria, a person with significant disability who does not receive treatment would still be classified as having a disorder. Yet the converse is also true: Their criteria would still admit those who seek treatment but do not experience significant disability. Even if this tautology were eliminated, their proposal is still premised on the idea that the presence of a disorder and the need for treatment go hand in hand, something other critics have already rejected.[9] By the logic of this proposal, the widespread expansion of psychiatric treatment in the late 1990s produced not only an increase in treatment but an increase in prevalence as well.

Another conservative approach is to focus on the number of disorders contained in the *DSM* rather than on the specific criteria for any single disorder. This approach is guided by some of the same ideas as other conservative approaches, especially the goal of reducing the estimated prevalence that conventional criteria yield. Concerned with identifying only the most serious symptoms, this approach encourages a focus on the most disabling disorders and eliminating from consideration disorders that are, on average, mild. Taking this proposal seriously, one would look at some of the research findings presented earlier and revise the *DSM* accordingly. Look at which disorders tend to be serious, look at which disorders tend to be mild, and include the former but not the latter. In light of the NCS evidence, this proposal would, among other things, preserve most mood disorders but eliminate most anxiety disorders. This approach implies another thing that is important to emphasize: that tightening the *DSM* is best achieved by thinking about specific disorders rather than broad concepts like clinical significance.[10] Although this proposal might radically trim the size of the *DSM*—many disorders would presumably be eliminated—it is more conservative than other proposals in the sense that it would preserve the diagnostic criteria for those disorders that remained in the manual.

Another approach would reduce the number of disorders contained in the *DSM* in a different way. It would limit the *DSM* to disorders that are serious in and of themselves or those for which the prognosis, absent treatment, is poor.[11] This approach, then, favors harmonization between what disorders are described in the *DSM* and what disorders clinicians are prepared to treat. It appears modest in intent, but in effect it would severely reduce the number of disorders contained in the *DSM*. This approach would also require a strong interplay between science and nosology, perhaps one much stronger than is presently possible. The "best" diagnoses would be those for which there is an established body of evidence indicating that the disorder has a chronic course and an effective treatment. Not all disorders, however, have established treatments or even strong evidence regarding their chronicity. This approach, for example, would likely eliminate many personality disorders as well as some specific phobias.

Proposals of this sort also have the potential to distort the interface between science and diagnosis. Knowing which disorders tend to be severe requires credible knowledge about the severity of those particular disorders. And only by naming and describing a disorder can we study it in the first place. The rest of medicine has made inroads against disease by first understanding the existence of those diseases. A treatment for HIV, for example, was developed only after the virus was recognized and became the focus of scientific (and political) attention. Psychiatric disorders differ from infectious diseases in fundamental ways, of course, but they are no less dependent on the light we choose to direct toward them. Psychiatric disorders are also stigmatized in ways that can diminish the prospects of a thoroughgoing research enterprise. At this stage of research on psychiatric disorders, restricting the *DSM* to disorders for which we have a treatment in hand might have the unfortunate consequence of foreclosing on the possibility of developing an effective treatment in the first place.

THE DIMENSIONAL APPROACH

Although these various proposals differ in their emphasis and approach, they all share an interest in preserving much of the *DSM*'s structure. Even proposals that would radically reduce the number of disorders contained in the *DSM* still preserve the manual's essential form. There is little in these proposals, then, that betrays a *radical* dissatisfaction. Other proposals highlight deeper flaws and insist on more fundamental revisions. For them, the core issue is the *DSM*'s reliance on *categorical* diagnoses. In these proposals, all the things critics see as "artificial" about the *DSM*—its rules, its lists, its counts—rest on the need to create categories from experiences. These proposals insist, instead, that psychological experiences are fundamentally *dimensional* and therefore do not lend themselves to neat categorization. If some critics argue that the *DSM*'s diagnostic thresholds have no empirical justification—something that is plainly true—others argue that there is no reason to maintain a threshold at all.

The dimensional approach has a number of defining features. First, it recognizes *degrees* of functioning, moving beyond simple classifications of present or absent and, in some cases, even from the idea of a disorder. In a dimensional framework, psychological functioning is assessed on a spectrum. Individuals suffer, for example, from more or less depression, anxiety, and phobia. Second, the dimensional approach assigns more significance to individual symptoms than entire syndromes. The idea is not necessarily that major depression ought to be discarded altogether. Instead, the idea is that major depression, as the *DSM* defines it, consists of multiple symptoms and that each of these symptoms should be considered in its own right. The idea is further informed by the notion that, whatever we think major depression is in nature, we classify it based on the presence or absence of specific symptoms. Information, then, is critical: It is best to respect fully the information that symptoms can provide (and, at a minimum, recognize the manner in which we assess them), rather than reduce that information to a single value based on a potentially flawed definition. Third, the dimensional approach views comorbidity very differently from the categorical approach. Rather than emphasizing the simultaneous presence of multiple disorders, the dimensional approach arrays individuals across multiple dimensions of functioning. Any relationship between those dimensions—say, alcohol use being positively correlated with depression—merely represents the presence of two types of symptoms, not the existence of two types of disorder.

Perhaps the strongest articulation of the dimensional approach rests on the idea that the *DSM* induces *reification*.[12] Reification refers to the idea of bringing something into existence and making it concrete, to the transformation of the abstract into the real. In the context of psychiatric disorders, however, the idea of reification assumes an especially critical edge, with the implication that reification is a fallacy. To critics, the process of reification renders psychiatric disorders "real," when they were never real to begin with. It obscures what ought to be transparent. And it creates permanence in something that is irremediably conditional. Those who emphasize reification begin by noting—as I have done—that the *DSM* is premised on expert judgment more than scientific research. They go further, though, in arguing that clinical utility—always a goal of the *DSM*—is not well served by categorical thinking. By taking a variety of symptoms and experiences and reducing them to a simple yes/no dichotomy, a categorical approach reduces information, even though science, clinicians, and patients would almost certainly prefer more. In addition, a categorical approach obscures important similarities between cases and muddles otherwise instructive comparisons. Two people might differ only by a single symptom, for instance, yet by the rules of the *DSM*, one person will meet the diagnostic criteria for a disorder while the other will not. By the same token, a categorical approach obscures the *set* of symptoms leading to a disorder. Because of polythetic criteria, two people with exactly the same diagnosis can still have very different symptom portfolios. They share a label but potentially little else apart from that.

It is instructive to think about the consequences of reification from the perspective of clinicians or patients, but its consequences are perhaps clearest with respect to research.[13] The *DSM* is used by the National Institute of Mental Health for funding research projects. The *DSM* is implicated in several ways in the process. Scientists seeking funding to study major depression, for instance, will propose to identify cases of major depression using the *DSM*'s diagnostic criteria. And in doing so they will usually describe—and, in effect, pledge—fidelity to established diagnostic instruments, such as the Composite International Diagnostic Interview. The scientific community, in turn, will evaluate the research in light of its contributions to the study of major depression, so defined. The *DSM* thus sets the terms of the debate. What is not codified in the *DSM* is, in effect, not studied. And what is codified in the *DSM* is studied in the strictest possible terms. Even symptoms that tend to occur naturally with a disorder will be disregarded if they are not included as part of the *DSM*'s formal criteria for that disorder.

The study of schizophrenia, for example, has suffered as a result of reification of this sort. The hallmark of schizophrenia is its so-called positive symptoms, including hallucinations and delusions. A number of effective treatments exist for these symptoms and, for purposes of diagnosis, these symptoms are seen as emblematic of the disorder. Yet clinicians also recognize other aspects of the disorder because they see them manifest in the patients they actually treat. In particular, they recognize that patients often also suffer from a variety of cognitive symptoms, including poor working memory. Unfortunately the pharmaceuticals traditionally used in treating schizophrenia are largely ineffective in treating these symptoms. And one explanation for this ineffectiveness is that pharmaceutical research has been tailored to the symptoms explicitly included in the *DSM*, and *only* those symptoms, leading to a discontinuity between the schizophrenia that is the subject of research and the schizophrenia that is the target of treatment. To be sure, things have changed over time, but the difficult history of this change only highlights the *DSM*'s hold. Addressing orphaned symptoms of this sort requires the concerted effort of scientists and funding agencies to think about the symptoms of the disorder apart from the *DSM* framework and to agree on a framework for studying them.

The same scientific inflexibility is consequential for more prevalent disorders as well. Attention deficit/hyperactivity disorder (ADHD) is common among school-aged children. The *DSM-IV* criteria for ADHD (used in much of the existing research) specify a threshold of six or more symptoms (out of a total of nine) across two symptom categories, symptoms related to inattention and symptoms related to hyperactivity-impulsivity. ADHD is a categorical disorder, premised on a threshold, but evidence suggests that both of its symptom types reflect continuous capacities with strong developmental trajectories—that is, children naturally move along both dimensions as they mature. Although some children might be delayed along the way, a delay in itself does not reveal abnormal brain development. In attempting to render a diagnosis, however, clinicians must contend with the *DSM* as it is written. They must also render a decision based on the symptoms they observe at the time. Unlike the situation with height and weight charts, clinicians are not provided with age-graded information for the normal pace of development in attention-related capacities. They are, instead, provided with fixed rules regarding symptom counts. And with these seemingly primitive tools they must make diagnoses that are enormously consequential for students.

Advocates for a dimensional approach believe it would achieve at least three things. First, the dimensional approach would better reflect the reality of mental illness. Second, even in the absence of a strong scientific understanding of the dimensionality of a disorder, it would allow researchers to study symptoms as they naturally occur rather than impose a rigid structure a priori. Third, it would indemnify the profession against some aspects of public skepticism. Dimensional measures do not lend themselves to deriving (potentially suspicious) prevalence estimates. If dimensional measures were used for evaluating suffering, there would be no basis for claiming that nearly half of all Americans have suffered from a psychiatric disorder at some point in their lifetime, just as there is no real basis for claiming that some percentage of Americans are too tall or short. To be sure, a dimensional approach would still be inconsistent with the rest of medicine, wherein a categorical approach prevails. But even here there are some physical disorders for which a dimensional approach is accepted and entirely operational. Hypertension, for instance, is a categorical diagnosis that represents blood pressure consistently in excess of 140/90. Yet doctors recognize that the relationship between blood pressure and the risk for cardiac events is, in fact, continuous and, furthermore, that the effectiveness of treatment can be evaluated in terms of moving someone up or down, not just moving someone below or above a diagnostic threshold. By the same token, type 2 diabetes is a metabolic disease and is diagnosed categorically, but average blood glucose is the metric for evaluating effective control of blood sugar, and it reflects a spectrum.

Table 4.1 provides two examples of a dimensional measure. The first is a measure of distress, and the second is a measure of schizophrenia. The measure of distress is especially popular. It is included in surveys such as the U.S. National Health Interview Survey, the largest and most regularly conducted survey of its kind. The instrument is known as the K-10, in reference to its creator, Ronald Kessler. In essence, the K-10 is a greatest-hits collection of questions culled from previous dimensional measures. In creating the

TABLE 4.1 EXAMPLES OF DIMENSIONAL MEASURES:
PART A. THE K-10 MEASURE OF NONSPECIFIC PSYCHOLOGICAL DISTRESS

THE FOLLOWING QUESTIONS ASK ABOUT HOW YOU HAVE BEEN FEELING DURING THE PAST 30 DAYS. FOR EACH QUESTION, PLEASE CIRCLE THE NUMBER THAT BEST DESCRIBES HOW OFTEN YOU HAD THIS FEELING. DURING THAT MONTH, HOW OFTEN DID YOU FEEL:

Tired out for no good reason?
Nervous?
So nervous that nothing could calm you down?
Hopeless?
Restless or fidgety?
So restless that you could not sit still?
Depressed?
So depressed that nothing could cheer you up?
That everything was an effort?
Worthless?

Note: Response categories consist of: all of the time; most of the time; some of the time; a little of the time; and none of the time.

Source: R. C. Kessler et al., "Short Screening Scales to Monitor Population Prevalences and Trends in Non-Specific Psychological Distress," *Psychological Medicine* 32, no. 06 (2002): 959–76.

PART B. DIMENSIONAL MEASURE OF SCHIZOPHRENIA

HOW OFTEN IN THE PAST MONTH HAVE YOU:

Felt that your mind was dominated by forces beyond your control?
Heard voices without knowing where they came from?
Had visions or seen things other people say they cannot see?
Felt that you were possessed by a spirit or devil?
Felt you had special powers?
Felt that you did not exist at all, that you were dead, dissolved?
Seemed to hear your thoughts spoken aloud—almost as if someone standing nearby could hear them?
Felt that your unspoken thoughts were being broadcast or transmitted, so that everyone knew what you were thinking?

Note: Response categories consist of: never; almost never; sometimes; fairly often; or often.

Source: Blair Wheaton, "Personal Resources and Mental Health," in *Research in Community and Mental Health*, ed. James R. Greenley (Greenwich, Conn.: JAI, 1985), 139–184.

instrument, Kessler and his team sought indicators of *nonspecific* psychological distress, that is, symptoms that may or may not correspond to a specific
psychiatric disorder and reflect "distress" generally rather than just anxiety
or depression or fear. Scales measuring distress generally cover a range of
symptoms, including those that are cognitive, behavioral, emotional, and
physiological. They also cover multiple disorders, in this case focusing on
symptoms consistent with depression and anxiety. In total, Kessler and his
colleagues identified eighteen such scales, each consisting of twenty or more
separate items, for a total of 612 questions.[14] From this pool, they identified
the items that best represented that concept of distress according to formal
psychometric tests. As is apparent in the figure, the items they settled on are
varied. Remarkably, though, all ten items are strongly correlated with one
another (a result reflecting the psychometric properties on which they were
selected). Although on their face the symptoms differ in their character—
some symptoms are somatic, whereas others are affective—these distinctions
are not *empirically* meaningful, and the items can be summed into a single
score without losing much information. The summed scale ranges from 0
(corresponding to experiencing all of the symptoms none of the time) to
40 (corresponding to experiencing all of the symptoms all of the time). Dimensional measures can be converted into categorical ones, if users decide
that a score above a certain threshold indicates a disorder, but dimensional
measures usually were not designed with that purpose in mind. And because they were not designed to show strict fidelity to the *DSM*, any decision about a threshold would not be drawn directly from the *DSM*'s rules.

The schizophrenia-related questions have a similar spirit. Of course, the
questions themselves are different from the distress questions, but the intent
is similar. The creators were interested in providing spectrum-related information for a disorder we might ordinarily regard as either present or absent.[15] These questions, too, are highly correlated with one another, although
some of the questions pertain to symptoms that are presumably more common than others. This difference is central to the approach: Schizophrenia
is a rare disorder, but some of its symptoms might not be. The creators
imagined, for example, that many people might feel their thoughts are beyond their control, and almost certainly more people than those that suffer

from schizophrenia. And the creators felt that knowing the frequency of this experience was scientifically important irrespective of whether the experience coincided with full-blown schizophrenia.

There are many other dimensional measures. Indeed, the sheer variety of dimensional measures reflects the ecumenical spirit of the enterprise. Advocates for a dimensional approach are less wed to any one definition in particular and more to the general idea that the *DSM* errs in assuming a categorical approach. In this vein, John Mirowsky and Catherine Ross—longstanding and compelling advocates for dimensionality—regard the science premised on dimensional measures as more "human" in its fidelity to lived experience.[16] To the extent that critics of the *DSM* like Mirowsky and Ross favor a manual at all, they envision something different. They envision an approach wherein clinicians assess their patients across a variety of spectrums, ultimately settling on a multidimensional assessment of the patient's overall mental health rather than a diagnosis. From there, clinicians could decide whether treatment was necessary and, if so, what treatment was effective for a particular set of symptoms.

THE NETWORK APPROACH

Other alternatives to the *DSM* share the same focus on symptoms but regard the underlying problem differently. These approaches begin with the idea that the *DSM* might be correct, at least in a limited way. They note that the symptoms of major depression, for instance, do in fact tend to co-occur. In this sense, the *DSM*, as a catalogue of symptoms, has organized its symptoms in a way that roughly approximates how they are actually present in individuals. Major depression looks, more or less, like it is described in the *DSM*. Where these approaches depart from the *DSM*, though, is in where they believe these symptoms originate. Recall in chapter 2 I discussed how the *DSM* assumes that symptoms are the product of an underlying disorder. In the *DSM*, symptoms are important, but only as signs of the thing we really care about. Symptoms signal a disorder, and once a disorder is properly identified, that disorder becomes the object of attention and the target of treatment.

Some approaches, though, push beyond the notion of symptoms as signs. They argue, in particular, for a greater appreciation of how some symptoms can cause others. Denny Borsboom and Angélique Cramer provide an especially compelling statement of what is referred to as the network approach and contrast it with the existing approach to psychiatric disorders.[17] Their idea appears simple—it is easy to envision how some symptoms might produce others—but it has strong implications and allows for a more integrative approach. They begin by asserting that the disease model does not work well for psychiatric disorders, even if it works well for other diseases. In this, they are not unlike some of the strongest critics of psychiatry, including Thomas Szasz, as discussed earlier. A brain tumor, for example, can produce headaches and poor eyesight. In this case, the tumor is the cause of the symptoms, and eliminating the tumor will alleviate the symptoms. The symptoms, then, are properly regarded as signs of the disorder, and they strictly denote the problem. Applying the same logic to psychiatric disorders, however, is misleading, as Borsboom and Cramer argue. For one, the symptoms of psychiatric disorders are *constitutive* of the disorder rather than *indicative*. One can have a tumor without headaches—and, in any case, more information is required to determine whether a tumor is present—but one cannot be depressed without feeling sad or losing interest in things. Furthermore, the latent entity behind psychiatric disorders is not well characterized, at least not as well characterized as a tumor. Although there are many proposals to improve the *DSM*, Borsboom and Cramer point out that these proposals fail to move beyond the question of what to do with symptoms. But the symptoms, they argue, are the opportunity.

Focusing on symptoms, the network approach proposes something very different and more fundamental. It encourages an appreciation of relationships among symptoms instead of the demarcation of a set of symptoms caused by a disorder. For example, rather than regarding major depression as causing sadness and indecisiveness (among other things), a network approach allows for the possibility that sadness can *cause* indecisiveness. Indeed, the network approach sees relationships among symptoms as a pervasive and underappreciated feature of psychiatric disorders. Such relationships are often part of the narrative patients construct, even though they are absent from the *DSM*. Sleep disruptions, for instance, might produce fatigue, which might produce problems in concentration, which might eventually produce all the symptoms necessary for a diagnosis of a major depressive episode. Examples of these pathways are represented in figure 4.1, representing the nine symptoms of a major depressive episode and one symptom of generalized anxiety. These pathways, the network approach insists, are easier to imagine than some poorly characterized entity producing all the symptoms of the disorder more or less simultaneously.

Being consistent with the *DSM*'s framework, the network approach does maintain a focus on symptoms, and although strictly speaking it violates theory neutrality, it does so in a quite limited way. The network approach does not require, for instance, that one accept a specific model of psychopathology, whether psychodynamic or genetic. Furthermore, something similar to the network approach is not entirely absent from aspects of the existing *DSM*. The *DSM* already posits some connections between symptoms, albeit of a limited and often implicit nature. For instance, the diagnostic criteria for a panic disorder require that a person change his or her behavior in light of panic attacks, implying that the latter causes the former (and if it does not, it is probably not a panic disorder). Similarly, in the diagnostic criteria for an obsessive-compulsive disorder the two essential components of the disorder

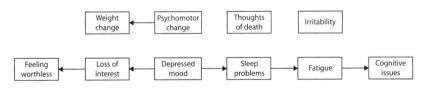

FIGURE 4.1 Network approach to major depression.

Source: Adapted from Denny Borsboom and Angélique O. J. Cramer, "Network Analysis: An Integrative Approach to the Structure of Psychopathology," *Annual Review of Clinical Psychology* 9, no. 1 (2013): 91–121.

are conveyed as part of a sequence. Compulsive behavior is assumed to alleviate partially the distress caused by an obsession. A network approach would expand and deepen these sorts of connections.

Advocates for the network approach see a number of additional advantages. For one, the approach allows for the possibility that different symptoms have different types of causes. Symptoms earlier in the causal chain might be caused by genetic factors, whereas those later in the chain might reflect the environment. In this way, the network approach avoids overinvesting in one type of cause over another. Furthermore, the network approach resists the idea that disorders are entities, even if it does not jettison the idea altogether. In the network approach, many symptoms can occur together, to be sure, but they are not presumed to be caused by a single underlying pathology. In addition, the network approach has the added benefit of formalizing what clinicians have already appreciated informally: that the same disorder can be manifest in very different ways from person to person, even among those people who share similar experiences. In this way, the network approach moves beyond the mere use of polythetic criteria to explode the concept of heterogeneity. In the network approach, the same five symptoms can appear differently in people depending on the sequence in which those five symptoms emerge. The *DSM* criteria are blind to this possibility, but the network approach is not.

The network approach also provides a different framework for thinking about comorbidity. The interpretation of comorbidity is complex, fraught, and often reveals, as much as anything, what the interpreter thinks about the *DSM*. Critics of the *DSM* argue, for example, that comorbidity is merely an artifact of the natural overlap between artificial diagnostic criteria. If two disorders share at least some of the same symptoms, those disorders are likely to be comorbid for no reason other than that, by definition, they have similar characteristics. Generalized anxiety and a major depressive episode, for example, share sleep problems, concentration problems, and fatigue.

The idea that comorbidity is an artifact of classification can be pushed even further. If we allow that one symptom can cause another, it is easy to envision pathways, through so-called bridge symptoms, that connect symptoms that are entirely unique to depression to symptoms that are entirely unique to anxiety. Figure 4.1 shows the symptoms of a major depressive episode but also presents irritability, a symptom of generalized anxiety. If fatigue can cause irritability, the comorbidity between depression and anxiety could reflect both the symptoms the two disorders share and the possibility that the symptoms of one disorder can cause those of the other. The *DSM*, in fact, sets the stage for pervasive comorbidity both by using some symptoms that cross disorders and by failing to allow for between-disorder causality. One network-based analysis of all the symptoms contained in the *DSM* revealed what network scientists refer to as a "small-world" phenomenon.[18] *DSM-IV* contains a series of symptoms that, although appearing in distinct criteria, can easily be connected with one another through a relatively small number of pathways. Just as there might be only six or fewer degrees of separation between you and anyone else in the world, there might be very few degrees of separation between the symptoms of one disorder and those of another, even disorders seemingly far removed. Indeed, this degree of association was found to be especially narrow between disorders that are, in fact, highly comorbid, including mood, anxiety, and substance abuse disorders. The network approach to classification would bring these connections to light.

CONSIDERING NORMAL AND ABNORMAL RESPONSES TO THE ENVIRONMENT

Although the network approach violates theory neutrality in a strict sense, some alternative approaches to diagnosis insist that the *DSM* must wrangle with the thorny of issue of whether a psychological response is appropriate to the environment. In these approaches, a better *DSM* begins with explicitly considering the causes of psychiatric disorder, especially the context in which they occur, and explicitly including them as part of the diagnostic criteria. What separates normal and abnormal, the argument goes, is not simply the severity of the symptoms per se but rather the degree to which the symptoms reflect a normal response to the environment. If sadness results from severe stress, for example, it should not be regarded as depression, because it reflects an expected and appropriate response. If anxiety results from a genuinely high-stakes situation, it should not be regarded as a phobia, because it can be interpreted as functional. According to this framework, false positives emerge when our diagnostic criteria are not crafted in ways that allow us to distinguish when symptoms are an expected response rather than an aberration.

Jerome Wakefield has done more than any other researcher (he is also a clinician) to formalize the ideas behind this distinction.[19] In particular, he defines mental disorder as a *harmful dysfunction*. In this framework, symptoms constitute a disorder only when two conditions are met, one of which invites cultural considerations; the other is more a matter of science. First, the symptoms must cause some identifiable *harm*. What constitutes harm will vary depending on social values and culture, as Wakefield allows, but the idea is that any disorder—in order to be considered a real disorder—must cause some harm to the person suffering from it. One might fear snakes, for example, but if that fear does not affect one's daily functioning, it should not be regarded as a psychiatric disorder. Second, the symptoms must reflect a *dysfunction*. Although the term dysfunction is general, the concept is specific, and Wakefield has a particular model in mind. For him a dysfunction occurs when an internal mechanism is not performing its intended function, as set by evolution. Of course, the notion of an "intended" function invites ambiguity (let alone an "internal" mechanism). For one, evolution has no intentions, which is easy enough to rectify as a matter of terminology but still betrays something about the original framework. Furthermore, it is difficult to discern the intended function of a system that evolved in the past but functions in the present. Wakefield acknowledges these difficulties, but he sees them as no especially significant challenge. Evolution has produced organs that serve vital and plain functions, including eyes that allow vision and ears that allow hearing. Blindness and deafness are medical problems because the eyes and ears are failing to do what they are supposed to do. Wakefield imagines something similar for mental processes and envisions a wide variety of internal mechanisms that intersect with psychiatric disorders. Many emotions, for example, are normal and serve a purpose, but when they fail to serve their function, they constitute a dysfunction. Discerning the function of psychological processes is, of course, more difficult than discerning the function of eyes, but there are frameworks for at least thinking about it in a thoroughgoing fashion.

Sadness, for example, could serve some evolutionary needs for a species, even if it is aversive for individuals. Randolph Nesse provides perhaps the most comprehensive account in this regard.[20] He argues that depressed mood can be adaptive in some circumstances. For one, depression can serve as an important social cue. Depression can signal to a friend that help is needed or to an enemy that a fight has ended, transcending the value of speech. Depression can also provide information to the individual or at least implicitly encourage different behavior. For example, depression might encourage disengagement from goals that have become unattainable and indicate that time and energy could be better directed toward other activities. Being thwarted in a career is painful, to be sure, but if the resulting sadness motivates the person to pursue a more satisfying career in another field, it has served a useful function. An important feature of Wakefield's dysfunction concept rests on its conditionality: Depression is only useful (or not) under specific circumstances. To the extent that it confers any advantage at all, it does so only when it is responsive to the environment. If it is not, it provides no information to the individual and does not signal anything useful to others.

The harmful-dysfunction approach also provides a way for thinking about symptoms that no longer serve their intended function. The approach does so by combining dysfunction with *harm*. Evolution is not the sole criterion. Evolution might produce behaviors that resemble the symptoms of a psychiatric disorder, but according to the idea of harmful dysfunction those behaviors will constitute a disorder only insofar as they cause harm. For instance, evolution might favor aggressive behavior because aggressive behavior promotes reproductive fitness when the environment is generally hostile, as it was for much of our evolutionary history. Similarly, a fear of snakes might be appropriate when venomous snakes do, in fact, pose a significant threat to foragers. Today, however, highly aggressive behavior and unwarranted fear might cause considerable harm.

On its surface, the harmful-dysfunction approach resembles other approaches that emphasize disability. The *harmful* part of harmful dysfunction is clear. Wakefield, however, distinguishes his approach by also emphasizing *dysfunction* and by highlighting some of the difficulties of definitions that rely on *harm*. According to Wakefield, any definition of disability requires a specific sense of what the disability is, but the concept is difficult to define on its own. Moreover, according to Wakefield, disability can result from even "normal" levels of psychological distress. On this point, Wakefield departs significantly from previous critiques. For instance, one could be distressed following the death of a loved one and, as a result, perform less effectively. This distress could then be considered harmful, but for Wakefield it does not constitute a disorder because there is no evidence the experience is a dysfunction. To the contrary, distress of this sort could reflect a psychological system that is working entirely as it should. Similarly, a child who steals candy has behavioral patterns that are demonstrably harmful (at least for those from whom he steals), but this does not constitute a disorder because the child has yet to develop the capacity to regulate his behavior.

The harmful-dysfunction approach necessarily considers the role of causes. It also elevates certain causes over others. Wakefield's emphasis on evolution, for example, increases the significance of genes for identifying dysfunction. Yet Wakefield emphasizes the role of evolution in bequeathing us with "normal" genes, those that give us emotions like sadness or fear. Moreover, he is quick to point out that his approach also considers other types of causes when it comes to evaluating whether something is dysfunctional. Wakefield considers Freud's theory of repression as an example, though he does so to illustrate how easily his approach can accommodate a range of ideas and not as an endorsement of Freud. Indeed, as a scientific framework, Freud's theory has not held up well, but if we accept one of his basic ideas— that we repress traumatic or shameful experiences in order to maintain mental health—the theory can fit within a harmful-dysfunction framework. Freud regarded repression as a mechanism that kept painful memories from reaching consciousness. Repression is not a symptom or even a problem, but when it fails, Freud argued, painful memories could reach consciousness in the form of neuroses. Viewed in terms of its purpose, repression illustrates an aspect of harmful dysfunction. Repression ordinarily works as a mechanism for maintaining psychological equipoise, but when it fails the resulting neurosis can be regarded as a dysfunction. If it is also harmful, it constitutes a disorder. One need not subscribe to Freud's view—Wakefield would argue that any psychological defense mechanism could play a similar role, and, indeed, science has discovered a variety of aspects to a healthy psychological immune system. The task of the scientist is simply to determine what a "functioning" system looks like, and, with this information, science can derive better diagnostic criteria.

The focal point of Wakefield's approach has been the bereavement exclusion. As discussed earlier, the *DSM* criteria for a major depressive episode have historically included a bereavement exclusion, allowing that the symptoms of depression might emerge as a normal part of grieving and so should not be regarded as indicative of a depressive episode, so long as the bereavement fits certain parameters. In *DSM-IV*, the period of normal bereavement was specified as two months. It is easy to see the attraction of this exclusion. There are perhaps few disorders for which the false-negative/false-positive tension is as acute. Furthermore, bereavement is part of normal experience. Most people will experience the death of a loved one at some point in their lives. Moreover, those who have experienced the death of a loved one know the pain it can cause. Indeed, the symptoms of bereavement overlap closely with the symptoms of a major depressive episode, including sleep disturbances, crying when waking, a loss of appetite, and a loss of interest. In this light, Wakefield regards the bereavement exclusion as an especially effective means of eliminating false positives. He only wonders why bereavement is the *only* identified instance of something that might cause sadness. Why not have other exclusions, especially if, given the bereavement exclusion, the *DSM* has already conceded that life events produce unhappiness? Why not also extend the exclusion to other disorders, which presumably are affected by the environment as well?

Wakefield has subsequently elaborated on how a scientific understanding of the causes of depression can be leveraged to define the disorder more sharply. For him, depression "without cause" is more emblematic of harmful dysfunction than depression "with cause," especially when it pertains to causes that fall squarely within the domain of everyday life. Depression following the death of a loved one, for example, has an explicable cause, and the resulting depression might serve some useful function, as when it compels others to bestow the grieving person with gifts or resources. Recognizing some of the difficulties surrounding the traditional with-versus-without-cause distinction, Wakefield and Horwitz provide three features of normal depression: It emerges in light of specific environmental triggers, especially loss; it tends to be roughly proportionate to the magnitude of the trigger; and it tends to dissipate when the stress subsides or when the individual is given sufficient time to cope.[21] A spouse might not return, but grieving will eventually end.

In this approach, depression becomes a disorder under specific circumstances, and, by the same token, depression without an apparent cause assumes special significance. Depression is indicative of dysfunction when it is occasioned by no apparent event. Under these conditions depression could serve no plausible function because it provides no relevant information. It does not signal any change in the environment or direct the person toward some behavior that might make the environment better. Moreover, when depression cannot be linked to any obvious *external* event, an *internal* change is naturally seen as the cause. For Wakefield, this idea casts a more credible sheen over the idea of psychiatric disorders as biological dysfunctions.

Although much of Wakefield's critique has focused on bereavement, his logic points to other exclusions that have the same character, and he has put some of his ideas to the test. Depression can result from many things, including marital dissolution, job loss, natural disasters, the rupturing of friendships, and financial problems. In one study, Wakefield and his collaborators explored what happened to a variety of people experiencing different loss-related events, including but not limited to bereavement.[22] If bereavement is special—as the *DSM* criteria seem to suggest it is—episodes of depression following bereavement should differ from episodes following some other loss. Wakefield and his colleagues showed, however, that episodes of depression were similar regardless of whether they were brought on by bereavement or something else. In this light, Wakefield and his collaborates concluded that there was no reason to focus only on bereavement. Other exclusions could be added because they have much the same effect.

In another demonstration of this idea, Wakefield and Schmitz used the likelihood of recurrence as a criterion for testing dysfunction.[23] They found that three sorts of exclusions led to better predictive validity; that is, in this case, they increased the ability of researchers to predict new episodes of depression in the future. They were: (1) excluding episodes of depression that lasted no longer than two months and did not include any severe symptoms, such as suicidal thoughts, psychotic symptoms, feelings of worthlessness, or psychomotor retardation; (2) excluding cases with five symptoms rather than the normal six, that is, raising the symptom threshold and thereby eliminating "mild" disorders; and (3) excluding nonmelancholic depression. In order to be considered melancholic, a depressive episode must have at least three of the following five symptoms: chronic fatigue, psychomotor retardation, agitation, decreased interest in sex, and slowed thinking. Wakefield and Schmitz showed that episodes of depression defined in this fashion did much better in predicting a later episode than depression defined using the conventional *DSM-IV* diagnostic criteria. Some exclusions were, however, more powerful than others. The identification of melancholic episodes, for instance, and the removal of brief episodes of depression were especially powerful in enhancing the ability to predict future recurrence. Another way to think about this issue is that the revised criteria proposed by Wakefield and Schmitz did better in identifying chronic cases of depression than did the standard diagnostic criteria—using the likelihood of recurrence as a criterion for evaluating validity elevates the relevance of chronicity. In effect, the standard diagnostic criteria yield a large number of episodes that remit in a short amount of time. Wakefield and Schmitz's enhanced criteria also, quite naturally, reduced the estimated prevalence of major depression.

MORE LUMPING AND LESS SPLITTING

Another approach to revising the *DSM* favors creating synthetic categories. Creating such categories, advocates argue, would retain the major goals of the *DSM* but yield a more coherent system. Some critics see the evolution of the *DSM* in terms of excessive splitting, that is, in terms of creating ever more narrow diagnoses, while losing sight of the many characteristics disorders have in common. This trend is related to reliability and so resonates with the kinds of criticisms raised regarding psychiatry in the pre-*DSM-III* era. As discussed earlier, the reliability of psychiatric diagnoses is greater for broad classes of disorders than for specific disorders. Thus, for example, there is usually agreement among clinicians regarding whether someone suffers from a mood disorder, even if there is disagreement regarding whether the disorder is unipolar or bipolar depression. If reliability is enhanced by casting a wider net, the *DSM* might benefit from consolidation. Some commonalities between disorders, though, cut across categories and so require more radical revisions. Clinicians appreciate, for example, that schizophrenia and obsessive-compulsive disorder frequently occur together, even though the two disorders belong to different categories. This has led some to propose a new schizo-obsessive dimension, which would encompass both.[24] Other *DSM* categories could be created to reflect different commonalities. In this vein, Steven Hyman points to three especially large clusters of co-occurring disorders: fear-based anxiety disorders, obsessive-compulsive spectrum disorders, and addictive and other impulse-control disorders.[25] In the same spirit, other scientists have proposed even more clusters. Paul McHugh, for instance, proposes four clusters based on shared characteristics and causes.[26] The themes behind these clusters are very abstract and even existential, but they still could serve as the foundation of a plausible organizing framework to otherwise distinct disorders. The first cluster contains brain diseases that have a direct relationship with neural processes, including, for example, Alzheimer's disease. McHugh characterizes these disorders as ones patients "have," based on an identifiable pathology. The second cluster contains disorders that are more psychological than neurological, characterized by who patients "are." These include disorders related to personality and disposition, including how strongly an individual responds to stress (and, thus, how prone they are to disproportionate reactions). The third cluster contains disorders involving maladaptive or fixed behaviors, such as drug addiction and eating disorders, characterized by what individuals are "doing." And the fourth cluster includes disorders that are bought on by events that thwart aspirations or endanger identities. The resulting experiences include grief, anxiety, and stress. The defining feature of these disorders is what individuals "encounter" and what those encounters mean to them. According to McHugh this synthetic approach helps return the focus of psychiatry not simply to the symptoms of disorders but also to their underlying causes and processes. His use of verbs to characterize the categories, while unusual, is, thus, intentional—the instinct to regard causes as essential to diagnosis is strong. He also argues that such an approach is already part of how many psychiatrists think about the disorders they find in their patients.

A similar approach also focuses on creating synthetic categories but uses a different architecture. Craddock and Owen propose what would perhaps be the most radical reorganization of the *DSM*.[27] Their approach emphasizes similarity at the level of symptoms and functioning rather than at the level of types of disorders. Nick Craddock and Michael Owen first posit the existence of five syndromes. They then array these syndromes on a single dimension according to their resemblance to one another. They propose a single spectrum that moves from mental retardation to autism to schizophrenia to schizoaffective disorder to bipolar/unipolar disorder, with each zone on the spectrum encompassing a host of disorders. The idea of a single spectrum is especially significant, both as a reflection of the science of psychiatric disorders and their phenomenology. The spectrum acknowledges that some disorders are, in fact, more likely to co-occur and thus can be thought of as residing closer in space. Mental retardation and autism, for example, are more similar to each other than mental retardation and unipolar depression and, therefore, are "closer" to each other. But Craddock and Owen envision an even deeper connection between adjacent disorders. They envision a growing contribution of neurodevelopmental issues as one moves to the left, toward mental retardation, and a growing affective contribution as one moves to the right, toward unipolar/bipolar disorder. They also propose that certain types of symptoms are more common in some parts of the spectrum than others. They focus on several types of symptoms: cognitive impairment; negative symptoms, characterized by the absence of something, such as a lack of emotional response; positive symptoms, characterized by the presence of something, including delusions; and mood swings, characterized by wide variation in affect. These symptoms, they argue, can be arrayed sequentially along the spectrum and imply some segregation. Cognitive impairment, for instance, is common in mental retardation, autism, and schizophrenia but not in bipolar/unipolar disorders. On the flip side, mood swings are common in schizoaffective disorders and bipolar/unipolar disorders but not in autism or schizophrenia. Positive symptoms might be the broadest category, spanning many disorders along the spectrum, but, even so, positive symptoms are not typical of mental retardation and, therefore, can still be said to occupy a defined space. Using this framework, clinicians would not make a diagnosis in the traditional sense. They would instead evaluate patients on each of the symptom classes and from this assign an individual to a point along the spectrum. Among the benefits of this approach is its simplicity. It involves reorganizing disorders that are already in place. Yet it radically reframes the idea of comorbidity and, indeed, of diagnosis. Rather than an individual suffering from various anxiety disorders, for instance, it would reclassify that individual as having a fear-based disorder, denoted by the place he or she occupies on the spectrum. Although their approach is far-reaching in many respects, Craddock and Owen are, in some sense, merely taking the phenomenological approach, which has existed for decades, to the next level: They are trying to organize formally what clinicians and researchers have observed already.

CONSIDERING THE CAREER OF A DIAGNOSIS

Proposals to revise the *DSM* are remarkably varied, ranging from mere tweaks to the existing criteria to more fundamental reimaginings of its entire taxometric apparatus. The range of proposals is remarkable. On the one hand, many proposals seek to combine disorders into larger categories, thereby rolling back much of the inertia since *DSM-III*. On the other hand, other proposals are based on a much finer level of granularity than is in place now. The network approach, for instance, focuses not only on symptoms rather than disorders but also on connections among symptoms, thereby greatly elevating the complexity of psychiatric classification. Harmful dysfunction, meanwhile, might retain some of the features of the *DSM* but would still require a much more detailed assessment of the circumstances surrounding symptoms, as would any approach emphasizing a contextual assessment. The fact that there is little consensus over even the basic direction that revisions should take suggests a more or less open field.

In later chapters, I will return to these proposals, especially when I discuss the contemporary science of psychiatric nosology. In that context, I will review what science has to say about the "best" and most scientifically defensible nosology, at least when the proposed nosology involves some testable propositions. Some proposals have, in fact, fared better than others. Some, though, are more amenable to testing than others. Before that, though, it is useful to think about what diagnoses actually *do*. What purpose do they serve? How are diagnoses made in actual practice? What effect, if any, does a diagnosis have on patients? How, if at all, has the publication of the *DSM* changed how the public thinks about mental illness? Questions of this sort are perhaps best thought of in terms of the "career" of a diagnosis. This concept is in reference to how diagnoses move through a field of users, from clinicians who deploy formal diagnostic criteria, to patients who receive diagnoses, to scientists who use diagnostic criteria to identify research subjects, to entire cultures that appropriate diagnostic thinking in order to understand behavioral problems.

These various actors might seem far afield of the discussion thus far. To this point, we have only discussed what diagnoses are in fact, as well as what some people might prefer them to be. Yet understanding how diagnoses are used is crucial to understanding the difficulty of constructing perfectly satisfying diagnostic criteria—in fact, it might help explain the persistence of widely varying preferences regarding what the *DSM* ought to be. The various actors that use the *DSM* operate with their own prerogatives. They have different interests and needs. And these interests and needs are not always in alignment. In fact, they almost never are. This lack of alliance is not a superficial matter. Much of my discussion surrounding *DSM-III* pertained to the criteria's *usefulness*. Certainly the authors of *DSM-III* emphasized the utility of clear and specific diagnostic criteria, especially for clinicians. And every version of the *DSM* since has emphasized this point in its prefatory content (and usually elsewhere as well). Yet what is regarded as most "useful" about the *DSM* varies a great deal between parties, so elevating the importance of pragmatic considerations often accentuates controversy rather than defuses it. The meaning patients derive from a diagnosis, for example, need not be the same thing as the meaning clinicians derive from it. Many stakeholders use the *DSM*, but few do so without imposing their own interpretative frameworks. Users disagree on the best way to understand severity, on how to evaluate causes, and what features of context are most important. Understanding how diagnoses are actually used, then, is important for interpreting ongoing controversies regarding the *DSM* and, indeed, the prospects for its revision. To this end, it is perhaps best to begin with clinicians (or, more broadly, clinical "professionals"). The *DSM* was written with their interests in mind, but even from the standpoint of how clinicians use the manual there are many complications.

5

HOW PROFESSIONALS USE DIAGNOSES

One of the motivations behind *DSM-III* was to encourage reliable diagnoses by providing more detailed diagnostic criteria. In effect, the goal was to rein in the subjective component of clinicians by implementing uniform guidelines. Yet despite the *DSM*'s emphasis on objectivity and standardization, clinicians remain steeped in the subjective and idiosyncratic. Part of this reflects their professional preferences. In their daily practice, clinicians hope to be interpreters rather than accountants. And they see their skill in terms of making inferences rather than applying rules. In this, clinicians are not unlike other medical professionals, who regard themselves as highly skilled practitioners. This in part also reflects their occupational demands. Clinicians are engaged in many tasks apart from diagnosis, and some tasks are seen as more significant than others. Clinicians see their role more in terms of providing treatment than in simply naming or describing a problem. In the same vein, clinicians hope to provide their patients with insights, not just labels. The *DSM* does not address these tasks directly, and, indeed, it actively eschews a few of them.

In this chapter, I review how clinicians and other professionals actually use—and occasionally misuse—diagnostic criteria. For all the debate and dissatisfaction surrounding the *DSM*, clinicians are remarkably adept at tailoring the *DSM* to their own needs. Despite the *DSM*'s effort to maintain theory neutrality, for example, clinicians routinely make diagnostic decisions based on what they believe is causing a disorder, not just on how that disorder appears on its surface. The *DSM* is pragmatic in intent, of course, but few people are as pragmatic as those who must actually implement what the manual stipulates. Clinicians do not have the luxury of waiting around for the best diagnostic criteria to materialize. They use what they are given—or what they are told to use—but more importantly they use clinical expertise. The work of clinicians prevents them from thinking about diagnosis in the pure way envisioned by the *DSM*.

This discontinuity between the *DSM* and clinical practice has another implication. Some of the criticisms of the *DSM* discussed earlier in this book pertain mostly to how the *DSM* is used in epidemiological research. Arguments regarding especially high levels of false positives, for instance, pertain mostly to prevalence estimates derived from survey instruments administered by lay interviewers. If clinicians, however, use the *DSM* in an adaptive fashion, the possibility of false positives might be much lower in clinical settings than in research settings. Once again, though, evaluating true cases of disorder depends on the standard used to evaluate disorders. Those who believe the *DSM* produces false positives because it is blind to causes might find reassurance in clinicians who are especially keen on the context surrounding symptoms, though it is important to discuss in detail what sort of prototype for psychiatric disorders clinicians might have in mind.

A caveat is necessary. People seek mental health treatment through a variety of sources. Many seek treatment through a general practitioner, a few see a psychiatrist, and still others see a psychologist or clinical social worker. I will use the term "clinician" generally, in reference to professionals who provide mental health services. As will be clear, however, I am occasionally referring to professionals with the power of prescription, effectively limiting my discussion to medically trained professionals such as psychiatrists or general practitioners. In general, though, many different professionals use the *DSM*, with many different treatment modalities, so it is worth thinking broadly whenever possible. Indeed, in the final part of this chapter I will discuss professionals who do not provide any kind of therapy and, instead, are involved in administration: They seek to determine who should be eligible or not for benefits, and they, too, use the *DSM* and should be considered.

THEORY NEUTRALITY IN PRACTICE

A key principle in the construction of *DSM-III* was theory neutrality, the idea that disorders ought not to be defined based on what causes them. The authors of *DSM-III* used this idea both as a way to allow many different professionals to use the manual and out of an accurate appreciation of the then-current state of the science. The causes of psychiatric disorder were not, in fact, well established. Yet a variety of studies indicate that clinicians use causal reasoning extensively when rendering a diagnosis. In itself this behavior is a departure from theory neutrality, but it is not at all inconsistent with how people think about and perceive the world generally. Individuals routinely draw causal connections between things and events, whether those connections are right or wrong. And they employ a variety of intuitions in doing so. Events happening earlier, for example, are seen as causing events happening later. Similarly, human behavior is usually seen as emanating from deep-seated motivations rather than from the circumstances people find themselves in.

Clinicians, too, instinctively look for causality in their patients' experiences. Nancy Kim and Woo-kyoung Ahn have performed a variety of experiments to illustrate how clinicians actually use atheoretical nosology. They take as their starting point the equal weighting the *DSM* assigns to symptoms within a set.[1] In polythetic criteria, symptoms within a set are usually granted the same weight: If five out of nine symptoms are necessary for a diagnosis, one symptom does not count more than another. Kim and Ahn reason, however, that if clinicians think in terms of causes rather than counts, they should not, in effect, weigh symptoms equally. Some symptoms should be seen as more important than others, especially if those symptoms are seen as causing others. Kim and Ahn further reason that *deeper* causes—those lying closer to the essence of the disorder—should be assigned a higher weight because they affect more things. If, for example, a distorted body image causes insufficient caloric intake and, in turn, extreme weight loss, then a distorted body image should count for more in the diagnosis of anorexia than insufficient calories or weight loss. By the same logic, symptoms that are causally connected to many other symptoms should be more important than symptoms that are isolated from other symptoms. And symptoms that do not fit neatly into an imputed causal theory should count for less than symptoms that do. Depressed mood, for example, should be more central to the diagnosis of a major depressive episode than, say, indecisiveness, especially if one believes depressed mood is the source of other cognitive and behavioral problems.

To test these ideas, Kim and Ahn provided clinicians with lists of symptoms and asked them to depict relationships among them. Clinicians were only instructed to draw *relationships*. They were not explicitly instructed to draw *causal* relationships. A relationship could simply mean that two symptoms were similar to each other, though clinicians were later asked to elaborate why they drew the relationships they did. To mitigate the influence of professional specialty or experience, Kim and Ahn focused on disorders that should be familiar to most clinicians, including anorexia nervosa, schizophrenia, a major depressive episode, antisocial personality disorder, and specific phobia. Their study demonstrated that some symptoms were, indeed, seen as more important than others and, furthermore, that those symptoms were regarded as more important because they were seen as causing others. In the case of depression, for instance, depressed mood was seen as especially significant because it caused suicidal ideation and behavioral problems. By the same token, some symptoms were downplayed precisely because they failed to fit neatly within a narrative structure. According to the *DSM* criteria for a major depressive episode, weight change and psychomotor problems are equally characteristic of depression as emotional symptoms, but in the study clinicians depicted these symptoms as isolated from others and, thereby, overlooked them. By the same token, a distorted body image emerged as the central symptom in the diagnosis of anorexia. Other symptoms, such as the absence of a period for three months, were seen as less important because they were related to body image only through other symptoms. The *DSM* was nonbinding in another way as well. Clinicians included other symptoms that were not part of the *DSM*'s formal diagnostic criteria but were relatively central to their own conceptions. Difficulties in intimate relationships, for example, were seen as central to major depression, connecting depressed mood and a lack of pleasure, even though interpersonal difficulties do not enter into the *DSM*'s formal diagnostic criteria.

Clinicians' intuitive mappings were not for lack of training. The tendency to impute a causal model did not reflect, for instance, an insufficient level of familiarity with the *DSM*. Indeed, there was remarkable consensus in the pathways clinicians drew, even for seemingly complex disorders such as phobia. Regardless of their experience, history, or clinical orientation, clinicians drew causal connections, and they drew connections that were very similar to those other clinicians drew. Clinicians may have been drawing on a general cultural tendency rather than something unique to their experience. In a separate study, Kim and Ahn found a similar pattern in the general public. Like clinicians, the public drew causal connections between symptoms and, thereby, saw some symptoms as more important than others. Furthermore, the public thought in more or less the same terms as clinicians. When asked to rank the symptoms of a major depressive episode, for example, clinicians and the lay public came up with very similar lists.

It is one thing to demonstrate that clinicians violate theory neutrality, but it is quite another to demonstrate the significance of this violation. After all, clinicians could regard some symptoms as more important than others but still render a diagnosis that is reasonably consistent with the *DSM*. Kim and another colleague also showed, however, that clinicians' causal models influenced how they treated their patients. In the study, clinicians were asked to evaluate two hypothetical patients. One patient was described as having symptoms that were central to the clinician's causal theory of the disorder, as revealed in the earlier exercise. The other patient was described as having symptoms that were more peripheral to their theory but still sufficient to satisfy the formal diagnostic criteria for the disorder. If clinicians were using the *DSM* criteria faithfully, they should diagnose both patients as having the disorder, regardless of how the symptoms were framed. Yet clinicians were far more likely to diagnose the patient whose symptoms matched their theory. Clinicians' causal models were also relevant for what treatment they recommended. Clinicians were more likely to regard specific treatments as effective if those treatments addressed the symptoms they presumed to be the underlying cause.[2]

Ideas about causes are used in other ways as well. In particular, a causal understanding is used to evaluate the severity of the disorder. In one study, clinicians were presented with hypothetical patients whose symptoms were described in different ways. When patients were described in terms of causally related symptoms (e.g., she has insomnia because she is stressed) clinicians were more likely to judge the patient as "normal" relative to when patients were described in terms of disconnected symptoms (e.g., she has insomnia).[3] In this way, causal descriptions appeared to foster understanding—it is easier to put yourself in the shoes of someone whose symptoms are described in terms of a narrative—and understanding appears to lessen the tendency to infer a mental disorder.

Clinicians appear to do much the same in routine settings. To the extent that they can derive a satisfying explanation for the patient's symptoms, they are more likely to regard the patient as normal. This tendency overlaps, of course, with the scientific debate regarding the bereavement exclusion. Not only do clinicians appear to respect bereavement as a reasonable exclusion, but they also appear to extend the same logic to other events. Clinicians apply the same thinking to, for example, divorce, job loss, and a serious injury, judging cases of depression as less serious when a plausible cause is evident.[4] Clinicians further apply the idea of a proportionate response, as proportionality fits squarely into their narrative focus. Clinicians are more likely to infer mental disorder when individuals are either greatly affected by seemingly minor events or are not affected at all by seemingly major events. Clinicians might be trained in lists, as the *DSM* requires, but they practice in prose.

MENTAL DISORDERS AS ESSENCES

Although clinicians resist the idea of theory neutrality in a variety of ways, there are other ways in which their thinking might still be in line with the *DSM*. Clinicians might still, for instance, subscribe to the view that psychiatric disorders represent *essences*. That is, they might still believe that disorders are either present or absent and, therefore, that disorders possess some kind of core, even if that core is not well understood. As medically trained professionals, psychiatrists recognize the essence of, say, cancer as indicated by the presence of specific invasive cells. By the same token, they recognize the essence of infectious disease as indicated by the presence of a pathogen. The *DSM* transposes this logic to psychiatric disorders, even though it makes no assumptions about what the underlying essence is. It presumes only that disorders that originate from the same cause should have the same symptoms. Even here, however, clinicians depart from the *DSM*. Experimental evidence suggests that clinicians do not "essentialize" psychiatric disorders in the way the *DSM* implies.[5] Clinicians, for example, do not see all patients with a psychiatric disorder as sharing something in common, at least in the same way as they see all patients with a physical disorder. There is something more essential, then, about cancer than there is, say, about generalized anxiety. Clinicians also do not believe that removing a single cause of a psychiatric disorder will cure the patient, as they believe will happen for some physical disorders if they remove a pathogen. In short, clinicians do not overwhelmingly regard mental disorders as all-or-none entities. Remarkably, though, the same studies also suggest that *novices* have a more essentialist view of psychiatric disorders than experts. Although experts and novices agree that physical disorders have essences, novices are more likely than experts to extend the same model to psychiatric disorders. There are a variety of ways to interpret this discontinuity. It could be that novices regard mental disorders as essences only because they have faith in the taxonomies described in the *DSM*. With experience or training, that faith in formal nomenclature might be eroded. I will take up the effects of the *DSM* on lay people and cultures in a later chapter, which lends some additional insight to this idea. Another interpretation is that experts are better able to appreciate that mental disorders have multiple causes, belying the idea of a single cause. This, too, could be a product of seeing many different kinds of major depression in patients. Regardless, though, this finding suggests a difference between how the *DSM* was conceived and what clinicians are taught through experience.

THE PRODUCTION OF UNRELIABILITY

These studies point to significant departures from the goals and principles of the *DSM*. Yet these studies are based largely on experiments. For all their benefits, experiments present a somewhat artificial situation, especially relative to the complexities of real clinical encounters with actual patients. In some experiments, for example, clinicians are presented only with lists of symptoms. These are designed to mimic the symptoms represented in the *DSM*, but they are far from representing a whole person. In other cases, clinicians are presented with hypothetical patients, about whom the clinician will only know what the researcher decides to depict. When presented with their actual patients, by contrast, clinicians are in a social interaction and are required to know the person as much as the problem. The clinician must ask questions. And their patients may or may not feel comfortable answering those questions. Clinicians' decisions will be only as good as the information their patients are coaxed into revealing. At the same time, the amount of information clinicians can obtain will depend on other factors, including, for example, how many times they have seen the patient. In experiments, the information clinicians receive is consistent, but in clinical practice it is not, and it is subject to lots of other considerations because little is entirely by design.

In light of these issues, some studies have explored what clinicians do in their everyday practices. Recall that the *DSM-III* field trials produced a reasonably high level of agreement in a somewhat artificial situation: Agreement was found between clinicians who were instructed to use the *DSM* criteria to evaluate the same patients. Research focusing on routine clinical decisions reveals much poorer agreement.[6] In these studies, clinicians are not instructed to use the *DSM*. Instead, they are instructed to make decisions as they normally would, after which the researcher evaluates the case based on *DSM* criteria and compares the two determinations. In one study of this sort, Shear and colleagues found kappas no higher than .33, much lower than the kappas found in the *DSM-III* field trials.[7] Furthermore, they found that clinicians were no better at evaluating more common disorders than less common ones. The kappa among anxiety disorders, for example, was only .12, despite the high prevalence of anxiety disorders. In short, familiarity with the disorder did not produce better decisions.

Part of this unreliability reflects what clinicians are looking for and when they are satisfied that they have found it. The *DSM* presumes comprehensiveness; that is, it presumes clinicians will ask about all the symptoms necessary to make an accurate diagnosis. The *DSM* was designed to provide clinicians with objective diagnostic criteria, but it was also designed as an instrument for directing attention: If you see these symptoms, for example, you might want to ask about these related symptoms. Yet studies find that clinicians ask about only half the symptoms the *DSM* suggests they should.[8] In short, clinicians do not use the *DSM* criteria completely. Furthermore, there are patterns in what parts of the *DSM* criteria clinicians focus on. In general, clinicians focus on those symptoms that will cement their initial impression rather than ask about the full variety of symptoms that might point them in the direction of a different disorder.[9] In this way, they fail to search for symptoms exhaustively. This tendency is consequential. Because they are not exhaustive in their evaluations, clinicians diagnose fewer disorders in their patients than a more structured *DSM*-based assessment would reveal.[10] Zimmerman and Mattia compared the diagnoses produced through unstructured interviews, the kind that occur in routine visits, with those produced through more structured interviews based on a script.[11] Patients assessed through structured interviews were diagnosed with significantly more disorders. Indeed, in structured interviews, more than a third of patients had three or more disorders, whereas in unstructured interviews less than 10 percent did.

Studies of this sort suggest several things. For one, they suggest that in surveys the *DSM* might produce very high prevalence estimates even though it does not in actual clinical practice. Moreover, these studies suggest that in clinical practice some disorders tend to overshadow others and that the dominance of certain disorders appears to be based on severity.[12] For example, clinicians routinely overlook generalized anxiety when presented with a clear case of major depression, assuming the former is less severe than the latter.[13] These two tendencies—the tendency to diagnose few disorders and to elevate certain disorders over others—occasionally work in opposing directions. The focus on diagnosing a single disorder occasionally leads clinicians to overlook other symptoms, even symptoms clinicians might otherwise regard as severe. One study, for example, found that structured interviews uncovered far more depression, hallucinations, hysteria, and suicidal thoughts than unstructured interviews.[14] These omissions are plainly not for lack of concern, but they do reflect the centrality of prototypes and the relevance of creating a narrative surrounding a disorder rather than merely rendering a series of impartial judgments about a string of disorders catalogued in the *DSM*.

DIAGNOSTIC WORKAROUNDS

These departures from the *DSM* reveal another important aspect of clinical practice. Clinicians receive a good deal of training, especially psychiatrists, who are trained in medical schools. Among the different professionals involved with providing treatment, we might expect psychiatrists to show the most fidelity to the *DSM*. Psychiatrists have the most specialized training. They are taught to recognize psychiatric disorders, and, to this end, they are trained extensively in formal diagnostic criteria. As medical professionals, they are also, of course, taught to recognize *physical illnesses*, so their acceptance of the idea of disease specificity is perhaps even stronger than their training in the *DSM* implies. Social workers, for instance, need not subscribe to the idea of disease specificity in order to think about psychiatric disorders generally.

Yet studies indicate that psychiatrists nonetheless feel ambivalent about the *DSM*. To understand this, it is important to appreciate the difference between the *role* of psychiatrists and their training, a difference sociologists in particular have highlighted. In general, medical professionals embrace the independence their occupation affords. Physicians are trained in much the same way from medical school to medical school, and, for this reason, there is a good deal of consistency in their approach. Yet physicians are also granted an extraordinary degree of professional autonomy and discretion. Few question the authority of physicians when it comes to their decisions regarding appropriate care. Moreover, within the field of medicine, personal experience and intuition are valued nearly as much as training and knowledge.[15] Indeed, this separates physicians from other health experts and grants physicians a special kind of authority. Scientists who study psychiatric disorders, for example, base their ideas on empirical research and the scientific method. Their knowledge is objective, and they are "experts" by any definition of the term. Clinicians use and respect scientific evidence, too, but their expertise is rooted in additional sources. Clinicians value the insights that can be gained from clinical practice. Clinicians learn based on experience, and this experience is, in some sense, interpreted and accepted by other clinicians as knowledge.

Evidence for this orientation is apparent in general medical settings, where studies have explored how physicians use other tools for standardization. Stefan Timmermans and his colleagues, for instance, have looked at the effects of evidence-based medicine on medical practice.[16] The goal of evidence-based medicine is to achieve better outcomes through the more uniform use of current clinical evidence in everyday medical practice. The approach relies on clinical practice guidelines, which provide step-by-step instructions regarding the diagnostic and therapeutic techniques with the best evidence behind them. Some feared such guidelines would cut against some long-standing features of clinical practice, even if those guidelines encouraged a focus on best practices. They might, for instance, push physicians away from a particularistic approach to patients toward a more universalistic one, they might limit the role of discretion and elevate the role of mechanical objectivity, and they might enhance concerns with cost control over a patient-centered approach. Timmermans finds, though, that physicians *adapt* to evidence-based guidelines. They use such guidelines—in much the same way that they consult the medical literature generally—but they do not feel beholden to them. And they often apply their own skepticism to the evidence upon which the guidelines are based.[17] This slippage between the intended and the actual is fostered in part by the basic recognition among physicians that evidence-based medicine can almost never be implemented without problems in individual cases. Similarly, other studies have found that physicians conduct their own informal clinical trials on their patients, preferring what they see in their own patients to what they read in published reports.[18] In short, the autonomy of physicians more or less prevails even in an environment that increasingly wants to encourage scientific standardization.

In this professional setting, the *DSM*, too, has a less than snug fit. The *DSM* does several things that are inconsistent with the culture of medicine. For one, in emphasizing standardization, the *DSM* seemingly eliminates the relevance of discretion. Furthermore, in describing symptoms that are observable to everyone, the *DSM* seemingly removes the need for interpretation or investigation. No technology, for example, is necessary to assess whether someone is sad. A diagnosis of heart disease, by contrast, requires clinical tests, some of which yield results that are difficult for a layperson interpret. With this in mind, Owen Whooley provides a different interpretation of how psychiatrists use the *DSM*, one that parallels in some ways how physicians use evidence-based medicine.[19] Whooley identifies three "diagnostic workarounds" that psychiatrists employ in an attempt to balance their clinical autonomy with the authority of the *DSM*. Perhaps the most dramatic workaround is the tendency to constrain the *DSM*'s vast universe of disorders to only a few especially useful categories. Recent editions of the *DSM* contain hundreds of discrete diagnoses, but the number of diagnoses psychiatrists use in routine practice is far smaller. Indeed, among the psychiatrists Whooley interviewed, some pared the vast manual to only three or four primary disorders. Of course, studies have shown that some disorders are, in fact, more common than others, but the practices Whooley uncovers are probably not an accurate reflection of the patients psychiatrists are likely to see. Other studies have reached a similar conclusion or, indeed, identified an even smaller set of routinely used diagnoses. The anthropologist Tanya Luhrmann, for example, identifies the centrality of schizophrenia, bipolar disorder, and major depression.[20] Within this small set of disorders, she further distills a small set of symptoms that psychiatrists focus on, including depression, psychosis, mood swings, and anxiety.[21] Whatever the exact number of diagnoses or symptoms psychiatrists actually use, one thing is clear: There appears to be little pressure among psychiatrists to use the

DSM to its fullest possible extent. Indeed, the practice of reduction represents a remarkable inversion of the goals of the *DSM*, given how the *DSM* sought to be maximally sensitive to all the symptoms clinicians are likely to encounter in their daily practices. Prevalence was not an especially important consideration. Disorders thought to be rare were still codified in the *DSM* in order to insure that all possible symptoms and disorders were registered. In principle, psychiatrists themselves could behave in ways that further this goal. And there is evidence that psychiatrists focus on what makes patients unique rather than what makes them typical. Yet when it comes to the simple act of diagnosis, Whooley and Luhrmann find nearly the opposite tendency. In the minds of psychiatrists, it would seem, diagnosis per se is not the appropriate place for registering the nuances of a case.

Psychiatrists also invert the usual practice of providing a diagnosis *before* deciding on a treatment. Luhrmann finds that some clinicians divide patients into two groups, those with traditional Axis 1 disorders, such as mood and anxiety disorders, and those with traditional Axis 2 disorders, including personality disorders. These categories reflect not only the symptoms patients have, as the organization of the axes implies, but how clinicians intend to treat the patients. Patients they think will benefit from medication are usually assigned to the first group, whereas patients they think will benefit from therapy are usually given to the second, even though depression, for example, has been shown to benefit from both medication and therapy. These patterns are revealing. Rather than a treatment recommendation following an appropriate diagnosis, which, in turn, is presumed to be based on an objective assessment of the symptoms a patient presents, a diagnosis appears to follow a discretionary judgment regarding the treatment, which is decided on relatively early in the process.

The distinction between diagnosis and treatment is muddled in another way. Treatment is occasionally used as a way to provide information regarding the disorder.[22] Because medications are indicated for specific disorders—otherwise their use is regarded as "off label"—psychiatrists occasionally use evidence on what medication works as a tool for understanding what a patient suffers from. For example, if a patient who appears to be suffering from bipolar disorder does not respond to medication intended to treat mood swings, the initial diagnosis can be revised. Similarly, medication is occasionally used as a tool for uncovering the primary disorder in situations where clinicians are presented with comorbidity (even though the *DSM* does not require it). If a patient is suffering from anxiety and depression but responds only to anxiety medication, the patient can be reconsidered as a case of a pure anxiety disorder.

The connection between diagnosis and medication is not incidental. Over the twentieth century pharmaceuticals have played an important role in refining diagnostic criteria for psychiatric disorders. Lithium carbonate, for example, helped clinicians further clarify their thinking about schizophrenia.[23] Lithium had already been shown to be effective in treating manic-depressive disorder, and because some patients with schizophrenia also responded well to lithium, clinicians wondered whether those patients might be suffering from a manic-depressive disorder instead. Other clinicians went a step further and argued that this positive response to treatment revealed the presence of a third disorder, one distinct from schizophrenia and manic depression.[24] Lithium is hardly an example of precision psychopharmacology, but it has long provided clinicians with a tool for refining diagnostic criteria.[25]

The usual diagnoses-to-treatment sequence is inverted in other ways as well. Although diagnosis is central to the clinician-patient relationship, there is a mundane reason for clinicians to assign a diagnosis: to get paid. The majority of mental health professionals seeks reimbursement from insured patients and so must follow the reimbursement rules set by insurers. As part of their billing process, insurers require a diagnosis. They are unwilling to pay for services for a disorder that does not exist or for a patient that does not merit such a diagnosis. Furthermore, the diagnosis often dictates the type and extent of treatment insurers are willing to pay for. Yet because psychiatrists appear to focus on treatment, the policies of insurers promote another kind of diagnostic workaround: To be reimbursed for the treatments they prefer, psychiatrists occasionally "fudge" their diagnoses, often in the direction of a more severe diagnosis.[26] Here, too, the behavior of psychiatrists reveals the dominance of treatment over diagnosis. Out of fear that a patient will not receive the treatment he needs, psychiatrists change the diagnosis, rather than reconsider the treatment. Even if a patient is below some diagnostic threshold, clinicians see little reason to deny treatment to someone they think will benefit from it. Indeed, at least one survey of clinicians found that the *primary* reason clinicians gave for using the *DSM* was to secure third-party payments, superseding any value they saw with respect to determining a treatment, arriving at a prognosis, or helping to conceptualize a case.[27]

One fear stemming from these workarounds, of course, is that psychiatrists will be prone to overdiagnosis. Their interest in providing treatment might blind them to the possibility that some symptoms do not warrant it. Yet some evidence indicates a more nuanced approach. Psychiatrists are not always interested in positively finding a disorder. Their interest in providing *care*—if not treatment per se—sometimes moves them in another direction. Psychiatrists appreciate the stigma surrounding many psychiatric disorders, especially severe ones. Psychiatrists also recognize that rendering a more severe diagnosis than the symptoms warrant could be jarring from the standpoint of patients, even if it is useful from the standpoint of insurers. In response to this tension, psychiatrists frequently turn to the "not otherwise specified" (NOS) category. As it was originally written in the *DSM*, the NOS category was intended for limited use and was designed for complicated cases that were severe but failed to match any *DSM* diagnostic criteria precisely. Among psychiatrists, however, the NOS category is used with other goals in mind. One such goal is allaying stigma. Stigma tends to inhere around specific disorders, especially those that have a strong public profile, such as major depression, schizophrenia, and, for different reasons, ADHD. The public has beliefs about these disorders and about the kinds of people who suffer from them. An NOS diagnosis—even one closely related to a more well-known disorder—does not have the same public resonance and presumably carries less stigma as well. In this way, having a generic developmental disorder, for example, is not received in the same way as having ADHD. At the same time, the NOS category allows for more professional autonomy and discretion and, therefore, coheres better with the culture of medicine. A standard diagnosis would necessarily link the case to a much larger body of research and, in some cases, to strong evidence regarding an appropriate treatment. An NOS diagnosis, though, allows a psychiatrist to *use* that empirical research, derived from disorders with a family resemblance to the one they are considering, without feeling *beholden* to that research. There is usually much less scientific guidance on treating NOS disorders than their standard counterparts.

The clinical use of NOS is based on a few other considerations, and these considerations, too, reveal important aspects of clinical practice. For one, NOS is used more frequently when the symptoms of a disorder involve more abstract concepts. This is especially true of personality disorders, which require judgments about whether someone's behavior is "self-defeating," whether a person is "dependent," whether attachments are "shallow," or whether an identity is "stable." When presented with ambiguous diagnostic concepts of this sort, clinicians resort to NOS with higher frequency. Occasionally, however, the use of NOS reflects the actual characteristics of the disorders the term describes. Verheul and Widiger argue that if the *DSM* criteria were deployed precisely, personality disorder not otherwise specified would, in fact, be the most common personality disorder.[28] Something similar is apparent with respect to eating disorders. In routine clinical settings, eating disorder not otherwise specified is the most frequently diagnosed eating disorder, surpassing anorexia nervosa and bulimia.[29] The symptoms of an eating disorder NOS resemble those of anorexia and bulimia but fall short of the thresholds required for either of those disorders. For example, the symptoms of eating disorder NOS often involve binge eating below the frequency required for bulimia or a weight that is slightly more than the limit set for anorexia.

Although these departures from the *DSM* generally reveal clinicians' concern about their patients, another consequence of not maintaining strict fidelity to the *DSM* is less benign. Not sticking to the *DSM* permits the influence of other nonclinical factors. There is evidence from experiments that clinicians consider the race and sex of their patients in ways that can lead to misdiagnosis.[30] Evidence for this tendency comes from controlled experiments similar to those described earlier, in which clinicians are presented with vignettes of hypothetical patients. In all cases, the symptoms are presented in a way that should facilitate a clear diagnosis—the patients have all the symptoms sufficient for a diagnosis. In addition, however, the race and sex of the patient is randomly varied. If clinicians evaluated the symptoms they were presented in the way the *DSM* envisions, the demographic characteristics of the patient should be irrelevant. Yet these studies reveal the importance of these characteristics. For example, even when presenting exactly the same symptoms, African Americans are more likely to be diagnosed with paranoid schizophrenia and whites more likely to be diagnosed with major depression. In addition, male psychiatrists are more likely to diagnose histrionic personality disorder in their female patients where they would diagnose antisocial personality in males.[31]

None of these departures from the *DSM*'s criteria means that psychiatrists find the *DSM* useless. As Whooley sees it, virtually all psychiatrists appreciate what the *DSM* does with respect to reliability. They also appreciate its value in affirming the medical model. Psychiatrists jealously guard their reputations as physicians. Yet psychiatrists are also aware that the *DSM* is provisional, that it awaits better scientific validation, and that it is open to revision. For this reason they feel comfortable rendering diagnoses that are equally provisional. Furthermore, the flexibility they display with respect to diagnosis is not at all inconsistent with how physicians make other decisions. Prognosis, for example, is also an important clinical task and is a natural extension of diagnosis. To know what something is implies knowing something about its course. Physicians have an interest in being accurate, both in diagnosis and prognosis, and patients appreciate honesty when it comes to understanding when their disease might be cured. Yet there is evidence physicians use prognosis in an instrumental fashion, just as they do diagnosis. In end-of-life settings, for example, prognoses tend to be optimistic, in part because physicians believe a more hopeful prognosis keeps the patient motivated.[32] A good prognosis, then, is not necessarily one that is accurate with respect to how long the patient will live—which is, in any case, probabilistic—but one that serves a positive clinical function. Something similar appears to happen with respect to psychiatric diagnosis. In psychiatric settings, a good diagnosis is one that best serves the patient without fundamentally distorting the nature of their suffering or the possibility of relief. Luhrmann, for instance, finds that clinicians will often substitute a diagnosis that has a better prognosis for one that has a worse one.[33] To be sure, distorting a diagnosis in this fashion is often easy to do in psychiatry, given how many common disorders share symptoms. Manic-depressive disorders, for instance, have a better prognosis than schizophrenia, although they share many of the same symptoms. Yet this distortion does, once again, reveal the significance clinicians grant to the case over the taxonomy.

INSTITUTIONAL PRESSURES ON DIAGNOSIS

The professional and interpersonal demands on psychiatrists are not the only thing influencing diagnosis. Much of the foregoing discussion was set in the clinical encounter: What happens when clinicians are presented with actual patients in routine settings? But despite being face to face, the clinical encounter is subject to a remarkably wide set of influences, including elements far beyond the mindsets of the two people involved. With this in mind, it is instructive to think about the *institutional* pressures that can also distort the *DSM*. These pressures are, to be sure, mediated through clinicians—in the end, clinicians render diagnoses—but they represent influences that cannot be dismissed out of hand. In fact, some of the most controversial psychiatric disorders are contentious precisely because they intersect with other institutions. What makes psychiatric disorders so troubling to some observers is how easily certain disorders can be contaminated by "external" influences, and, of course, the universe of "external" influences is wide. We should be clear about how these influences operate and what might blunt them.

THE CASE OF ADHD

Perhaps the most prominent current example of institutional pressures over diagnosis is the use of stimulants in the treatment of attention deficit/hyperactivity disorder (ADHD). Stimulants are an effective treatment for ADHD, and ADHD is not a rare disorder. ADHD is among the most common psychiatric disorders diagnosed in children, especially among students.

Critics, though, see an overreliance on psychiatric medications and an explosion of inappropriate diagnoses. Moreover, they see the use of stimulants as a strategy for improving academic performance rather than treating a disorder. One researcher calls the use of overuse of stimulants "a very real problem."[34] The charge of overdiagnosis, though, is generally difficult to adjudicate. One might debate the validity of the *DSM*'s criteria for ADHD, but if a child meets those criteria, their diagnosis is at least not in excess of that standard. Yet the case for overdiagnosis is perhaps clearer in the case of ADHD than other disorders. About one in ten school-aged youth are diagnosed with ADHD, and about 70 percent of those who are diagnosed take medication.[35] The apparent need for treatment, then, is generally quite high. Yet the prevalence of ADHD varies considerably over time and across geographic regions. For example, the diagnosis of ADHD increased a remarkable 42 percent between 2003 and 2011. Furthermore, ADHD appears to be especially prevalent in certain neighborhoods, inviting questions about whether the disorder is found by clinicians or is, instead, fabricated by parents.

Evidence in this regard is suggestive but not conclusive. It is one thing to believe that stimulants are overprescribed and quite another to show the circumstances under which overdiagnosis occurs. King and colleagues look for traces of overdiagnosis using seasonal patterns in prescription filling.[36] Their intuition is straightforward. There is little reason to believe that ADHD takes a break over the summer, but students certainly do. Psychiatric disorders are generally chronic or at least prone to recurrence, and so they should not systematically appear in one season only to disappear in another. Moreover, if we regard ADHD as a serious disorder, one involving clinically significant impairment, it should be treated consistently throughout the year to prevent any further complications. Yet King and colleagues show that parents are far more likely to fill their children's prescriptions when school is in session than during the summer recess. Moreover, they show that students of higher socioeconomic status are more sensitive to this seasonal pattern—the gap between their summer and school-year prescription filling is larger than it is for students of lower socioeconomic status. Stated differently, lower socioeconomic status students with ADHD are more likely to take their medication year round, whereas higher socioeconomic status students take medication only when it matters most with respect to performance.

This pattern can be interpreted in a variety of ways. It is possible that lower-socioeconomic-status students simply have more severe cases of ADHD than higher-socioeconomic-status students and, therefore, require more consistent treatment. Yet King and colleagues find the same pattern regardless of the type of ADHD that is diagnosed. Furthermore, they find that students with the weakest symptoms are the most likely to have their prescription filled only during the school year. In addition, prescribing is responsive to state policies in ways that suggest test performance is the driving force. High-stakes testing is stressful regardless of where a student lives, but some states have policies that heighten the stakes. In some states, for example, schools are rated based in part on average test scores. Although these policies matter for testing, they presumably do not matter for the prevalence of ADHD. Yet King and colleagues find that prescriptions are more likely to be filled during the school year in states where test scores are more consequential.

Although evidence of this sort suggests that students are taking stimulants to enhance test performance, a lingering question pertains as to who is responsible for this behavior. There are obviously environmental influences at play that are beyond the responsibility of clinicians, parents, or students. It is possible, though, to winnow culpability a bit. King and colleagues check, for instance, to see whether certain physicians are prescribing more stimulants to higher-socioeconomic-status parents. Some physicians might be more responsible than others in the sense that they are more willing to prescribe medication and, thus, are sought out by especially motivated parents. In principle, these physicians could be identified and sanctioned by those who wish to curtail overdiagnosis, much like removing a bad apple can preserve a batch. Yet King and colleagues find little evidence that only certain physicians are responsible for excess prescribing. They find, instead, that patients and physicians work together in overprescribing. The average physician—not an extraordinary physician or an especially bad actor—appears to be at least partly responsive to the requests of parents. Other studies have corroborated this interpretation, although these studies also identify a rationale among parents that blends an implicit strategy for improving testing performance with an explicit concern about side effects. In particular, parents of children diagnosed with ADHD see themselves as stewards of their child's disorder. Parents report that they alone are responsible for when their child does or does not take medication and, further, that they see little value in taking medication when the social benefits of doing so are minimal.[37] For these parents, limiting medication to the school year is seen less as an acknowledgment that they are providing their child with an academic enhancement than as evidence that they are being responsible in their use of a powerful drug.

Students and their parents are hardly the only people caught up in the ambiguity surrounding psychiatric diagnosis and treatment. There is also evidence that adults might try to secure secondary advantages for themselves. The U.S. Social Security Disability Insurance program is a valuable program that has grown increasingly controversial. The program provides disability insurance to former workers. To receive benefits under the program, a person must have worked in a job during at least five of the last ten years and, crucially, to have a physical or mental condition that is expected to last at least a year and prevent them from working. The program has grown enormously over time.[38] The percent of working-age adults receiving benefits nearly doubled between 1985 and 2006, increasing from 2.2 percent to 4.1 percent. This increase reflects a number of factors, but a simple rise in the prevalence of disability is not one of them. In fact, disability has been steadily declining over time. The increase, instead, appears to be driven by changes in how disability is defined.

Over time, the nature of the disability insurance program has changed in complex ways. Support for the program has waxed and waned. In 1980, federal legislation made eligibility much more difficult, resulting in the loss of benefits for many recipients and, very quickly, a sharp public outcry. In 1984, Congress reversed course. They substantially liberalized the screening process, allowing far more beneficiaries than was possible when disability was defined strictly in terms of a person being "totally and permanently" unable to work. Under the revised definition of disability more consideration was given to impairments in work brought upon by changes in *functioning*, a sharp difference from defining disability in terms of the inability to work brought upon by *illness*. In addition to its definition, the process of determining disability also changed. Assessments shifted to the testimony of an applicant's physician rather than evidence from an in-home examination conducted by someone else. These changes in the process were consequential. The program expanded rapidly, including far more beneficiaries than it had before. Furthermore, the composition of illnesses among beneficiaries shifted. In 1983, the two largest categories of illness were heart disease (21.9 percent) and cancer (16.8 percent). In 2003, the two largest categories were musculoskeletal disorders (26.3 percent) and mental disorders (25.4 percent), together composing more than half of all awards.[39]

All this perhaps invites suspicion about the motives of claimants and, not unrelatedly, the value of admitting mental illness to the category of disabling conditions. It also invites concern over the growing obligations of the Social Security Administration to a greatly expanding pool of potential awardees. The life expectancy of those with mental disorders and musculoskeletal problems exceeds that of those with heart disease and cancer. Furthermore, the age of onset for most psychiatric disorders is much younger than for heart disease or cancer, implying a much longer expected duration of benefits. As with ADHD, though, adjudicating responsibility is very difficult. Psychiatric disorders can, in fact, be disabling, and, indeed, they often are. Furthermore, some of the most common disorders, like major depression, are especially disabling. Even so, some evidence points to the relevance of benefits-seeking behavior over the presence of disorders. Studies find that around 30 percent of adult males over the age of forty-five who are applying for disability insurance would have worked were it not for the availability of benefits.[40] Furthermore, the fact that subjective symptoms are now considered relevant has changed the assessment process in ways that favor diligence. The process is increasingly adversarial, open to the advocacy of nonmedical experts whose testimony does not rest on any external sources of material verification, like a blood test. Many applicants who are initially denied benefits later appeal, with an eventual success rate of around 75 percent.[41]

Responsibility is even more difficult to adjudicate given that other forces have conspired to increase the lure of benefits. Economists refer to the "replacement rate" of disability insurance in reference to the value of disability benefits relative to potential labor-market earnings.[42] In the disability insurance program, a recipient's benefit is based on past earnings, adjusted for the average expected growth in those earnings, as based on previous trends. This has important implications. If actual earnings for low-wage workers increase at a slower-than-expected rate, the relative value of disability payments increases quickly. This, in fact, has happened over time as income inequality has increased. For men in the lowest income bracket, for example, disability insurance can now replace over 50 percent of their earnings. The value of disability payments has also increased because of a decline in other potential sources of income. Applications for disability tend to increase when unemployment is high and decrease when it is low.[43] Those who are unemployed for a long period of time might ordinarily seek benefits from other income sources within the larger welfare system, but these, too, have deteriorated.[44] In this way, disability insurance has emerged to fill a multidimensional gap. It has become a partial replacement for welfare payments generally and, at that, provides more generous benefits over a longer expected timeframe, given that standard welfare is only considered temporary assistance. Disability insurance has also become a relatively more attractive source of nonlabor income for those struggling in low-wage labor markets.

As a statement about what psychiatric disorders are, the *DSM* is certainly caught in the middle of these economic and policy trends. On its own, though, it provides almost no insight relevant to disentangling these external influences. The *DSM* stipulates that symptoms must be clinically significant, but it says little about how much disability is expected with each disorder. Furthermore, the *DSM* says little about the interface between a person and his environment, which is critical for thinking about the issue of disability. In the above case, disability refers to the inability to work in a job someone held before. Some facts regarding psychiatric disability are clear. The disability associated with psychiatric disorders is, indeed, quite pronounced, including with respect to employment. For every hundred workers, psychiatric disorders are associated with six lost days of work per month and thirty-one days of diminished productivity.[45] Yet there is no easy way to determine the amount of disability without relying on a patient's testimony or inferring an average level over large samples. By contrast, the disability associated with some physical diseases is clear from the nature of the disease itself and would apply to almost every case. Those who have lost their legs, for example, cannot ambulate on their own. In the case of psychiatric disorders, though, the evaluation of disability is more indirect and belies any simple categorization or rule. Indeed, disability is more common among the disorders that are the most subjective in nature, including mood and anxiety disorders. Mood disorders, for example, are associated with twenty-five work loss days per hundred workers with the disorder. Projecting this to the entire U.S. population, there are approximately four million work-loss days per year because of mood disorders.[46] Further complicating matters, the disability associated with psychiatric disorders is often stronger among those who have the most to lose from accepting disability payments. Psychiatric disorders force more work cutback among highly paid professionals, including engineers and lawyers, than among janitors, manual laborers, or heavy-machine operators. In general, though, psychiatric disorders do not discriminate on the basis of occupation. Although those with a psychiatric disorder are somewhat overrepresented in service occupations, they are in fact found across the entire occupational spectrum.[47] There is no easy way to write diagnostic criteria that would provide a one-to-one mapping linking the disorder a person has to his work-related disability.

THE CASE OF PTSD

Post–traumatic stress disorder (PTSD) presents similar problems, although it perhaps renders the conflict between different stakeholders even more acute. As a diagnosis, the credibility of PTSD is, at least at this moment in history, almost unequivocal. It appears "real" in both cause and consequence. Although most war veterans do not suffer from PTSD, combat experience is a leading contributor to PTSD among men. Very few people doubt the reality of the disorder, especially those who have witnessed its toll. Yet there have been remarkable trends surrounding disability compensation associated with PTSD. Well after the conclusion of the Vietnam War, the number of Vietnam veterans receiving compensation for PTSD increased greatly. Between 1999 and 2010 the number receiving benefits nearly tripled, increasing to about 15 percent of veterans.[48] Although these veterans received benefits for a variety of conditions, the fraction receiving benefits because of PTSD grew precipitously. This increase is difficult to explain in terms of PTSD itself. It could reflect a delayed onset of symptoms, but the same pattern was not observed earlier for Korean War veterans, and PTSD was probably more common following the Korean War than the Vietnam War.[49] A close look at the characteristics of new beneficiaries suggests something similar to what is occurring with respect to disability benefits more generally. Among other things, veterans who receive benefits have lower levels of education than veterans who do not apply for them, suggesting, once again, a close alignment between socioeconomic opportunities and the appeal of benefits.

In this case, though, changes in the *DSM*'s diagnostic criteria for PTSD probably also played a role. PTSD is unusual among psychiatric disorders in that its diagnostic criteria specify a precipitating cause: The trauma is presumed to stem from a specific event. Yet the parameters of the precipitating event have changed between editions of the *DSM*. In *DSM-III*, the authors plainly had in mind severe traumatic events experienced directly by the person suffering from the disorder. The diagnostic criteria for the disorder referred to the "existence of a recognizable stressor that would evoke significant symptoms of distress in almost everyone."[50] In *DSM-IV*, the definition of a traumatic event was expanded, with the criteria stating that "the person experienced, witnessed, or was confronted with an event."[51] This revision expanded the number of potential traumatic events a great deal, but such an expansion was not without scientific merit. The intuition that only major events experienced directly by the person could cause PTSD was inconsistent with evidence showing that PTSD had no obvious dose-response relationship with the putative severity of traumatic events. The evidence, instead, showed that PTSD reflected the characteristics of the people who experienced a trauma more than the characteristics of the event.[52] For example, among men exposed to traumatic events at some point in their lifetime, only about 8 percent develop PTSD, suggesting most people cope effectively even with traumas we would almost certainly agree are severe. Although combat is regarded as among the most important contributors to PTSD, a study of Gulf War veterans found no difference in the number of days spent in a war zone between those suffering from PTSD and those not suffering from the disorder.[53] Other studies have found similar patterns. A study of tortured political activists in Turkey, for example, found no relationship between the number of episodes of torture and the severity of the activist's symptoms.[54] Even if we focus only on those who have PTSD and, therefore, on those who might have some preexisting risk for the disorder, the relationship between the amount of their suffering and the precipitating event is complex. The single most important factor in predicting the severity of PTSD appears to be how emotional the person was before the event rather than the nature of the event itself.[55] In a study of Vietnam veterans suffering from PTSD, researchers likewise found that personality characteristics and not the characteristics of combat accounted for most of the variation in symptoms.[56] Another study found that extensive exposure to combat in Vietnam had no stronger relationship with PTSD than minimal combat exposure. The severity of PTSD was better predicted by the personality and resilience of the solider.[57] The authors of *DSM-IV* also appear to have had empirical justification for including indirect exposure to events. Studies suggest that witnessing trauma or learning about it at second hand can lead to PTSD, much like direct exposure.[58] If we are concerned about the overdiagnosis of PTSD or about sufferers seeking secondary gain through disability benefits, there is little in the characteristics of trauma per se that will allow us to distinguish the truly sick from the malingering or the exaggerating. In any case, the *DSM* itself is unable to provide clear guidance.

THE ACCURACY OF DIAGNOSIS
IN PRIMARY-CARE SETTINGS

A variety of pressures shape how clinicians use the *DSM*. Clinicians are moved to render an inaccurate diagnosis for several reasons, sometimes to secure better treatment, sometimes to avoid stigma, and sometimes to secure payments. Although diagnoses made in this fashion can be considered "incorrect" from the standpoint of the *DSM*, they can also be characterized as motivated inaccuracies: Clinicians use the "wrong" diagnosis in order to serve some purpose they regard as professionally overriding. Patients still receive the right treatment, for example, even if the diagnosis is not completely accurate. Among critics, of course, these pressures invite fear of overdiagnosis and overtreatment: Clinicians might be so attuned to treatment that they produce far too many false positives. Yet there are also pressures that lead clinicians to overlook disorders altogether. Indeed, in routine settings clinicians can miss psychiatric disorders nearly as much as they detect them. It is important, then, to consider clinicians' decisions with respect to *both* sensitivity and specificity, that is, the potential for false positives and false negatives.

Several studies have examined how well general practitioners identify depression. The focus on general practitioners is intentional. The modal pathway to treatment for psychiatric disorders is through a general practitioner, but general practitioners often have less expertise in the treatment of psychiatric disorders and, at a minimum, are not specialists. Perhaps the most comprehensive study of this kind looked at diagnostic outcomes in 50,371 patients.[59] The researchers focused on "unassisted" decisions, meaning the decisions of physicians unaided by diagnostic instruments or supplementary education. Among the patients included in the analysis were 5,534 true cases of depression, as revealed through structured interviews independent of the physicians' determinations. Of these true cases, general practitioners only identified about half. This percentage varied depending on how the patient was assessed. Assessments based on case notes, for example, were less accurate than those based on in-person assessments. Assessments also varied depending on the patient's demographic characteristics. Older patients with depression were more likely to be detected than younger patients with depression. On the flip side, general practitioners also ruled out depression among those patients who did not have depression. Here, too, they did so imperfectly. Among patients *without* depression, 81 percent were accurately diagnosed as not having depression.

Putting these numbers together suggests a considerable amount of misdiagnosis in routine doctor-patient encounters. These figures can be extrapolated to larger populations based on what we assume the base rate of major depression is among those visiting a physician. Assuming a prevalence of around 20 percent, general practitioners should be able to diagnose accurately 75 percent of their patients: 65 percent of patients would be correctly diagnosed as not having depression, whereas 10 percent would be correctly diagnosed has having depression. Although these calculations suggest that *most* people will be correctly diagnosed, they also imply that 15 percent of patients will receive a false positive diagnosis and that 10 percent will receive a false negative. In other words, false positives outnumber true positives by 50 percent, in part because the number of truly nondepressed patients is large. Concerns about overdiagnosis are most pronounced when a disorder is rare. If only for this reason alone, critics are correct instinctively to fear overdiagnosis. If a larger fraction of patients is depressed, however, the possibility of overdiagnosis quickly recedes.

We should be careful about impugning physician practices based on observational studies. False positives are not only a product of overzealous physicians. They also reflect how physicians consider the idea of *risk*. Patients at a higher risk for depression are more likely to be diagnosed with the disorder, even when their current symptoms do not warrant it. What appears like a false positive from the standpoint of the *DSM*, then, might reflect a clinician inferring what could happen next with a patient rather than what is happening now. Furthermore, studies of false positives and false negatives are largely blind to issues of *certainty* because they depend on categories. A diagnosis of depression might seem solid when it appears in a clinical record, but recording an official diagnosis does not mean a clinician is confident in her decision. Other studies suggest a good deal of uncertainty just below the surface. When given an opportunity to indicate whether a diagnosis is definite, possible, or unclear, for example, clinicians report being unclear about a diagnosis at about the rate expected given the number of false positives clinicians produce.[60] In some instances, physicians might be complicit in overdiagnosis, but it is generally not for lack of insight. In addition, the fact that physicians occasionally overlook depression does not mean a depressed patient leaves the office with no diagnosis at all. General practitioners diagnose and treat other medical conditions, of course, and about half of those who suffer from depression also suffer from another medical condition.[61] Treating that other condition might very well treat depression, too, as in the treatment of pain, which is strongly related to depression. Altogether the behavior of physicians with respect to diagnosis reflects a not unreasonable approach given their professional role and how they see their obligations. In most cases, they make accurate diagnoses, and when they err, they err on the side of cautious false positives. This behavior can be understood in terms of an ethic of care. Physicians are acting on what they presume are the patient's best interests.

Drawing attention to the role of clinicians is important in another respect. The *DSM* encourages abstract thinking. The actual work of clinicians, however, centers on the concrete. Lists of symptoms are immaterial, but clients are real. All of the above suggests that clinicians toggle between these two styles of thought more or less successfully. Clinicians use the *DSM*, but they treat the patient. There is evidence, however, that clinicians shift their thinking in subtle ways when moving between the two.[62] This, too, points to a gulf between the *DSM* and clinical practice. In particular, symptoms are interpreted differently by clinicians, depending on how they are framed. When presented with abstract symptoms (e.g., "this disorder is characterized by feelings of worthlessness, with unrealistically negative self-evaluations"), clinicians are more likely to regard the symptoms as biological in origin, and, for this reason, they are more likely to recommend medication.[63] But when presented with the same symptoms expressed in terms of a person and his behavior (e.g., "Chris believes that he is incompetent at his job, despite excellent performance evaluations"), clinicians are more likely to regard the symptoms as psychological in origin, and, as a result, they are less likely to recommend medication. This split tendency has a number of implications. For one, it suggests that clinicians will be less likely to recommend medication the more familiar they are with a case, and, in this sense, the tendency to overdiagnose could be tempered by time. It also suggests a discontinuity between what clinicians accept as a matter of science and how they behave in actual practice. Clinicians might accept, for example, that psychiatric disorders are influenced by genes. Indeed, the scientific literature on psychiatric disorders is presented in ways that encourage abstract thinking and, therefore, according to this study, the literature encourages an emphasis on biological causes. Yet when presented with actual clients, clinicians might infer a different set of influences and depart from what they have learned from scientific sources. Because clinicians must reason about actual people, not just data, the distance between the science of psychiatric disorders and the practice of clinicians is quite large.

USING THE *DSM*

Clinicians use the *DSM* in a way that betrays the limits of the manual's authority. Their departures from the *DSM*'s formal nomenclature are not willful distortions of the manual's goals, necessarily. When clinicians search for causes as much as symptoms, for instance, or when they blend decisions regarding treatment with judgments regarding diagnosis, they do so because they are presented with unique people rather than abstract entities. They also depart from the *DSM* with considerable professional acumen in the sense that they overlay the manual's rules with their own insights. In short, clinicians fill the cracks left by the *DSM*, but they do not appear to do so in opposition to the manual's goals. The *DSM* was written, after all, with clinical relevance in mind.

In addition, there are limits to how much the *DSM* can arbitrate questions of overdiagnosis. The *DSM* often becomes the focal point of critics concerned with medicalization, the process whereby nonmedical problems get defined as medical ones. And, to be sure, the *DSM* provides critics with a convenient target.[64] It is easy to see the *DSM* as a tool for inflating medical authority, especially given the *DSM*'s growing size and the expanding range of its concerns. For some of these problems, it is easy to envision a fix. It is relatively simple, for example, to move a diagnostic threshold a bit higher or to drop a controversial diagnosis altogether (though, of course, these moves require the will to do so). Yet when it comes to diagnosis, the *DSM* does not act alone, and this points to the limits of the *DSM*'s influence. For example, the secondary gains that might come from receiving a psychiatric diagnosis, such as disability benefits, reflect not only how we choose to define a disorder but also the value of those benefits relative to an alternative. The vast majority of those who meet the *DSM*'s diagnostic criteria for a psychiatric disorder will never seek treatment, let alone any sort of disability benefit. And most of those working-aged adults who meet the diagnostic criteria for a disorder are, in fact, employed.[65] Furthermore, there are limits to how accurately a text that is used for diagnosing disorders can speak to concerns regarding the impact of those disorders in the lives of those suffering from them. An abstract document like the *DSM* only speaks indirectly to the context in which psychiatric disorders are actually experienced, and it invites the input of other authorities.

The influence of the *DSM* is also limited by the nature of the disorders it seeks to characterize. Formal diagnoses are ultimately made in a social interaction, and the clinical encounter involves both clinicians and patients. The clinician asks questions and infers what the underlying problem is, using the *DSM* as a guide (if not a script). The patient, meanwhile, answers those questions and presents the symptoms that most concern him. A lingering question, though, pertains to this other side of the encounter. How, if at all, do patients use the *DSM*? More generally, how has the public been influenced by the *DSM*'s approach? Concerns about the *DSM*'s diagnostic criteria are usually not limited to how the *DSM* influences psychiatry or scientific research for good or for ill. Some are concerned that the *DSM* also shapes how the public views mental illness and that the *DSM* encourages the public to interpret ordinary problems in living as medical ones. The next chapter explores the more complicated question of how patients use the *DSM*.

6

HOW THE PUBLIC USES DIAGNOSES

How the public thinks about mental illness is often regarded as an afterthought to debates about nosology. If diagnosis is a matter of medical authority, how relevant is the public's opinion? The issue can be cast narrower still: Do we need to think about the *public* when what we really care about are *patients*?

Yet it is critically important to understand what the public thinks about mental illness and, by extension, the *DSM*. Diagnoses are laden with complex moral and normative significance, and these dimensions are not addressed directly in the *DSM*. To those who receive a diagnosis, however, the meaning of a diagnosis is critical, and patients are quick to fill in the blanks left by diagnostic labels. For one, diagnoses shape how patients view themselves, moving them from someone who is experiencing deep sadness, for instance, to someone who is suffering from a major depressive episode. Furthermore, patients respond to their diagnoses in ways that can make their condition better or worse. Indeed, one could argue that, in the first instance, public beliefs matter more than what a clinician decides because people usually seek a diagnosis only after they decide they have a problem. Moreover, their decision to seek a diagnosis is often prompted by the encouragement of others, thereby elevating the importance of public beliefs generally.

By the same token, some critics fear that the widespread availability of the *DSM* might encourage uninformed lay diagnosis and, thereby, create more demand for psychiatric services than is necessary. Indeed, the latent demand for diagnostic information is potentially quite strong: The public might be hungry for diagnoses as a way to explain suffering and latch onto the *DSM*'s apparent medical authority as a way to understand everyday sadness and fear. Perhaps worse still, some fear that the *DSM* can *create* the very disorders it merely seeks to describe. The authors of the *DSM* were well aware of these issues and shared the same concerns. Among those who emphasize the damaging effects of diagnostic fads most strongly is Allen Frances, the chair of the *DSM-IV* task force.[1] Concern over psychiatric epidemics is partly premised on the idea that an informed public is a dangerous one. By creating new disorders, the *DSM* creates new idioms for people to express their distress, thereby creating new experiences from virtually whole cloth. Sadness and fatigue have long been among the most common physical complaints. The issue, though, is how these complaints are interpreted. When the public is aware of the concept of *major depression*, they might grant these experiences more significance than they would otherwise. The public might interpret them as symptoms of a disorder and, if sufficiently well informed about diagnoses, they might be more sensitive to the remaining symptoms of depression as well.[2] Even short of this kind of sensitivity, it is possible to envision ways in which the creation of diagnoses can adversely affect how those suffering from psychiatric disorders are seen by others. This brings us to the labeling debate. Some argue that labels play a powerful role in shaping the risk for mental illness, including Thomas Scheff, who famously argued that labels create disorders.[3] Labels are essentially superficial markers intended only to describe something, but they are also difficult to remove, apparent to others, and highly consequential. Even short of arguing that labels cause mental illness, it is possible to trace other negative effects of labeling, if, for instance, patients internalize the stigma that comes with their diagnosis.[4]

Public beliefs are also relevant to revising the *DSM*. Whatever classification system is devised, that system will be filtered through the beliefs and experiences of the public. Although the *DSM* is authoritative for many purposes, there is a refractory aspect to mental illness that is not as apparent for other physical illnesses. The *DSM* cannot, by force of will, move the public entirely in its favored direction. Those who advocate for a more genetic approach to psychiatric classification, for instance, often presume that if the public also endorsed a more genetic view, then some of the stigma attached to mental illness would dissipate. This optimism, however, overlooks the many layers to public beliefs about mental illness, and, in fact, there is little evidence that a genetic model dissolves stigma. In the previous chapter, I discussed how the *DSM* is used (and misused) by clinicians. In this chapter, I will discuss how the *DSM* is used (and misused) by the public. And, as before, I will elaborate the implications of the public's standpoint for understanding the *DSM*'s influence.

PUBLIC BELIEFS ABOUT MENTAL ILLNESS

Because it is so tempting to *guess* what the public is thinking—everyone is, after all, a member of the "public"—getting accurate scientific data is important. One of the best sources of data on public beliefs is the General Social Survey (GSS), a long-running, nationally representative survey that is still conducted mostly in person despite the migration of most public-opinion surveys to online platforms. The survey began in the 1970s and is ongoing. In 1996 and 2006 the GSS asked a series of questions about mental health. Because the GSS asked these questions in exactly the same way at both times, it is possible to explore trends in public beliefs without fear that any apparent trend only reflects changes in how a question was asked. The GSS has many other benefits.

The design of its questions is one of the GSS's most important features. The GSS is hardly the first survey to ask questions about mental health, but it used an especially innovative approach: It asked a series of questions about a person described in a short vignette as suffering from the symptoms of various psychiatric disorders. The vignettes depicted a person suffering from one of three psychiatric disorders, based on *DSM* criteria, as well as a person suffering from ordinary emotional ups and downs. The person described as suffering from alcohol dependence, for instance, was described as having to drink more to get the same effect, as trying to stop drinking, as growing agitated when trying to quit, and as being unreliable with his/her family. The person described as suffering from a major depressive disorder, meanwhile, was described as waking up with a heavy feeling, as not enjoying things as usual, as struggling with even simple things, and as having difficulty concentrating. Similarly, the person described as suffering from schizophrenia was depicted as believing others were talking about him/her behind his/her back, as losing the drive to participate in usual activities, as becoming preoccupied with his/her own thoughts, as skipping meals, and as hearing voices.

Although the symptoms depicted in these vignettes were sufficient for a *DSM* diagnosis, the person was not labeled in the vignettes as having a mental illness. They were not described as suffering, for example, from "major depression" or "schizophrenia," even though all the symptoms they were depicted as having were sufficient for such a diagnosis. This strategy is important for reasons that will become apparent. It allows researchers to assess beliefs about mental illness rather than beliefs about a label. Labeling theory presumes a difference: What the public thinks when told a person suffers from schizophrenia might differ from what it thinks about a person who has the symptoms of schizophrenia. Those who believe diagnoses are stigmatized are, in effect, asserting that a label carries negative connotations that stretch beyond the symptoms alone. To presuppose a diagnosis, then, is to distort how the public thinks about mental illness, and, as a matter of research strategy, it is important to evaluate beliefs about mental illness apart from other influences. In the same spirit, the race, gender, and education of the person in the vignette was varied randomly, so as not to conflate beliefs about alcohol abuse, for instance, with beliefs about men.

Respondents were asked a series of questions about the person described in the vignette. Table 6.1 shows the basic findings.[5] The table has many dimensions, but among the most important is evidence for the ascendance of a disease model. Americans are increasingly likely to regard the symptoms described in these vignettes as indicative of a mental illness. Although even in 1996 most Americans regarded schizophrenia and depression as mental illnesses, these percentages grew over the following decade. In the same vein, when asked whether the person described in the vignette should seek treatment, Americans are more encouraging. The percentage endorsing psychiatric medication is especially strong in 2006. At the same time, fewer

TABLE 6.1 TRENDS IN BELIEFS ABOUT MENTAL ILLNESS, 1996 TO 2006, GENERAL SOCIAL SURVEY

	SCHIZOPHRENIA		MAJOR DEPRESSION		ALCOHOL DEPENDENCE	
	1996 (%)	2006 (%)	1996 (%)	2006 (%)	1996 (%)	2006 (%)
Nature of disease:						
A mental illness	85	91	65	72	44	50
Normal ups and downs	40	37	78	67	60	61
Caused by:						
Chemical imbalance	78	87	67	80	59	68
Genes	61	71	51	64	58	68
Bad character	31	31	38	32	49	65
Way raised	40	33	45	41	64	69
Recommend treatment:						
Physician	72	87	78	91	74	89
Psychiatrist	90	92	75	85	61	79
Psychiatric medication	76	86	71	79	40	53

Source: Adapted from Bernice A. Pescosolido et al., "'A Disease Like Any Other'? A Decade of Change in Public Reactions to Schizophrenia, Depression, and Alcohol Dependence," *American Journal of Psychiatry* 167, no. 11 (2010): 1321–30.

people believe disorders are the result of the usual ups and downs of life, suggesting a growing distinction between what Americans regard as normal and abnormal suffering. In short, even when nothing about the symptoms has changed, Americans increasingly regard those symptoms through the lens of disease.

The time span covered by the GSS is fortuitous and lends itself to further insights.[6] During this time period, direct-to-consumer marketing of psychiatric pharmaceuticals grew enormously. Televised advertisements of prescription drugs only became possible in 1997, with the publication of new guidelines by the Food and Drug Administration. The GSS data correspond, then, to the year prior to the advent of television advertising for pharmaceuticals and nearly ten years after. This span allows the GSS to speak to the effects of direct-to-consumer advertising, and this feature is enhanced by the variety of disorders depicted in the GSS. The vignettes describe disorders that are the subject of a great deal of advertising, such as major depression, as well as disorders that are not, such as schizophrenia. Viewed in this light, the GSS reveals something important about the effects of advertising: The percentage of Americans recommending treatment increased for *both* schizophrenia and depression, despite the difference in exposure through the media. Pharmaceutical advertisements appear to have been a tide that lifted all boats. The public plainly recognizes a distinction between schizophrenia and depression, as is apparent in other beliefs, but thinking about biological causes with respect to one behavioral problem appears to spill over to others.

HOW IS INFORMATION ABOUT DIAGNOSIS USED IN THE CLINICAL ENCOUNTER?

If the public accepts a biomedical model in the abstract, does that mean they also seek medical treatment when they are sick? As noted already, the vast majority of people who meet the diagnostic criteria for a psychiatric disorder do not seek treatment of any kind. This is true even when including many different types of providers, such as psychiatric specialists, general practitioners, and social workers. It is also true even for the most severe psychiatric disorders. Although the likelihood of using services certainly increases the more severe a condition is, a large number of those with the most serious disorders still do not seek treatment. The public is more aware of psychiatric disorders than they were in the past, and they are certainly more aware of the many ways disorders can be treated, but this has not resulted in a public that is especially willing or able to seek treatment.

Part of the explanation for this is the public's complex set of beliefs about the causes of psychiatric disorders. The public accepts biomedical causes, including chemical imbalances and genes, but they also accept environmental causes, such as stress. This is relevant to their likelihood of seeking treatment. When presented with especially strong information that a disorder is environmental in origin, the public is unlikely to endorse treatment. In this way, judgments about treatment are based less on symptoms than on causes. By the same logic, judgments about normality are based less on the degree to which symptoms are serious than on how easily they can be explained. Both of these considerations depart from the *DSM*. However, as discussed in the previous chapter, they are consistent with how clinicians, too, view psychiatric disorders. Recall that one criticism of the *DSM* is that it is blind to causes when it really ought to embrace them. Some critics of the *DSM* encourage an approach that distinguishes disorders with and without cause, preferring that only the latter be regarded as genuine. The public appears to use a similar theory when evaluating symptoms. When people are able to provide a plausible explanation for a symptom, they are more likely to regard that symptom as normal, an inference referred to as the "understanding-it-makes-it-normal" effect.[7] In the case of psychiatric disorders, the public holds the reasonable view that stress can cause psychiatric disorders, so learning about a precipitating event, such as a job loss, leads people to interpret depression as more ordinary than they would if it had no apparent cause.[8] The public, much like professionals, feels compelled to explain psychiatric disorders.

The emphasis on causes is consequential, but it is even more complex than it appears. It betrays an overwhelming emphasis on *existential understanding*. In the same fashion as many clinicians, the public uses a narrative thought process in evaluating mental illness, and, for this reason, the public sees causes that are "deeper" as more indicative of a dysfunction. In an experiment similar to the vignette strategy used in the GSS, Kim and LoSavio presented college undergraduates with hypothetical patients exhibiting a variety of abnormal behaviors consistent, again, with a formal psychiatric disorder.[9] In some instances, though, the students were also presented with information about events precipitating those behaviors. As expected from the "understanding-it-makes-it-normal" effect, Kim and LoSavio found that information about causes was critical to how students evaluated the disorder. When presented with information about a precipitating event, students reported less need for treatment. This was only the case, however, when the event was seen as outside of the individual's control. When the individual was seen as responsible in some way (e.g., the divorce happened because she cheated on her husband), she was seen as more in need of treatment than if the same event was seen as outside her control (e.g., the divorce happened because her husband cheated on her). Strictly speaking, the public might not blame people for mental illness—the GSS data are encouraging in this regard—but it still uses the idea of responsibility for differentiating superficial and real symptoms.

The public also elevates the significance of some symptoms over others. In particular, the public regards symptoms that cause other symptoms as stronger signals of a genuine disorder.[10] In the case of major depression, for example, depressed mood is regarded as more important than indecisiveness, brooding, or even suicidal thoughts because a depressed mood is seen as causing the other symptoms and, therefore, as primary. This mindset, too, reflects an instinct to explain rather than simply to label. Yet it introduces a paradox with respect to treatment and a potential wedge between the patient and the clinician: When symptoms appear related to one another they are interpreted as both indicating that a psychiatric disorder is present *and* as a reason to forego treatment. At least in the mind of the public, those things that lend coherence to diagnostic criteria are also those things that mitigate against a medical approach.

This framework for thinking about causes might be appropriate from the standpoint of a public struggling with how to understand abnormal behavior, but it is also an unusual way to view disease. It suggests an alignment between how the public evaluates normality and whether it recommends treatment, even though the standard disease model posits no necessary connection between the two. We know that smoking causes lung cancer, for example, but we can treat lung cancer regardless of whether it was caused by smoking or not. By the same logic, being an inexperienced cyclist can provide a plausible explanation for why someone falls off a bike, but that fact does not eliminate the need to set the resulting fracture. If "normal" is interpreted as "common"—which is an even simpler heuristic than the one the public employs—it still implies nothing about the need for treatment. High blood pressure is common among those over fifty, but it is no less worthwhile to treat for being ordinary. When it comes to psychiatric disorders, though, the public aligns judgments about normality with assessments about the need for treatment. If something is normal, it is not worth treating. This alignment is especially consequential because it is apparent regardless of other considerations that are ordinarily relevant to determining whether treatment is necessary, including how severe the symptoms are. Pushing the logic further suggests that for the public even *severe* depression might not be worth treating if there is a plausible explanation for it.

Overall the public's mindset promotes a conservative approach. Because the public appreciates how the social environment can produce the symptoms of a psychiatric disorder, it has a variety of plausible explanations available to them. Few disorders would seem to be truly without cause or at least without a deep cause. Evidence for a conservative approach is apparent in actual treatment-seeking behavior. Even if we focus only on people who regard their symptoms as serious, there is little evidence they aggressively seek treatment. In general practice settings, for example, patients routinely present at least *some* symptoms of depression, but few patients explicitly seek a diagnosis of major depression.[11] Even after mentioning their symptoms to a doctor—something that might ordinarily indicate that patients are concerned about their symptoms—patients resist the idea that they might be suffering from a psychiatric disorder.

Kravitz and colleagues explored a particularly controversial aspect of treatment seeking, the influence of patients' explicit requests for name-brand antidepressants.[12] Their research strategy involved the use of confederates who were provided with a script to be used during a physician visit. Confederates were asked to present the symptoms of either major depression or an adjustment disorder with depressive symptoms. They were then instructed to do one of three things: request a brand-specific medication, request a general medication, or make no explicit request. Altogether the confederates made 298 visits. Although the appointments were arranged under false pretenses, physicians involved with the study rarely suspected the confederates were not real patients, and the effects of the confederates' requests were very real. Among patients presenting major depression and asking for a general medication, 75 percent received a prescription, compared to 31 percent among similar patients who made no request. Interestingly, prescribing rates were lower (53 percent) among those who made a request for a specific medication, although these patients often did not get exactly what they asked for. In the case of major depression, for instance, 27 percent of those who asked for Paxil received it, whereas 26 percent received something else. Prescribing was generally lower among those presenting with an adjustment disorder than among those presenting with depression, which was expected given the lack of consensus regarding how adjustment disorders should be treated. Nevertheless, requests for medication were as consequential for adjustment disorders as they were for depression. In the case of adjustment disorders, brand-specific requests had a greater effect than general requests, suggesting that specific requests matter more when the clinical value of a prescription is unclear. In the case of major depression, by contrast, physicians are probably aware that generic medications are as effective as name-brand medications.

A general interpretation of these patterns is that patient requests are quite powerful but that physicians—especially when properly informed about the value of a medication—still serve as gatekeepers regarding which medication works best. The integrity of the process is preserved in another way as well. Patients appear to accept the recommendations of their physicians, even after making an explicit request. One observational study, for example, found that only 15 percent of those patients whose requests were not met would consider terminating the relationship with the physician and that only 25 percent would try harder to persuade him or her.[13]

The backdrop to this level of physician authority is patient trust, another important element in the ecology of diagnosis. The public still regards physicians—especially their *personal* physicians—as the expert in matters of diagnosis. More than fifty years ago, Talcott Parsons famously laid out the conditions for this level of trust, noting above all the competence gap between patients and providers.[14] Although trust in physicians has declined somewhat over time, the vast majority of Americans still have enormous faith in their personal physician, and most Americans do not feel compelled to seek a second opinion.[15] For their part, physicians are still driven by a profound sense of professionalism. Although there is evidence that physicians occasionally accommodate the requests of patients, there is little evidence that they abrogate their authority altogether.

DOES THE *DSM* CREATE FALSE EPIDEMICS?

There are safeguards to overdiagnosis embedded in the doctor-patient relationship, but one lingering fear is that mere awareness of a disorder can help create the disorder itself. In this case, physicians provide less of a safeguard because the symptoms are generated or apprehended entirely by patients. This is a strong argument, but it has softer forms. Modern forms of the argument, for instance, are embedded in the idea of "fad diagnoses," which suddenly rise in prominence with little obvious basis in nature. Older forms of the argument focused on the negative effects of labeling. In the original labeling theory, Thomas Scheff argued that labels create the very disorders they were meant to describe.[16] Of course, this is a strong statement, and subsequent elaborations of the idea have been far more modest. The modern idea of false epidemics, for instance, does not assert that labels themselves create disorders. It only asserts that diagnoses are, under some circumstances, too broadly applied. Yet it is important to understand labeling theory and its evolution as a backdrop to understanding how the *DSM* might create diagnostic fads.

Scheff argued that being labeled creates the conditions necessary for developing a disorder. In labeling theory, the backdrop to psychiatric disorders are behavioral and emotional symptoms. These symptoms are common, according to Scheff, although for most individuals they are fleeting and will pass with time. Being labeled, however, sets the individual on a different course. If, for example, two people are both experiencing the same symptoms of depression, only the person who is labeled will develop major depression in full. This happens because the label implicates the person's identity in a way the symptoms alone do not. The label sets a series of reactions in motion: Once a person is labeled, his behavior becomes organized around the diagnosis; other people begin to treat him differently, consistent with the label; and his identity eventually crystallizes around that of someone suffering from "major depression" rather than someone experiencing transitory symptoms. This process works because people carry expectations regarding psychiatric disorders, including what they mean and what other people think of people who suffer from them. In this setting, a label takes these abstract expectations and suddenly makes them personal. What was once merely an abstract understanding of a psychiatric disorder suddenly becomes an insight into the person's identity. Labeling theory is related to the idea of a self-fulfilling prophecy but differs in an important respect. In labeling theory, the process that creates a disorder does not depend entirely on the individual. How other people respond is just as relevant. If, for instance, other people fear those with mental illness, those who are labeled mentally ill experience social rejection, which is itself a risk factor for a psychiatric disorder.

In these arguments, there is no mistaking Scheff's critique of psychiatry. Scheff explicitly argues that, in the absence of a label, the symptoms of a psychiatric disorder will not stabilize. Furthermore, Scheff argues that the symptoms of mental illness should not be interpreted as indicating a disorder—they are common, they are normal, and they are transient. In this way, mental illness *as an illness* is entirely an artifact of the label. It has no reality otherwise. Scheff's theory has another aspect. Instead of seeing mental illness in terms of medicine, Scheff interprets psychiatric disorders in terms of social control. Society creates rules and laws to regulate what it regards as deviant behavior, but, his argument goes, there is always a residual category of unusual behaviors and thoughts. The symptoms of mental illness are not crimes, exactly, or even bad manners, yet they are still seen as abnormal and worthy of discipline. For Scheff, then, psychiatric disorders were created in order to control behaviors that society regarded as deviant but for which it had no other means of regulating.

Labeling theory, at least in its strongest form, has not fared well. Critics of the idea have argued that mental illness, especially serious mental illness, cannot be explained by labeling. Critics have also pointed out that those suffering from psychiatric disorders rarely report the sort of social rejection Scheff had in mind.[17] On the contrary, a label occasionally invites sympathy rather than scorn. In a similar vein, some have charged that much of the stigma surrounding mental illness, such as it is, comes from the *symptoms* of mental illness rather than the label per se. Those with schizophrenia, for example, are avoided because their behavior is disturbing, not because they are known to be schizophrenic. The label itself is incidental.

Some aspects of labeling theory, though, live on. And labeling theory was not entirely incorrect in its basic idea that labels can be powerful. Modified labeling theory reformulates the impact of labels in a more fruitful (and modest) direction. Bruce Link and colleagues begin with the idea that labels do, in fact, matter.[18] They argue that when a person is labeled, public beliefs about mental illness suddenly become relevant in a way that those beliefs were not before. Some of these beliefs might be positive, and some might be negative, but, whatever else, they are suddenly significant when a person is diagnosed. The dilemma for someone who has been labeled, then, is how to respond to these beliefs and expectations, and Link and colleagues show that many people who are labeled respond *as if* they will be rejected. Some, for example, try to hide their diagnoses, becoming more secretive in the process. Some go even further and withdraw from social interaction altogether, fearing they will be found out. These behaviors, in turn, are actual risk factors for additional symptoms. Social isolation, for example, can increase the risk for major depression. Furthermore, the strain of trying to conceal a diagnosis can undermine confidence and self-esteem. In these ways, people who have been labeled are vulnerable to new episodes of a disorder not because the label alone prompts vulnerability but because the label changes the person's behavior in detrimental ways.

The differences between labeling theory and modified labeling theory are important to emphasize. Link and colleagues do not argue that labels are the primary cause of mental illness. And they certainly do not argue that mental illness is a myth. If, according to modified labeling theory, someone is suffering from the symptoms of a psychiatric disorder and they are not labeled, those symptoms are still real, and they might eventually develop into a chronic disorder. The ideas of modified labeling theory are also more consistent with contemporary science. They are consistent, for example, with what we know about the genetic determinants of psychiatric disorders. The claims of modified labeling theory are limited in their scope and do not prohibit an allowance for genetic causes. Link and colleagues argue that if a person suffering from a psychiatric disorder is not labeled, there are no consequences *that stem from labeling*. Other risk factors, including genetics, still matter. Furthermore, the impact of a label hinges on the idea of *stigma*. Labeled persons withdraw from social life, for example, because they expect to be rejected, not because the label alone conveys something negative. This allows for an important contingency that was not apparent in labeling theory. If there were no stigma surrounding psychiatric disorders, being labeled would not be consequential. Modified labeling theory also empowers individuals far more than labeling theory. In labeling theory, individuals are in effect beholden to the larger culture and unable to change it. When labeled, individuals begin to imagine what others will think of them and act accordingly. Furthermore, labeling theory assumes individuals accept the label as true. Modified labeling theory, by contrast, allows for the possibility that those who are labeled might not accept the diagnosis, that they might try to address the stigma surrounding their condition, and, at a minimum, that they might not absorb the label as a key feature of their identity.

Perhaps because of these various contingencies, modified labeling theory has fared much better in empirical research than labeling theory. The theory has been tested in studies that follow individuals over time, comparing the experiences of those who were and were not labeled. Studies of this sort have uncovered several things.[19] First, they have revealed that those who suffer from psychiatric disorders have mixed feelings about their diagnoses. Labels are not entirely bad. Some patients feel that a label was essential to receiving treatment, and other patients report that a label allowed them to realize they had a problem. Yet the evidence also suggests that many people who have been labeled expect to be rejected. They report, for example, that other people would think less of them if they knew about their diagnosis. This inference, in turn, leads to behaviors that do, in fact, worsen their condition, much as modified labeling theory anticipates. A question remains, though. Modified labeling theory was developed over twenty years ago. Is there still a significant stigma surrounding psychiatric disorders? Might the cultural conditions that upheld the effects of labels in modified labeling theory no longer obtain?

THE STIGMA OF PSYCHIATRIC DISORDERS

The GSS is, again, the best data to study stigma, this time with supplementary data from 1950.[20] In 1950 and 1996, survey respondents were asked: "When you hear someone say that a person is 'mentally-ill,' what does that mean to you?" Although this is a very general question allowing an open-ended response, it is an appropriate way to gauge the range of things Americans consider "mental illness" and the degree to which their conceptions match those in the *DSM*. Researchers documented at least two important patterns. For one, Americans' understanding of what mental illness is has widened over time. In 1950, the two most commonly described disorders pertained to psychosis and some combination of anxiety and depression. In 1996, fewer people mentioned these specific disorders, but not because they no longer regarded them as disorders. Rather, respondents nominated a host of other disorders, too. About 35 percent mentioned psychosis, about the same percentage mentioned depression and anxiety, and another 20 percent mentioned a variety of other nonpsychotic symptoms. Twice as many people— about 16 percent relative to 7 percent—mentioned social deviance, something the *DSM* had explicitly sought to curtail in its definition of mental disorder. In addition, about twice as many people mentioned cognitive impairment of some kind. In short, understandings of what mental illness is have become more varied than they were in the past.

Given the expansive definition of mental illness, it is tempting to infer that stigma has declined. If when the public thinks about mental illness they are more likely to think of cognitive impairment, for example, and somewhat less likely to think of psychosis, perhaps they are also less likely to think of those with mental illness as dangerous. This is not the case, however. The percentage also mentioning violent symptoms in their descriptions increased from 7 percent to 12 percent. Even disorders that have long appeared dangerous were seen as more dangerous in 1996 than earlier. In 1950, for example, about 13 percent of those who described psychosis also described violence, but in 1996 this percentage increased to just over 30 percent.

There are other ways to gauge stigma. In the social sciences, stigma is often measured in terms of *social distance*. Social distance refers to the willingness of one person to interact with someone else. More reluctance (or "distance") implies more stigma. The presumption is that one of the key manifestations of stigma is being unwilling, for example, to work with someone who suffers from a psychiatric disorder. The GSS included a battery of social-distance questions in both 1996 and 2006. Responses to these questions are presented in table 6.2.[21] The questions pertain to a variety of

TABLE 6.2 TRENDS IN DESIRED SOCIAL DISTANCE FROM MENTAL ILLNESS, 1996 TO 2006, GENERAL SOCIAL SURVEY

	SCHIZOPHRENIA		MAJOR DEPRESSION		ALCOHOL DEPENDENCE	
	1996 (%)	2006 (%)	1996 (%)	2006 (%)	1996 (%)	2006 (%)
Unwilling to:						
Work closely with	56	62	46	47	72	74
Have as a neighbor	34	45	23	20	44	39
Socialize with	46	52	35	30	56	54
Make friends with	30	35	23	21	35	36
Marry into family	65	69	57	53	70	79
Dangerous toward:						
Self	81	84	73	70	78	79
Others	54	60	33	32	65	67

Source: Adapted from Bernice A. Pescosolido et al., "'A Disease Like Any Other'? A Decade of Change in Public Reactions to Schizophrenia, Depression, and Alcohol Dependence," *American Journal of Psychiatry* 167, no. 11 (2010): 1321–30.

potential interactions with the person described in the vignette, from simply having the person as a neighbor to having the person marry into your family. In this way, the questions are designed to be sensitive to the full range of potential encounters. Americans might be willing to socialize briefly with someone who has delusions, for example, but draw the line at working with him.

One common assumption is that social distance has declined over time. The reasoning is simple: If Americans are increasingly familiar with mental illness and are adopting a more biomedical approach, perhaps they are also more willing to associate with those with mental illness. The actual trends, though, are mixed, and much depends on the specific disorder. Social distance directed at people with schizophrenia has increased, while social distance directed at people with depression has decreased. For alcohol dependence, the direction of the change depends on the specific aspect of social distance being considered, suggesting a complex approach/avoidance calculation. Altogether these data prove at least one idea wrong: Americans are not becoming uniformly more tolerant of psychiatric disorders.

Paradoxically, the explanation for these mixed patterns lies in the ascent of a more scientific approach to mental illness. In particular, the rise of a genetic model has pushed public opinion in two directions simultaneously. Earlier I showed that more Americans endorse a genetic model of mental illness. Some mental health advocates have welcomed this as good news, assuming that the stigma surrounding psychiatric disorders was born of ignorance. In particular, they reasoned that stigma was rooted in the idea that mental illness was not "real" in the same way as other illnesses and, therefore, assumed that Americans' negative attitudes might fade as they accept a more biological approach. Unfortunately, however, genetic arguments carry more complex connotations. On one hand, a genetic basis for mental illness implies that the illness is not the fault of the individual suffering from it. In the past, a not unreasonable assumption was that people were intolerant of depression because they regarded it in personal terms. Those suffering from depression, the argument went, were revealing a character weakness, not a physical problem. Similarly, those who abused alcohol were regarded in terms of bad choices and not in terms of addiction. Certainly other illnesses have benefited from being understood in genetic terms. Americans are tolerant of those who suffer from Down syndrome or at least do not blame people for the disorder. If the same mindset was applied to depression, the assumption was that tolerance would increase. Related to this is the connection the public often makes between identifying the genes for a disease and finding a cure. If depression is a biomedical problem and not a matter of personal weakness, the assumption goes, an effective treatment may be possible. On the other hand, genes have some less sanguine connotations. For one, a genetic basis for disease implies a deep-seated cause. Although the individual suffering from a genetic condition might not be responsible for his condition, the presence of faulty genes reveals a more fundamental defect than would be implied if his depression were regarded as only a product of stress. Indeed, genes can easily extend stigma from the sick to the healthy. Even if an individual is not currently depressed, having the genetic risk for depression implies she might develop the disorder in the future. The strongest statement in this vein comes from those fearing the emergence of a new kind of "genetic essentialism," wherein individuals are reduced to their genes.[22] Under some conditions, knowledge of genetic risks can accentuate perceived personal responsibility rather than mitigate it. Learning that one is "at risk" for a genetic condition perhaps obligates the individual to do more to prevent it.[23] In this vein, Rose argues that genes are creating new responsibilities for managing risk and to see health as the product of prudence, choice, and responsible action rather than chance.[24]

Reconciling these competing views is not straightforward. It involves considering all the other beliefs people hold about mental illness. And, indeed, evidence indicates that genetic arguments have mixed consequences, depending on the disorder. In the case of schizophrenia, genetic arguments decrease tolerance. In the case of depression, though, they increase tolerance.[25] The explanation for this divergence revolves around what other beliefs genetic arguments intersect. In the case of schizophrenia, genetic arguments enhance how threatening the symptoms appear. If those with schizophrenia are almost always regarded as dangerous, their symptoms become even more alarming if those symptoms are also regarded as genetic. In the case of depression, however, the symptoms of the disorder are interpreted in a different way. If the individual is not seen as responsible for her depression, she is more likely to be regarded as sick and, therefore, sympathetic. In short, the rise of a biomedical model is not a cure-all for stigma. It will not elevate tolerance like a rising tide lifting all boats. Genetic arguments introduce new concerns even as they alleviate others.

An emphasis on genes has another implication that is equally troubling. The rise of a genetic model affects how people see *themselves* as much as how they see others. In particular, when individuals with symptoms of depression believe their condition reflects genes, it can lead to a self-fulfilling prophecy. When made to believe their depression is caused by genetic factors, patients are more pessimistic about their prognosis and less likely to regard their disorder as malleable.[26] Similarly, individuals who are told that they carry a gene for alcoholism are more likely to regard themselves as unable to avoid drinking.[27] Although educating patients about the importance of environmental influences can restore optimism among those with risky genes, findings of this sort suggest that most people regard genetic arguments in a rather blunt and unconditional fashion.

DO LABELS MATTER FOR PUBLIC BELIEFS?

The research on public beliefs discussed thus far leaves one important question unresolved. Recall that the GSS used the *DSM* as a guide for its vignettes. The vignette depicting depression, for instance, includes all the symptoms necessary to meet the diagnostic criteria for a major depressive episode. Yet the person in the vignette is never described as suffering from "major depression." In short, the person is not explicitly labeled. This is a potentially important omission, even if a scientifically justified one. If we believe labels matter, the label itself might change how people interpret the symptoms presented in the vignettes. If labels matter above and beyond the symptoms, for example, then the label "schizophrenic" might decrease tolerance even more than the symptoms alone. This might be the case in depression as well, especially if the person is perceived as "normal" up until the point they are explicitly labeled as being disordered.

Other studies have looked at the effects of labels, using the vignette design but adding a label to some of the descriptions. In this vein, Link and colleagues employed a vignette in which they varied the presentation of the person along two dimensions.[28] First, in some vignettes the person was described as being in a psychiatric hospital two years earlier because of "problems he was having." The vignette then described his current symptoms. In another vignette, the same person was described as being hospitalized for back problems. Second, Link and colleagues varied how severe the disorder was. In one vignette, the person was described as having normal fears and concerns, mixed with occasional bouts of anger. In another vignette, though, the person was described in stronger terms. He was described as banging his fists on the table, storming out of meetings, and occasionally threatening coworkers.

Using this experimental design, Link and colleagues found that labels do indeed matter, but in conflicting directions. When a label is applied to a person who has relatively mild symptoms, the label *increases* tolerance. Respondents presented with the vignette were more willing to interact with someone who had been in a psychiatric hospital than with the same person described as having been hospitalized for back pain. As the symptoms grew worse, however, the labeling effect was reversed. When presented with severe symptoms, respondents were *less* tolerant of the person who had been labeled than the person who had not. In the first case, the label appears to have evoked a helping response. The person in the vignette attracted sympathy and was, in effect, cut an "extra break" for his flare-ups. In the second case, though, the label accentuated fear. For the same behavior, a person known to have been in a psychiatric hospital was seen as more dangerous and unpredictable. This finding can be interpreted in tandem with the earlier findings regarding genes. Being angry at coworkers is not uncommon, but seeing anger through the lens of a label transforms outbursts into symptoms and, thus, moves the person closer to being considered sick rather than upset.

RESISTING AND AVOIDING LABELS

Altogether these studies present a complex picture, but they still provide evidence that labels can, in fact, make things worse. These studies also provide little assurance that stigma is declining and, in this way, might encourage even more caution when it comes to applying labels. Yet the power of labels is not overwhelming. Even if we accept that there is some stigma surrounding psychiatric disorders, stigma does not always undermine well-being. When labeled, some people choose to resist the stigma of their disorder, seeking, for example, to persuade others of their normality.[29] Still other people refuse to believe that the stereotypes surrounding their illness are true of themselves, even if they recognize that other people might accept these stereotypes as accurate.[30] Understanding how people resist labels is just as important as understanding how they are affected by them.

Sue Estroff and colleagues followed 169 patients with severe mental illness over time, focusing on how they grappled with the meaning and significance of their diagnoses.[31] Even in the case of severe and persistent mental illness, Estroff found a range of responses. She uncovered an especially sharp distinction between self-labeling and a formal diagnosis. In principle, the two could be the same: Patients might vary in how they *interpret* their disorder, but if a professional says they have schizophrenia, they at least accept that diagnosis as accurate. Estroff, however, found a gap: She found that only 23 percent of patients agreed they were "mentally ill," and this percentage changed very little the longer patients were hospitalized.[32] Patients routinely normalized even their most severe experiences. Psychotic episodes, for example, were referred to using the more benign language of a "fantasy."[33] Other symptoms, meanwhile, were regarded as something everyone experiences at least occasionally. Even when patients recognized their symptoms as real and serious, those symptoms were seen as something apart from who they were. Patients further distinguished between the emotional aspects of mental illness and the cognitive aspects. When patients distanced themselves from being "mentally ill," they did so in reference to the idea that mental illness consists of cognitive impairment. They saw their own disorders in terms of emotions, which they regarded as part of regular everyday experience and not necessarily characteristic of sickness.[34] This distinction was particularly strong in the case of mood disorders. Those with depression made few references to clinical nomenclature or even to the word "illness." They instead spoke of depression's emotional aspects, including sadness and loneliness.[35]

A good deal of research has focused on the effects of professional labels. That is, research has focused on what happens after the individual has been diagnosed by a *clinician*. In thinking about false epidemics, however, it is important to consider whether and how individuals label *themselves*. Although there is evidence the public is more sophisticated about what mental illness is, there is also evidence that members of the public are hardly eager to apply diagnostic labels to themselves. In the same vein, there is also evidence the public actively eschews the medical model when it comes to explaining personal experiences.[36] Accepting the presence of a clinical disorder comes slowly, if at all. In the 1950s, a now classic study explored wives whose husbands were suffering from schizophrenia.[37] The study documented the wives' difficulty in recognizing the disorder and provided an especially vivid example of the idea that "understanding it makes it normal." The difficulty in recognizing the disorder was not because wives failed to understand their husband's behavior but precisely because they understood their husbands so well and could easily call to mind other explanations. Behaviors that were clearly a departure from how their husbands had behaved in the past, for example, were attributed to situational factors, such as a stressful job. Other symptoms were downplayed as simply an aspect of their husbands' personality. Growing anxiety and fear, for instance, were attributed to how they had always been nervous. Although from a clinical standpoint their husbands were clearly suffering from schizophrenia, wives resisted the interpretation until it was absolutely unavoidable.

Much has changed since this study, but even now the process of recognizing a psychiatric disorder in others is complex, fitful, and hesitant. Part of this complexity stems from what people believe about mental illness. Recall from earlier in this chapter that while a growing number of Americans are willing to attribute the symptoms to mental illness to genetics, the percentage that attributes psychiatric symptoms to the normal ups and downs of life is nearly as high. For the public, then, the line between sick and well is indistinct, and there is very little evidence people jump the line with ease or certainty. Furthermore, when explanations other than sickness are possible, those explanations tend to be employed first.

Taking this point further, one way to think about the issue of lay recognition of psychiatric disorders is in terms of the explanatory frameworks available to the public. The symptoms of psychiatric disorders are, in many cases, simply more extreme aspects of everyday behavior, and when trying to account for their daily experience, people have a variety of credible explanations available to them. Consider, for example, the case of sadness. People suffering from depression can explain it in terms of recent experiences, they can explain it in terms of personality, or they can explain it in terms of a psychiatric disorder. The medical model is perhaps the latest explanatory framework in the mix, but it is not the *only* one, and when it comes to explaining suffering one framework usually cannot dominate another. Even as the public increasingly accepts a medical model, for example, other explanations for psychiatric disorders have not faded from relevance. Because individuals are generally motivated to see themselves and others as normal, any hint that they might be sick will be considered alongside other explanations. This tendency to seek balance among alternative frameworks is so strong that even when individuals become patients in a psychiatric hospital they resist the label "mentally ill," as Estroff's work makes clear.

DISEASE SPECIFICITY AND THE PUBLIC

The *DSM* was written with disease specificity in mind. It was guided by the idea that psychiatric disorders have a specific manifestation and can be characterized accurately by their symptoms. The *DSM* was further guided by the idea that psychiatric disorders are manifest in typical ways across patients. For this reason, the authors of the *DSM* saw no loss in describing major depression in ways that could be separated from the individual suffering from it. The public, however, interprets and absorbs psychiatric diagnoses very differently. For one, the public regards causes as more important than symptoms. Indeed, for the public, the context surrounding symptoms is critical. The public also thinks of psychiatric disorders in terms of narratives, blending considerations of the person, his symptoms, his past, and his environment, and thereby eschewing the abstract approach favored by the *DSM*. There is certainly little evidence that psychiatric disorders are interpreted *uncritically* by the public. Diagnoses filter through the public's beliefs and experiences in ways that blunt the influence of the *DSM*. Can the same be said of scientists? How do scientists—as creators of facts and purveyors of sober interpretations—use the *DSM*?

7

HOW SCIENTISTS USE THE *DSM*

So far I have focused on how various parties use psychiatric diagnoses, and I have emphasized the ways in which those parties depart from the *DSM*. There are far fewer departures, however, when it comes to how scientists use the *DSM*. Scientists are bound by the rules of the *DSM* in a way clinicians are not. Their profession demands it. In order to obtain a grant or publish a study, scientists must assure funders and editors that the subjects of their study were selected in a standardized fashion, based on firm psychiatric nomenclature. Adherence is self-reinforcing in the sense that scientists also expect this of one another. When scientists study major depression, for instance, they want reassurance that every other scientist studying the disorder is talking about the same kinds of people. Everyone they categorize as depressed should meet the diagnostic criteria for a major depressive episode. Science demands replication, and only with a common set of terms and instruments is it possible to reproduce previous findings.

The *DSM* certainly facilitates this, but therein lies the problem. The *DSM* both sets the terms of the debate and imposes the limits. Sometimes these limits are straightforward, as when they pertain to the obsolescence of diagnostic criteria. With each new edition of the *DSM*, the instruments researchers use to identify mental illness are necessarily revised, too. Past research—even fundamentally important research—can be rendered outdated simply because the *DSM*'s diagnostic criteria have changed enough to create effectively a new disorder or identify a different population. At other times, though, the *DSM* can misdirect scientists in ways that stretch beyond the continuous revision of the *DSM*. If the *DSM* fails to list symptoms that actually occur frequently in certain disorders, those symptoms receive little or no scientific attention.

It is worth exploring in detail how scientists use the *DSM*. It is also worth considering the pros and cons of maintaining strict fidelity to the *DSM*. The balance between the two is more complex than the intuition that "if the criteria are wrong, the research is wrong too." Furthermore, the fetters of the *DSM*, such as they are, cannot be lifted simply by granting scientists more flexibility. The departures from the *DSM* that I have discussed thus far are, in some ways, benign. They can be interpreted as motivated as opposed to fickle, and they are driven by professionalism more than perfidy. Clinicians, for example, are interested in providing care, and thus they put treatment ahead of diagnosis, to the point that the two tasks begin to blend. By the same token, patients are interested in understanding, so they use a diagnosis only as a point of entrée, to the point that they consider causes tantamount to symptoms. In these ways, clinicians and patients suspend firm diagnostic thresholds and maintain, at best, a tentative adherence to the *DSM*. For scientists, though, fidelity to the *DSM* is both necessary and misleading—something scientists themselves are acutely aware of. Steven Hyman served as the director of the National Institute of Mental Health—clearly one of the most preeminent leadership positions in the field—from 1996 to 2001. The NIMH is responsible for funding much of the mental health research in the United States and so sets much of the scientific agenda. Reflecting on his experiences, Hyman acknowledges that the *DSM* has "exerted enormous influence both for good and ill," but he ultimately emphasizes the ill, in no uncertain terms. He characterizes the manual as an "epistemic prison," one that has trapped researchers as its "cognitive prisoners."[1] These are bold claims, but they are not off base. For scientists, the *DSM* presents something of a paradox. It often forces scientists to study highly unusual cases of mental disorder even as it attempts to facilitate typification. It has also sparked a tremendous amount of research, but at the same time it has limited much of what can be achieved. And it has invited more scientists to study the topic of mental illness even as it has systematically excluded certain types of investigations.

To understand the role of the *DSM* in research it is useful to take a step back and think about research conducted *prior* to *DSM-III*. In the context of discussing the development of *DSM-III*, I discussed the unreliability of clinical diagnoses—that clinicians, looking at the same person and observing the same symptoms, could still produce very different diagnoses. It is indeed disconcerting when psychiatrists cannot render the same diagnoses or even recognize the well when looking for the sick. For patients, too, it can be unsettling when their diagnoses seem to change simply when they switch providers. In the context of scientific research, though, the issue of unreliability is not as easily indexed or so plainly bothersome. If pre-*DSM-III* researchers lacked common diagnostic criteria, they at least shared some basic terms. Researchers studying schizophrenia in the United Kingdom, for instance, presumed that researchers studying schizophrenia in the United States were investigating mostly the same thing. This turned out not to be the case. The diagnosis of schizophrenia was applied to a much wider variety of conditions in the United States than in the United Kingdom, leading to very different research conclusions.[2]

In principle, science need not be so concerned with reliability. Reliability is critical to clinicians and patients, but scientists are not in the business of providing care or even of deeply understanding the situation of individual cases. For this reason, it is possible to envision high-quality science without something like the *DSM*. In writing a research report, scientists are obligated to describe the key characteristics of their subjects as well as what they are trying to explain. So long as the subjects are clearly and completely described and the dependent variable well articulated, it should be transparent to readers what exactly the scientist is studying. Good research does not require absolute fidelity to any particular definition of a psychiatric disorder.[3] It only requires detailed description and a well-motivated target. Furthermore, there is no need to presuppose disorder per se. It is possible to study, for instance, the consumption of alcohol—as in the number of drinks someone consumes in a day—without studying alcohol abuse. It is possible, too, to study sadness without considering all the other elements contained in the diagnostic criteria for a major depressive episode. One can even study delusions without invoking schizophrenia. Among researchers, the choice of what to study and how to study it is ordinarily a scientific one, and it is a choice for which there is considerable flexibility and professional autonomy.

Yet the *DSM* has been so influential as to claim authority over the lingua franca of mental disorders and, in turn, to control the execution of research studies. After the publication of *DSM-III* (as well as its even more fine-grained revision, *DSM-III-R*), journals and funding agencies began requiring not only greater specificity in describing research subjects but also demanding more fidelity to the diagnostic criteria outlined in the *DSM*. This imposes a burden on scientists, but the demands of the *DSM* were not, in fact, hard to meet. Indeed, because a variety of measurement instruments were developed and promulgated in light of *DSM-III*, this task was straightforward. With instruments in hand, scientists found it easy to implement the *DSM-III*'s rules. Yet the ascendance of the *DSM* had a shadow side that was less easily addressed. Furthermore, in the ensuing enthusiasm for specific and useful diagnostic criteria, this shadow side was not readily perceived or appreciated. It became apparent only over time and, even then, only with extraordinary scientific attention. Understanding the epistemic blinders of the *DSM*, as Steven Hyman has described them, requires an appreciation of the organization of science and its interface with clinicians and patients.

THE NEGLECT OF NATURALLY OCCURRING SYMPTOM PROFILES

DSM-III introduced a gap between what disorders are studied and what disorders are common. Ordinarily it might make sense to focus on the disorders and symptoms that are especially prevalent. And, in the abstract at least, the *DSM* could be a useful tool for this task. Properly constructed, the *DSM* could highlight symptoms that tend to occur together in a typical way. Yet the *DSM* systematically directs attention away from disorders that are, in fact, quite frequent. Within many diagnostic categories, for example, the "not otherwise specified" (NOS) designation represents the most common disorder. For clinicians, this is of little concern. When presented with complex cases, clinicians turn to the NOS designation because no other category describes the case accurately. One could even argue that this practice demonstrates that clinicians are so faithful to the *DSM* that they will appropriately select the NOS category rather than shoehorn a complex case into a more traditional diagnosis. Yet scientists almost never study NOS disorders. Precisely because disorders of the NOS type are so heterogeneous and poorly characterized—in effect, the NOS designation is a residual category—they do not lend themselves to scientific study. This has consequences.

Eating disorder NOS provides a good example. The diagnosis is used extensively by clinicians but almost never by scientists.[4] Indeed, in outpatient settings, the frequency of eating disorder NOS exceeds that of anorexia and bulimia by a ratio of more than two to one, although scientists studying eating disorders almost always study anorexia or bulimia. The symptoms of eating disorder NOS resemble those of anorexia and bulimia but are just below the threshold for either disorder or represent a mix of the two. The blended nature of eating disorder NOS does not, however, make it a *mild* disorder. The rate of recovery from eating disorder NOS is low, and its consequences resemble those of anorexia and bulimia.[5] The issue, then, is not that clinicians are overdiagnosing a mild subthreshold disorder. Instead, the issue is a poor interface between scientific and clinical applications of the *DSM*. One explanation for the low rate of recovery is simply a lack of scientifically tested treatments. Almost no study tests treatments among eating disorder NOS patients, so clinicians are left struggling to develop appropriate treatment protocols based on what science knows about the other eating disorders.[6] Although an eating disorder NOS might very well represent a different kind of eating disorder and so might benefit from being studied directly, studying the disorder on its own is discouraged by an insistence on studying "standard" *DSM* disorders.

To be sure, science is not altogether unresponsive to this problem. In some cases, scientists have deliberately studied "subthreshold" disorders, under the assumption that people whose symptoms fall just below a diagnostic threshold are "without a disorder" in only a superficial sense. Scientists have also recognized that the *DSM* overlooks things that are important to clinicians. Minor depression is an especially good example. One formal definition of "minor depression" is having at least two but not five of the symptoms required for a diagnosis of a major depressive episode.[7] Minor depression of this sort is very common in primary care settings. Physicians must deal with it routinely, and its presence can complicate the treatment of other illnesses, including, for example, heart disease. Furthermore, on its own, minor depression can lead to disability, much like major depression. Yet minor depression *is* different, at least from a clinical perspective. It does not respond to treatment in the same way as major depression. Psychiatric medications, for instance, are less effective for minor depression than major depression.[8] Moreover, minor depression receives very little attention from scientists. To the extent that it is studied at all, it is studied in a haphazard way.[9] And this reflects the lack of a crisp and authoritative set of diagnostic criteria. Research on minor depression is ad hoc precisely because the disorder breaks from the standards of the *DSM*, leaving scientists to deploy their own definitions. It is much easier, then, for scientists to study major depression than minor depression. Pincus and colleagues provide a concise summary of research on subthreshold disorders in saying that "a *laissez-faire* approach has resulted in a 'tower of Babel' with regard to understanding the nature of these conditions."[10] What Pincus and colleagues describe with respect to the study of subthreshold disorders could easily be applied to the study of *all* psychiatric disorders prior to the publication of *DSM-III*, but their comment is notable for laying bare the problems the *DSM* has still failed to address.

In a similar way, the *DSM* illuminates but averts the issue of comorbidity. As discussed earlier, the form of the diagnostic criteria contained in *DSM-III* paved the way for uncovering high levels of comorbidity.[11] Using *DSM-III*, scientists discovered that comorbidity is the norm rather than the exception. Yet paradoxically science has mostly avoided studying comorbidity itself. The structure of science emphasizes the study of *disorders* rather than the study of *people with disorders*. Following the logic of disease specificity, scientists seek prototypes of disorder, which need not reflect how that particular disorder is actually manifest in the people who suffer from it. In order to study major depression, for instance, researchers routinely exclude patients whose depression is accompanied by another disorder, despite the frequency of comorbidity. This is especially true in clinical trials. Drugs are approved—if they are approved at all—for the treatment of specific disorders, and they are evaluated in trials that test their effectiveness among those suffering from that disorder. In practice, then, testing the effectiveness of a drug for a certain indication requires identifying research subjects who suffer *only* from that disorder, but eliminating comorbid cases can produce highly unusual samples. One study found that only 5 percent of patients who met the lifetime criteria for a major depressive disorder did not also meet the criteria for an anxiety disorder.[12] Moreover, patients with pure disorders respond differently to treatment than those suffering from comorbid disorders. When a major depressive episode is comorbid with another disorder it responds less well to antidepressants.[13] The reasons for this are not well understood and cannot be well understood until comorbidity itself becomes a sanctioned topic of scientific curiosity.

The *DSM* prevents the development of effective treatments for other reasons as well. For one, the *DSM* inhibits researchers from uncovering shared pathological features. The *DSM* classifies disorders on the basis of surface characteristics. Other areas of medicine began in much the same way but have since evolved into a greater emphasis on clinical and biological tests. This, in turn, has led to a more synthetic approach to the study of seemingly disparate diseases.[14] In oncology, for example, research began by studying cancers according to their site, such as lung cancer, breast cancer, and prostate cancer. But adopting a more synthetic approach has proven more fruitful. For example, research on one type of breast cancer with an especially bad prognosis (associated with a human epidermal growth factor) led to the development of a treatment (an antibody therapy) that was effective not only for this type of breast cancer but also for cancers located in other sites, including ovarian, lung, and gastric cancers.[15] Those cancers, it turned out, shared common pathological features, previously unrecognized.

The *DSM* has also led to the neglect of certain *symptoms*, if not *disorders*. Overall, schizophrenia is among the more intractable psychiatric disorders. Some medications, though, are effective in treating what are called the "positive" symptoms of the disorder, namely hallucinations and delusions.[16] Furthermore, these medications have improved, with consecutive generations providing more effective relief with fewer side effects.[17] The so-called first generation of medications was developed in the 1950s, and the second generation was developed in the 1980s, with generally better efficacy. Yet neither generation treated the *cognitive* symptoms of schizophrenia, and no other pharmacological agents were developed with cognitive symptoms in mind.[18] Although the *DSM* criteria for schizophrenia make no mention of cognitive symptoms, much of what makes the disorder disabling is, in fact, related to cognitive impairment.[19] Eventually this omission was addressed, but only through extraordinary means and not through a revision of the *DSM* itself. In 2004, the National Institute of Mental Health convened a workshop with the Food and Drug Administration with the goal of developing clinical trials for medications specifically targeting schizophrenia's neurocognitive symptoms. The workshop also called for the development of measures to assess cognitive impairment in schizophrenia, something that was not emerging given how closely scientists hewed to the *DSM*.

In addition to misdirecting science occasionally with respect to missing symptoms, the *DSM* also influences how well scientists are able to address the symptoms that actually are included in the diagnostic criteria. The *DSM* sets the clinical targets for treatment. It does so at the level of disorders, but the pharmaceutical industry generally finds it easier to narrow its target and focus on specific symptoms. The end result is medications that may be effective in treating individual symptoms—and sometimes very common and disabling ones—but less effective in treating an entire syndrome. This tendency is accentuated by how clinicians prefer to prescribe medications. In general, clinicians' therapeutic approach emphasizes the use of one catch-all medication rather than "combination" therapy. In the case of psychiatric disorders, though, few drugs are truly effective in treating all the elements of a disorder.

The history of psychiatric pharmacology does not suggest an eventual refocus. Innovation in the field has generally happened because of serendipity as much as science.[20] The therapeutic effects of lithium salt, for example, were discovered in the late 1800s and applied to a variety of ailments, but they were rediscovered in the 1940s as a treatment for mood and bipolar disorders. Even then, however, the actual mechanisms for these effects were not discovered until much later. Other psychiatric medications, meanwhile, were initially developed with very different illnesses in mind. Iproniazid, for example, was developed to treat tuberculosis but was later shown to treat the symptoms of depression.[21] Still other drugs were developed with one mental disorder in mind but were later shown to be effective for another. Drugs for the treatment of schizophrenia, for example, have been shown to be effective in treating depression. In general, though, scientists studying indications for one disorder are not alert to potential crossovers. In using the *DSM*, they are encouraged to think in terms of discrete and independent entities. At the same time, even the most effective pharmaceutical agents work for reasons that are not always clear. Later-generation drugs target specific neurotransmitters, including especially serotonin (e.g., Prozac), but even these seemingly targeted drugs also affect other neurotransmitters through secondary processes, calling into question what exactly the active ingredient is. The disconnect between targets and disorders is even deeper, though. Although molecular targets such as neurotransmitters are correlated with the symptoms of psychiatric disorders, they have not been shown to play a role in their pathophysiology.[22] Targeting serotonin, for example, might treat some of the symptoms of depression, but there is little evidence that a deficit in serotonin is the cause of depression. For these reasons, the evolution of psychiatric medications is only superficially progressive. There are far more psychiatric medications today than there were in the 1950s, but apart from a gradual improvement in side effects—which, to be sure, is not an insignificant accomplishment—many of these medications are no better than their earlier progenitors.[23]

At times the role of the *DSM* in directing research has been so strong as to discourage scientists from innovating at all. Some major pharmaceutical companies, including GlaxoSmithKline and AstraZeneca, for example, have announced their intentions to cut back on efforts to discover new psychiatric pharmaceuticals.[24] Their decision is remarkable from the standpoint of science but perhaps even more from the standpoint of business. The potential market for such drugs is enormous. Psychiatric disorders are very prevalent, and there are many as yet untapped markets, including developing market economies. Furthermore, there is no existing pharmaceutical agent that is so effective as to dominate the treatment of any disorder completely. The decision of these pharmaceutical companies to cut back on discovery makes sense, however, because it is not based on market opportunities. Instead, it is based on the structure of the underlying science. Apart from a few molecular targets identified in the 1950s, there are few validated targets around which drug manufacturers can develop new products.[25] And, of course, the *DSM* itself does not provide scientists with these sorts of targets. Indeed, if anything, the *DSM* dilutes molecular targets even further. Clinical trials are beholden to the *DSM*, but the *DSM* only provides lists of specific behaviors, thoughts, and emotions. Without validated biomarkers mapped to these symptoms, pharmaceutical companies have a difficult time evaluating the effectiveness of drugs. Moreover, it is unlikely that any psychiatric disorder is entirely homogenous at a biological or neurochemical level.[26] In this context, pharmaceutical companies must either develop drugs that treat the disorders as they are described in the *DSM* or develop their own psychiatric taxonomies that lend themselves to cleaner targets. In the case of the latter, though, pharmaceutical companies are unlikely to secure FDA approval. As GlaxoSmithKline's chief executive Andrew Witty put it when explaining his company's decision not to pursue drug discovery related to depression, anxiety, and pain—a triumvirate of common experiences—"we believe the probability of success is relatively low, [and] we think the cost of attaining success is disproportionately high."[27] In recent years, many pharmaceutical applications to the FDA have only been to approve old drugs for new indications.[28]

THE DIFFICULTIES OF REVISING THE *DSM* FOR PURPOSES OF RESEARCH

All this raises the question: Why not come up with more scientifically useful diagnostic criteria? Perhaps the greatest limitation of the *DSM*, though, is that it even forestalls the development of alternatives. At this point, the hegemony of the *DSM* is not for lack of awareness of its limitations. Scientists are acutely aware of the weaknesses of the *DSM*, and they sometimes behave in ways that reveal the classifications they might prefer. The American Psychiatric Association is aware of these limitations, too. In the introduction to *A Research Agenda for DSM-V*, published by the APA, the authors acknowledged virtually all of these problems.[29] They expressed concern over researchers' "slavish" adherence to the *DSM* criteria, which "may have hindered research in the etiology of mental disorders," among other things.[30] They further acknowledged that viewing the *DSM*'s disorders as entities is "more likely to obscure than to elucidate research findings."[31] Yet despite these known limitations, the *DSM* fosters no real alternative. Scientists, too, are implicated in the process. Scientists devote little attention to the issue of taxonomies per se. They instead study specific disorders, building their reputations around limited parts of the *DSM*. Few scientists study disorders in a synthetic fashion and, from the standpoint of research funding, there is little incentive to do so. To be sure, the *DSM* is revised, at least periodically. Furthermore, the role of the scientific literature in these revisions has increased over time. Most agree that *DSM-5* is more "scientific" than *DSM-III*, in part because they think the right scientific experts were brought on board, as will be discussed later. Yet the evolution of the *DSM*, such as it is, did not arise from a process wherein the APA explored all the alternative taxonomies available to them and admitted only the best ones, regardless of what came before. Diagnostic criteria are almost never tested against one another. The criteria from the latest revision simply supersede those from the last.

This is not entirely a matter of apathy. There are difficult tradeoffs, especially once we consider all the different interests at stake. It is difficult to envision revisions that would facilitate better research without also diluting some of the other goals of the *DSM*. Specific criteria facilitate better research—from the perspective of science, *DSM-III* is vastly superior to *DSM-II*—but greater specificity also increases the number of people who do not fit neatly into a diagnostic category. This, in turn, increases the number of people who are relegated to the rarely studied NOS category. The same tradeoffs apply to the problem of comorbidity. Although there have been efforts to develop taxometric hierarchies, such that one primary disorder can supersede a secondary one, a comprehensive hierarchical system is almost impossible to operationalize given the large number of disorders the APA wishes to include in the *DSM*. Introducing a hierarchy would require relegating some disorders to a lesser status, and, at present, there is little scientific basis for doing so. Disorders are positively correlated. The presence of any disorder increases the likelihood of any other disorder, meaning there are few empirical guidelines for reducing the number of diagnoses in an unambiguous way.[32]

Revisions to the *DSM* are also difficult because virtually any change, no matter how small, is consequential. Indeed, even simple changes in *wording* can result in big changes in what the diagnostic criteria identify. Slade and Andres, for example, compared the diagnostic criteria for generalized anxiety disorder in *DSM-IV* and ICD-10.[33] On their face, the two taxometric systems resemble each other, and, in fact, they yield almost identical prevalence estimates in a general population. In both cases, for example, the prevalence of generalized anxiety disorder is around 3 percent, implying some consistency at the level of diagnostic criteria. Yet when employed simultaneously in the same population, the two systems identify very different people. Fewer than half of the cases diagnosed in one system are also diagnosed in the other. There is no obvious reason why the two criteria would identify different groups, although there are some seemingly slight differences between the two that, in effect, matter a great deal. The ICD criteria, for example, require autonomic arousal (e.g., palpitations, trembling), whereas the *DSM* criteria do not. In addition, the ICD criteria specify that a generalized anxiety disorder should not occur in the context of certain other disorders, including a panic disorder, phobic anxiety disorder, obsessive-compulsive disorder, or hypochondriacal disorder. Both criteria list worry as the primary symptom, although the *DSM* specifies that the worry must be "excessive." All these differences would seem to be superficial, especially in the context of a rare disorder for which few people would even seem to have the main symptoms, let alone the secondary ones. Yet the two systems still identify very different groups.

Evidence that the *DSM* distorts scientific research is clear, but for some critics the influence of the *DSM* is even more nefarious. Critics envision effects of the *DSM* at the level of entire cultures. They imagine the manual has created such a powerful and reified view of psychiatric disorders that, even if its criteria are occasionally resisted by scientists or ignored by clinicians or transmuted by patients, its underlying ideas are accepted with little resistance by the larger society. They suspect, for example, that the *DSM* creates categorical thinking regarding psychiatric disorders. In this way, it might encourage people to think about depression as an entity even if there is no scientific basis for doing so. By the same token, the *DSM* might encourage people to explain unusual behavior in terms of *sickness*, when, in absence of the *DSM*, they might think about deviance in more varied and ultimately more tolerant ways. These are big and provocative claims, of course, but they have some implications that can be explored empirically. The next chapter turns to evidence for large-scale cultural effects and looks at a critical facet of reification.

8

HOW CULTURES USE DIAGNOSES

At the broadest possible level entire cultures use psychiatric taxonomies. This chapter will discuss how the concepts described in the *DSM* become part of our everyday vocabulary and ordinary explanatory framework. At least in this respect, diagnoses are probably not benign. In everyday language, diagnoses are deployed, almost instinctively, in order to understand unusual behavior. "He's crazy" is an insult, to be sure, but it's also an explanation. It means his behavior is not just undesirable but sick. Diagnoses draw an equivalence between psychiatric disorders and medical disorders, insisting we regard both through a medical lens. By this logic, behaviors can be regarded as diseases that can and sometimes should be treated. A medical framework even taints how "normal" behaviors are interpreted, insofar as regarding something as "abnormal" implies knowing something about when it is not.

In using the term *culture*, I also have in mind the portability of ideas, especially how one particular culture, the culture of the United States, exports its ideas about mental illness. Although thinking about public beliefs—as I did in an earlier chapter—provides a window on culture, the beliefs of individuals are not the same as the orientations of a culture. Individuals hold a wide variety of beliefs, based on many different influences, but to think about a *culture* is to think about *shared* perspectives and assumptions, the foundational concepts that form the background around which individual beliefs are shaped.

How is it possible to study culture defined in this way? Moreover, how is it possible to study the influence of the *DSM* on culture? One method is to select from a culture's most significant written artifacts and look for changes in word or concept usage corresponding to changes in formal diagnostic nomenclature, as in the publication of a new version of the *DSM*. Tracing such changes reveals how, if at all, a culture appropriates a new concept.

With this in mind, I will present a quantitative analysis of word counts drawn from millions of digitized books published over a time span encompassing the publication and revision of the most significant editions of the *DSM*. The set of books is contained in the online collection of Google Books, referred to as the Google Books corpus.[1] The corpus is large and growing. The books contained therein were drawn from over forty libraries, including some of the largest libraries in the world. The corpus includes academic titles and more popular titles, meaning it covers both arcane science and bestselling fiction. The corpus also provides a sufficiently long timeframe to assess the influence of the *DSM*. It includes books published from 1600 to 2008 (although the consistency of the search tool is highest only through 2000). Although cultures have chewed over the concept of mental illness for centuries, the mid- to late twentieth century provides the critical years for evaluating the impact of the *DSM*.

In one sense, the Google Books corpus is a tool that takes the basic idea of content analysis to another level. The corpus—amounting to over five hundred billion words—cannot be read or comprehended in its entirety by any one person, but it can be searched and parsed electronically for words, phrases, and parts of speech that are emblematic of significant themes. Content analysis has long been used by social scientists to explore the meaning of language over multiple forms of expression. Google Books permits a version of content analysis that is both superficial and deep. Books reflect the choices of authors regarding what topics and concepts are significant. Books also reflect the decisions of authors regarding what words best express an idea. Patterns in word choice can be telling. The use of certain words rather than others can reveal progression in an underlying concept. Furthermore, the use of certain articles, such as *a* or *the*, can reveal the implied meaning of a term, especially how broad or specific the concept is. And trends in the frequency with which a certain word is used can reveal whether a concept is becoming more or less significant over time. In these ways, the application of Google Books to the study of the *DSM* is quite direct. Searching for relevant terms, such as "generalized anxiety disorder" (and allowing for differences in things like capitalization and plural versus singular forms), can yield important clues about how relevant a concept is as well as locate the point in time at which that concept emerged. If the *DSM* is culturally effective, we should see growth in the frequency with which a diagnosis is mentioned, corresponding approximately to when the term first appeared in the *DSM*. We should further see especially large changes corresponding with *DSM-III*, changes larger than those associated with earlier versions (or even later versions, in some cases). In the corpus search engine, the frequency of use is calculated by dividing the number of instances in which the word or phrase appears in that year by the total number of words appearing in books published that year. With the data normalized in this fashion, it is possible to evaluate trends accurately, even though the number of published books has increased over time and though the use of any single word relative to the total number of words in books will almost always be small, sometimes very small.

The Google Books corpus becomes an even more powerful tool when words and phrases are compared. Through comparisons it is possible, for instance, to see how quickly old diagnoses are retired or replaced by new ones. In a way, the twilight of a diagnosis—the amount of time it takes for a diagnosis to disappear fully from the lexicon—provides a test of the authority of the *DSM*. One fear surrounding the *DSM* pertains specifically to this issue. Critics assume a mismatch between culture and the manual: Culture evolves much more slowly than the pace at which the *DSM* is revised. Diagnoses can be eliminated from professional practice but still linger in the larger culture. And culture, then, has a memory for things the *DSM* might just as soon forget. The lag between a revision in the manual and a cultural change is, therefore, informative. Of further value is the ability to search for terms using Google Books within specific segments of the corpus. For instance, it is possible to search within fiction only, thereby excluding scientific manuscripts and zeroing in on the question of whether psychiatric jargon has become sufficiently salient to enter as themes in products of the imagination.

Although the Google Books corpus is an unprecedented tool, it is not without limitations. It allows users to detect patterns that they might not have been able to detect before, but books are only one facet of culture. And, at that, books are perhaps unusual. Books are written about topics that interest book writers and book readers, and "book people" might not reflect the larger culture in which they live. Furthermore, books themselves are not entirely representative of written language. A corpus of *books* is not the same thing as a corpus of e-mails, letters, tweets, or newspaper articles. Furthermore, *written* language—let alone *published* written language—is not the same thing as spoken language. We might assume that the written word and spoken word are closely related, but presumably the words written in published books are more disciplined in their production. In this chapter, I am attempting to uncover patterns in how people use psychiatric terms, but books provide only an imperfect window on everyday use among all people. Despite these limitations, though, the content analysis of books can be helpful in revealing the impact of the *DSM*.

THE *DSM* AND THE LEXICON OF DISORDERS

The first way to think about the influence of the *DSM* is simply to look at the number of times the manual itself is mentioned. Figure 8.1 presents several trends, the first for references to the "Diagnostic and Statistical Manual" (searched also using the acronym "DSM"). References to the *DSM* have increased over time, though not in perfect sync with the release of its editions. The first edition of the *DSM* was published in 1952 and the second in 1968, but neither edition seemed to attract much attention. The *DSM* was rarely mentioned from 1960 to the late 1970s, befitting its neglect among professionals, scientists, and certainly the general public. The strongest take-off point is in 1980, when *DSM-III* was published. And, indeed, references to the *DSM* grew exponentially thereafter, far exceeding any trend before it. Furthermore, the acceptance of the form of the *DSM*, as published in its third edition, hardly meant there was an eventual plateau in references

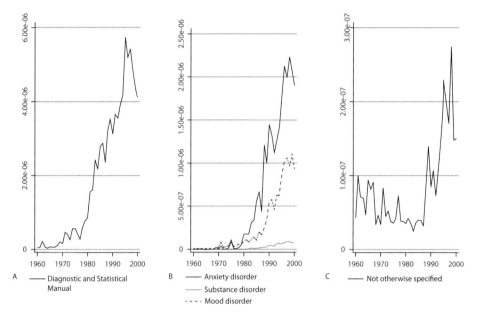

A — Diagnostic and Statistical Manual

B — Anxiety disorder
.... Substance disorder
- - - Mood disorder

C — Not otherwise specified

FIGURE 8.1 Google nGram frequency of basic DSM terms.

to the manual. Each subsequent edition appears to have produced still another spike.

References to the disorders contained within the *DSM* have increased as well. The second panel presents three disorders, all of which have increased in prominence over time. The disorders differ in their levels of appearance, to be sure, but references to each began to increase at approximately the same time, corresponding, again, to the publication of *DSM-III*. The fact that there were earlier editions of the *DSM* suggests that the promulgation of specific criteria—rather than the existence of any criteria at all—is the driving force behind this increase. Whatever else *DSM-II* achieved, it did not elevate the cultural significance of the disorders it contained. The third panel presents the same issue in a different way. The graph presents appearances of the phrase "not otherwise specified." As discussed earlier, this phrase is significant because it represents an important facet of *DSM-III*'s classification philosophy. Not only does the *DSM* name specific disorders through its criteria, but it also sets the terms for discussing disorders that fall outside those criteria. Specificity creates *disorders* but also creates *boundaries*. The phrase "not otherwise specified" was used at a relatively constant rate from 1950 until the early 1980s, but in the mid-1980s it began to increase sharply. It is difficult to attribute this to anything other than *DSM-III* and especially *III-R*, when the specific language of "not otherwise specified" was adopted. To be sure, the phrase could be applied to other topics—its use is not limited to psychiatry and applies also, for example, to a type of lymphoma—but since 1985 the most popular word preceding "not otherwise specified" has been "disorder," as in "mood disorder not otherwise specified," "eating disorder not otherwise specified," and "personality disorder not otherwise specified." As a spark for discussing psychiatric disorders, then, *DSM-III* is powerful and consolidating. It provides clarity and demands fidelity among users—and it appears to have received it.

These graphs also demonstrate the speed with which new disorders are adopted. The uptake of the *DSM*'s lexicon is, in fact, quick, suggesting a strong demand side. It suggests an audience hungry for the terms, rules, and concepts the *DSM* provides and, therefore, an audience desiring something *new*. But we should also think about the flipside of creation—how quickly disorders are *destroyed*. One crucial question for those who revise the *DSM* is not only what disorders to include or revise but also what disorders to retire or subsume. In this regard, the authors of the *DSM* envision a precise degree of influence: They assume the *DSM* will be used faithfully by professionals who will adapt when terms are no longer preferred. Yet at the level of culture, critics of the *DSM* do not assume as much: They fear growth by accretion. Once a diagnosis is created, it might be much harder to extinguish that disorder within a culture than it might be among professionals. The concept of "hysteria," for instance, is hardly used by professional psychiatrists, but it remains popular in at least some segments of the lay lexicon.

Figure 8.2 presents four panels. The first two show disorders that were revised sequentially over time. The first panel presents disorders related to sexual orientation.[2] In 1973, the American Psychiatric Association Board of Trustees passed a resolution to remove homosexuality per se as a disorder

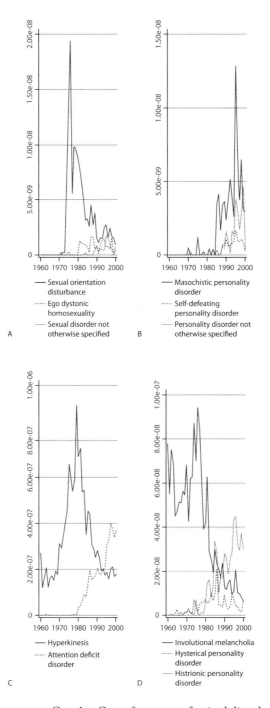

FIGURE 8.2 Google nGram frequency of retired disorders.

from *DSM-II* (which was initially published in 1968 but reprinted in 1974). They replaced it with something more conditional, a diagnostic category of "sexual orientation disturbance," defined as those whose sexual interests were directed toward people of the same sex *and* for whom this desire was a source of distress. That category was reclassified again in *DSM-III* as "ego-dystonic homosexuality," in reference to a mismatch between sexual desire and personal acceptance of that desire. Although the *DSM* was, in effect, moving toward an even more circumspect diagnosis surrounding homosexuality, the controversy regarding the diagnosis was growing. The revision used in *DSM-III* elicited considerable disagreement regarding the precise language the manual should adopt. It also occasioned more general controversy about why the APA was focusing on homosexuality at all. In *DSM-III-R* this revised category, too, was eliminated, replaced by a general category of "sexual disorder not otherwise specified," under which one example (among three) was "persistent and marked distress about one's sexual orientation."[3] Figure 8.2 shows the cultural consequences of this gradual refinement. Each successive term rapidly reached a peak in frequency, followed by nearly as rapid a decline, dating approximately to when the specific term was eliminated or revised. The most recent period is characterized by the slow growth of the "not otherwise specified" designation, but the frequency of that designation's use is still less than that of at least one earlier retired diagnosis. Overall, books are responsive to revisions in the *DSM*, albeit with a lag. Older disorders are difficult to discard altogether.

A not entirely dissimilar controversy surrounds masochistic personality disorder. This one disorder, in fact, involves two. Masochistic personality disorder and self-defeating personality disorder are largely regarded as synonyms, although masochistic personality has a longer history and more controversial connotations. Neither disorder appeared prior to *DSM-III-R*, although the terms were used regularly in psychoanalytic practice. Given this association with psychoanalysis, the authors of *DSM-III-R* approached the disorders with trepidation. In *DSM-III-R*, self-defeating personality appeared in an appendix of disorders that were thought to be in need of further study.[4] In that context, the manual noted the history of the disorder and its connotations. It noted that the disorder had been called masochistic personality disorder in earlier editions but that "the name of the category has been changed to avoid the historic association of the term masochistic with older psychoanalytic views of female sexuality." The disorder was not included in *DSM-IV*, although those who use the *DSM* could still consider it a "personality disorder not otherwise specified." In the context of personality disorders, the "not otherwise specified" designation refers to features of the personality that cause clinically significant distress or impairment, and one could easily envision a variety of "self-defeating" habits that do exactly that. In these ways the *DSM* sought to set the precise terms of the debate, but it is difficult to eliminate disorders that clinicians still find useful or disorders for which the political forces aligning against them are not as strong as they were against the inclusion of homosexuality. Panel B shows some dynamics in the favored term, especially the preference for "self-defeating" over "masochistic," but neither disorder has disappeared altogether.

The remaining panels show disorders that are less controversial. The third panel shows the replacement of "hyperkinesis" and "hyperkinetic" with "attention deficit/hyperactivity disorder." In this case, the older terms were simply replaced when moving from *DSM-II* to *DSM-III*. The third panel shows a sharp drop in the use of the former and an increase in the use of the latter. A similar process is apparent for two disorders that were not renamed but discarded. Hysterical personality disorder was included in *DSM-II*, as was histrionic personality disorder. In *DSM-III*, the category of histrionic personality disorder was retained, but hysterical personality disorder was not. *DSM-III* states, however, that "in other classifications this category is termed Hysterical Personality."[5] The move away from "hysterical" was attributable to the connotations of the term, if not from a widespread appreciation that the form of anxiety it represented did not exist.[6] The category of "involutional melancholia"—a type of mood disorder that includes features of paranoia—was included in *DSM-II*. It was removed from *DSM-III*, although the manual's index still includes an entry for the term, referring readers to major depression as an alternative. The panel shows the slow descent of "involutional melancholia," starting long before the publication of *DSM-III*. These panels show that, when presented with an alternative, authors tend to assume the new language and discard the old. But when older disorders do not align perfectly with revised disorders, the descent of older disorders tends to be slow, perhaps reflecting how those disorders, such as involutional melancholia, are still regarded as distinct by some parties even if they are not formally recognized as such. The same is true of hysterical personality, wherein the retirement of the previous disorder had been slowed by the value some professionals still see in it, despite its connotations. All this raises more questions: Exactly how far does the *DSM*'s authority stretch? And in what directions? Furthermore, how much has the *DSM* exceeded the bounds of the authors' original intent?

DIAGNOSING VERSUS TREATING DISORDERS

The *DSM* is a powerful tool for creating disorders and, under some circumstances, for destroying them. But the *DSM* is fundamentally a tool for *diagnosis*. And, in this regard, the intentions of the *DSM*'s authors are narrow. The *DSM* is intended to provide guidance for diagnosis, not treatment. The *DSM* provides some information on course and associated characteristics, befitting its "statistical" name, and, furthermore, the existence of a disorder perhaps implies the disorder is worthy of treatment. Yet the *DSM* does not, in fact, dictate anything regarding the correct way to treat a case. It is unclear, though, whether the *DSM* has been received by its audience in such a neutral and descriptive way. A cultural analysis is revealing not only for showing how the *DSM* creates the lexicon of disorders but also for showing how disorders are discussed and, in effect, what purpose the newly created nouns serve as aspects of language. One question to ask in this regard is whether most of the discussion surrounding psychiatric disorders pertains to diagnosis or treatment.

Figure 8.3 shows trends for different verbs preceding specific psychiatric terms, including "treat" and "diagnose" (and, to represent present participles and gerunds, "treating" and "diagnosing"). Two things emerge from these figures. First, mentions of both treatment and diagnosis increased rapidly

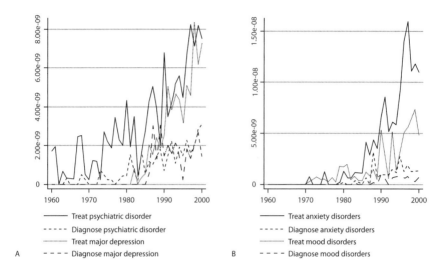

FIGURE 8.3 Google nGram frequency of treating versus diagnosing disorders.

around 1980, coinciding with the publication of *DSM-III*. Prior to 1980 clinicians were certainly interested in treating psychiatric disorders and had tools available for doing so. In fact, there were many references to treating psychiatric disorders prior to 1980. Yet robust discussions of treatment appear to have emerged only in tandem with a more cohesive discussion of specific diagnoses. As antecedents to specific disorders, references to "diagnose" and "treat" increased sharply around 1980 and continued to accelerate thereafter. As with the other trends documented thus far, it is difficult to attribute these increases to anything other than *DSM-III*. The timing is not consistent with major treatment innovations, for example. In the case of major depression, many of the most important innovations—or at least the development of most popular pharmaceuticals—happened well after 1980. Prozac, for instance, was approved in 1987. There was an increase in references to "treatment" around that time, to be sure, but so too was there a sharp increase in 1981. The second panel shows the same analysis for the two most prevalent categories of disorder in *DSM-III*: anxiety disorders and mood disorders (based on a refinement of the *DSM-II* category of "neuroses"). Both trends suggest a rapid evolution. The expansion of the lexicon of disorders created by *DSM-III* started in the theme of diagnosis but quickly moved to treatment (even though the scientific literature regarding the question of validity remained unsettled, as will be discussed shortly).

THE *DSM* CREATES NEW ENTITIES AND NOT JUST NEW SYMPTOMS

Thus far the findings suggest that the cultural effects of the *DSM* stretch beyond the intentions of its authors. There is other evidence that the significance of the *DSM* has spilled its bounds. Recall a theme discussed earlier. The *DSM* is primarily a classification system applied to lists of diverse symptoms. In this sense, the *DSM* creates—or at least solidifies—the idea of symptoms as signs. According to the *DSM-III*'s structure, symptoms have little relevance on their own and must be interpreted as part of a set— they are clues about the underlying problem, but because they represent only partial traces, they should be interpreted in light of other signs. One lingering fear, though, is that *DSM-III* achieves the framework of symptoms-as-signs only by a sleight of hand: that it creates *entities*—or at least the appearance of entities—only from a mix of *attributes*. By cataloging the symptoms of a major depressive episode, for example, the *DSM* creates a new *thing* that is different from the sum of its parts, and, over time, that thing might become reified as a bona fide medical entity.

How can we discern reification at the level of culture, which is where, in the end, critics think it resides and exerts its most significance? To the extent that the *DSM* creates entities from symptoms, the verbs that precede the names for disorders and symptoms should change. When a mental illness is seen as an entity, individuals will declare, for example, "I *have* depression," not just "I *am* depressed." In the case of *having* a disorder, the disorder is an object separable from the individual and, therefore, appropriate for use following a possessive. To say "I *am* depressed" is to make a different statement: "I am depressed" is merely a statement about experiencing an emotion, one that was, of course, named long before *DSM-III* came along. Depression presents an especially useful example. In the case of depression, claiming that one has a symptom—feeling depressed—which could be interpreted as a sign of a disorder, is far removed from claiming that one has the disorder itself. The statement "I am depressed" can plainly be made without referring to a psychiatric disorder. From a lexical perspective, not all disorders allow for this. Schizophrenia, for example, is a disorder, but "schizophrenia" or "schizophrenic" has no alternative meaning that might turn up in ordinary conversation apart from a disorder. To be sure, one can say someone or something is "schizophrenic," but this term is usually used incorrectly in the sense that it refers to a split personality and not to the symptoms of schizophrenia as a disorder, and, in any case, this usage still stems from the term's clinical meaning. The *DSM* provides many instances, though, of disorders that have more precise corollaries in popular speech, allowing us to discern more accurately whether disorders are increasingly seen as entities rather than as descriptions of symptoms.

Figure 8.4 presents several tests of this idea. The first explores "have depression" versus "am depressed." There are other verbs that could be used to test the idea of reification, but I focus on these words because they are the ones most likely to be used in reference to people rather than things. Markets, for instance, can be depressed. The phrases are also revealing in and of themselves. The phrase "have depression" has no meaning unless depression is regarded as a proper object. The phrase "am depressed" can simply refer to a mood. Saying "I have depression" has different connotations than "I am depressed." Although both phrases have become more popular over time, "have depression" increased markedly after 1980. The two phrases were used with near-equal frequency by 2000, although prior to that "am depressed" exceeded "have depression."

A different way to explore the same idea is to look at compound phrases. The term "anxiety disorders" represents a class of disorders created by the *DSM*, but "anxiety symptoms" are merely the elements of those disorders, of

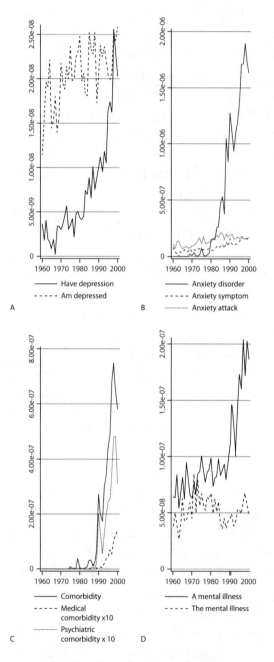

FIGURE 8.4 Google nGram frequency of psychiatric entities.

which an "anxiety attack" is perhaps the most well known. The second panel presents a graph of all three phrases. Both "anxiety attacks" and "anxiety symptoms" were used with approximately the same frequency for half a century, increasing only a small amount. With the publication of *DSM-III*, however, their use was suddenly dwarfed by that of "anxiety disorders." Furthermore, the use of "anxiety attacks"—although plainly derived from a psychiatric concept—declined somewhat in the mid-1980s, suggesting that the symptoms of anxiety, even the most prominent and well-known one, were being slowly subsumed by the category.

If the *DSM* is truly creating entities, there should be a parallel increase in the frequency with which books mention *multiple* disorders. That is, there should be an increase in references to "comorbidity" as a particular way to characterize the presence of many symptoms. This possibility must be weighed, though, against the broader definition of the term. The definition of "comorbidity" is very general. It refers only to the presence of one or more additional *diseases*, not necessarily one or more additional psychiatric disorders. Hypertension can be comorbid with diabetes, for example, just as major depression can be comorbid with generalized anxiety. Indeed, in hospital settings, comorbidity among medical conditions is quite common, and the expected prevalence of medical comorbidity should increase as the population gets older and lives longer. In the end, comorbidity is a simple concept. Appreciating its presence only requires acknowledging at least two distinct diseases. And long before *DSM-III* there was evidence that psychiatric disorders presented in groups. Yet prior to *DSM-III* this was only an impression. Psychiatric comorbidity per se was difficult to evaluate because the diagnostic criteria contained in the *DSM* did provide the right resolution. It did not create sharp boundaries. A primary disorder—one encompassing all others—was easier to envision and render as a diagnosis. One potential consequence of *DSM-III*, then, was to increase the prominence of psychiatric comorbidity as a concept. Panel C presents a graph of three terms: "comorbidity," "psychiatric comorbidity," and "medical comorbidity." It shows the rapid growth in references to comorbidity, propelled, in particular, by the concept of psychiatric comorbidity. References to comorbidity grew enormously in the mid-1980s. Moreover, prior to this, the phrase "psychiatric comorbidity" was essentially unknown, even though many sorts of disorders did, in fact, exist in *DSM-I* and *II*. Although they are not presented in the graph, some additional terms point to the centrality of psychiatric comorbidity to the issue of comorbidity generally. For instance, a wildcard search of the most frequently used words preceding "comorbidity" revealed that in the last year of the series it was "psychiatric" comorbidity by a wide margin. By the same token, the most frequently used words following "comorbid" were "anxiety," "depression," and "substance." Although general medical comorbidity is not unusual in treatment settings, none of the most commonly comorbid medical disorders—hypertension and diabetes, for example—exceeds the frequency of mentions of comorbid psychiatric disorders.

A more general test of the idea that the *DSM* creates entities is possible if we consider articles. As a part of speech, articles are very important. Articles, for example "the" and "an," are among the most frequently used words used in everyday conversation. They are part of the "glue" that holds a sentence together.[7] But their significance stretches far beyond sturdy grammar and coherent thought. Psychologists have studied the connection between personality and the words people use and have shown that articles are very important in revealing who people are.[8] In addition, articles have important implications regarding the meaning and interpretation of a noun, especially whether that noun is understood in the same way by both writer and reader (or speaker and listener). In this vein, "the" is a definite article, in reference to a noun that both the reader and writer have a shared understanding of. By contrast, "a" is an indefinite article, in reference to a noun that has yet to be specified. The difference between definite and indefinite articles is relevant to understanding changing conceptions of mental illness. Mental illness can be described in a variety of ways. Among the three terms regularly used to describe the concept, "mental illness," "psychiatric disorder," and "mental disorder," "mental illness" is the most common. Yet the use of the term took a sharp dive in frequency beginning sometime shortly after 1980, before making a recovery in the early 1990s. One explanation for this pattern is the changing way authors were writing about the topic. With the publication of *DSM-III* there was suddenly much greater emphasis on *specific* mental disorders rather than the more general category of being mentally *unhealthy, ill,* or *disordered.* To describe something specifically is also to insist that it not be described generally. Whatever else the *DSM* does, it provides a complete lexicon for describing all mental disorders and, in return, demands appropriate specificity among parties discussing them.

The fourth panel puts these ideas together. It presents trends for two phrases: "*a* mental illness" and "*the* mental illness." To interpret the significance of these trends, it is useful to imagine two cultures and how those cultures would talk about mental illness. In a culture where the idea of mental illness is regarded generically, as simply a term for describing behavior that is not healthy, references to "the" mental illness should prevail. In that culture, a shared understanding of mental illness—no matter how broad—is implied, and, even if specific disorders are recognized, the referent behind mental illness is sufficiently obvious to require no other article. But in a culture where there are many mental illnesses, each with its own specific features, and where there is great respect for such distinctions, references to "the" mental illness lose relevance. A reference to "the" mental illness requires a shared understanding of exactly what disorder is being discussed, but, absent some context, no shared understanding is to be had, as there are a variety of mental illnesses available for use. References to "a" mental illness, by contrast, should be more harmonious with a culture that appreciates psychiatric disorders as specific, unique, and distinguishable. References to "a" mental illness leave the specific disorder unspecified, referring only to the possible presence of an illness, but, in being indefinite, references of this sort respect specificity. The graph shows that the frequency of these two phrases has indeed shifted. Both phrases were used with growing frequency from 1930 until about 1975, suggesting a growing awareness of mental illness as a concept. After the publication of *DSM-III,* though, the use of "the mental illness" declined, and the use of "a mental illness" increased. Indeed, the increase in "a mental illness" from 1980 to 2000 far exceeds the entire increase prior to that period.

PSYCHIATRIC DISORDERS HAVE STRONG
SEMANTIC GRAVITY

The foregoing suggests that at the level of culture *DSM-III* succeeded in creating disorders from symptoms. Relative to symptoms, the disorders themselves are discussed with growing frequency, slowly eclipsing the discussion of symptoms. These effects are important, but the *DSM* is more than a catalogue of *nouns*. In addition to diagnostic terms, the *DSM* provides a rich compendium of verbs and adjectives, which have meaning both in conventional English usage and in psychiatric nomenclature. In the context of discussing the cultural impact of the *DSM*, it is useful to explore how these words, too, are shifting in meaning because of the semantic gravity of the *DSM*. We might not assume the influence of the *DSM* is so strong as to infiltrate how we talk about action generally, but the idea of reification suggests a certain amount of appropriation and overshadowing, that is, that the concepts in the *DSM* can eventually dominate other connotations.

Figure 8.5 illustrates this idea. It does so using popular terms and expressions, beginning with some nouns. The first two panels present ratios of the use of a psychiatric phrase, one that has a specific designation within the *DSM*, relative to the use of an element of that phrase that could be used in reference to many other ideas. "Depression," for example, can be discussed on its own, but "major depression" connotes a specific psychiatric diagnosis. The panel presents other examples of similar whole-to-part pairings, in these cases pairings that would be expected to be used frequently: "major depression" relative to "depression," "anxiety disorder" relative to "anxiety," "panic attack" relative to "panic," and "compulsive disorder" relative to "compulsive." The root words vary in the specificity of their meaning, and so the ratios will vary in their levels. "Depression," for example, is not restricted to a psychological state. As a noun, it can denote everything from economic slumps (e.g., the Great Depression) to meteorological formations (e.g., tropical depression). "Compulsive" is multifaceted as well, albeit in a different way, denoting irresistible behavior stemming from unwanted urges and, thus, conveying behavior that might be unhealthy. The term also,

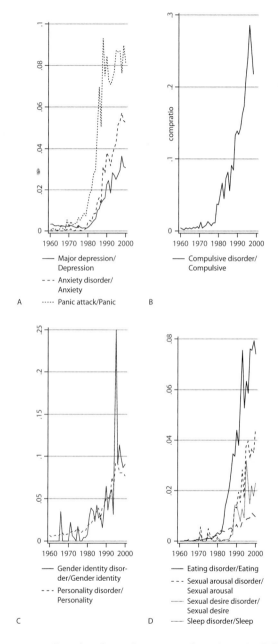

FIGURE 8.5 Google nGram frequencies describing the DSM's semantic gravity.

however, has a more prosaic meaning, describing something that is captivating, as in "compulsive" viewing of a television program.

Despite the potentially broad meaning of these terms, each is increasingly tied to its connotations with respect to a psychiatric disorder. The ratios of the phrase to the part have grown. This is especially the case for "compulsive," for which more than 20 percent of the usage of the term occurs when paired with "disorder." This is less the case with the other terms, although these terms, too, are frequently paired with a disorder. As many as one out of every twenty references to anxiety, for example, is in reference to an anxiety disorder, and around 3 percent of references to depression are to major depression.

It is one thing to show that the *DSM* increasingly overshadows the meaning of concepts such as compulsion and depression, which have some natural overlap with symptoms, but the *DSM*'s influence is so pervasive that it also overshadows even more neutral terms. Both "gender identity" and "personality," for example, are seemingly unaligned terms. To be sure, gender identity can be controversial when, for example, there is debate over extending legal protections to transgender people. Gender identity is also the subject of a critical branch of social science. But academic debates of this sort can plainly be separated from what we regard as *illness*. We can and should be able to discuss gender identity without invoking the possibility of a medical problem. Personality, too, is merely a descriptive term. It refers to characteristic patterns in behavior and thought, and the term can be used in an entirely positive fashion. Personality is often, for example, one element of a dating profile, used as an opportunity to showcase desirable characteristics. But panel C shows how both "personality" and "gender identity" are increasingly paired with the term "disorder." To think about personality is increasingly to consider a personality disorder. Similarly, gender identity is increasingly tied to how the term is used in the *DSM*: "gender identity" is paired with "gender identity disorder" in as many as 25 percent of instances.

Perhaps the strongest case for the semantic gravity of the *DSM* can be made by pitting psychiatric terms against their most elemental behavioral counterparts. Some aspects of the *DSM* are, as this book has emphasized, the stuff of life. There is no question that sleep, sex, and food are necessary to the perpetuation of humanity. To be sure, they are also related to psychiatric disorders, but in a specific and seemingly limited way (certainly the authors of the *DSM* would hope as much). The *DSM*, for example, contains a category of eating disorders, including, therein, the well-known disorders of anorexia and bulimia. But *eating* itself is an ordinary behavior. Similarly, sexual desire and sexual arousal are familiar human experiences. They both characterize a category of disorder as well, but on their own these experiences need not imply *illness*. People talked about sex and sexual desire well before the *DSM* came along. The same applies to *sleep*. The *DSM* contains a category of disorders related to dysfunctions in sleep, but sleep itself is not a problem. In fact, sleep is the desideratum and is almost always a daily activity. The fourth panel presents the ratio of these terms expressed as disorders relative to their root terms: "eating disorder" (including its plural form) relative to "eating," "sleep disorder" relative to "sleep," "sexual arousal disorder" relative to "sexual arousal," and "sexual desire disorder" relative to "sexual desire." If the publication of *DSM-III* simply happened to coincide with a greater interest in sleep, sex, and eating, these ratios would not change much over time, as both the numerator and the denominator would increase apace. For example, something of this sort could happen in the wake of a sexual revolution, providing grist for a variety of authors, adopting a variety of standpoints, as well as a greater demand for books about sex among readers. Similarly, if a culture is simply increasingly open to talking about sexuality, and this, too, happened to coincide with a revision of the *DSM*, the ratio need not change. The fourth panel, however, suggests that each term is increasingly appended to a disorder. Remarkably, eating disorders show the strongest such pairing, with over 7 percent of references to "eating" involving eating disorders of some kind.

Another explanation for these patterns is simply the growth in psychiatry as a discipline. Earlier I argued that *DSM-III* transformed how psychiatry conducted research, allowing scientists to publish more (and perhaps better) research. It is possible, then, that these graphs say less about the impact of the *DSM* on *culture* than they do about the impact of the *DSM* on (book-publishing) *science*. To be sure, this would not be an inconsequential effect of the *DSM*, but it would be a different kind of effect. One way to explore this distinction is to think about the scientific literature in particular. Figure 8.6 shows a graph for references to the top four psychiatry journals: the *Archives*

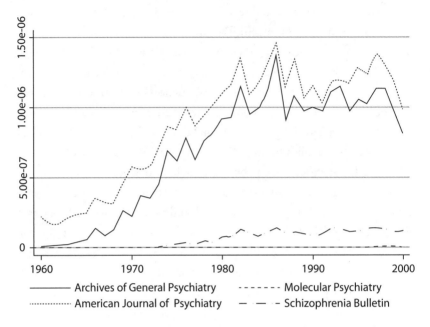

FIGURE 8.6 Google nGram of the growth of psychiatric research.

of General Psychiatry, *Molecular Psychiatry* (which only began publishing in 1997), the *American Journal of Psychiatry*, and *Schizophrenia Bulletin*. The shape of this curve is very different from those presented thus far. Whereas references to specific psychiatric disorders accelerated after 1980 and continued to grow through 2000, references to the most prominent psychiatry journals hit a plateau after 1980. Because of *DSM-III*, psychiatric research may have become more consolidated, respected, and well funded, but the growth of psychiatric research does not explain the cultural trends documented thus far.

THE USE OF PSYCHIATRIC TERMS IN FICTION

It is possible, however, to provide an even stronger test of cultural effects. So far all the trends I have discussed pertain to the entire English-language corpus of Google Books. But what happens when we focus on *fiction*? Fiction, of course, appropriates concepts from the larger culture. And fiction has long dealt with suffering, yearning, and anxiety, which are some of the basic elements of mental illness. But fiction is certainly not beholden to formal psychiatric nomenclature. It can consider suffering, for example, without also discussing a major depressive episode. Hamlet is a particularly famous representation of what we might now regard as someone suffering from a major depressive episode, but Shakespeare, of course, did not use modern clinical nomenclature, nor would he have likely felt compelled to use it if it were available at the time. Scientists are perhaps bound to a taxometric framework; artists certainly are not.

The use of psychiatric terms in fiction, therefore, represents an especially strong test of the suffusion of psychiatric concepts through the general culture. Figure 8.7 presents three illustrations of the impact of the *DSM*. Once again, the timing of the trends is particularly important, in this case because the base rate of references to explicit psychiatric terms still remains low. As before, the publication of *DSM-III* in 1980 is assumed to be a watershed moment, and, indeed, it appears to have been. The first panel begins with terms that might appear in fiction to describe any number of things but also happen to describe psychiatric disorders. The list includes, among other things, "depression" and "anxiety." In general, the use of these terms has been fairly consistent over a fifty-year period, albeit with some decrease in the word "anxiety" and some increase in the word "distracted" and "trauma." The use of the far more general word "mood" has changed very little.

The second panel shifts to words and phrases with more definite roots in psychiatric nomenclature. The words parallel those presented in the first panel in the sense that they add modifiers or the word "disorder" to the root. Yet the second panel presents very different trends from the first. The overall frequency of these phrases is less than the frequency of the root term, but all of the phrases increased sometime after 1980. The compound "attention deficit," for example, essentially never appeared in fiction until after 1980, after which it increased steadily. The most frequently used phrase in the set is "post-traumatic," which was used very infrequently until 1980, after which it grew sharply. References to "major depression" also increased around the

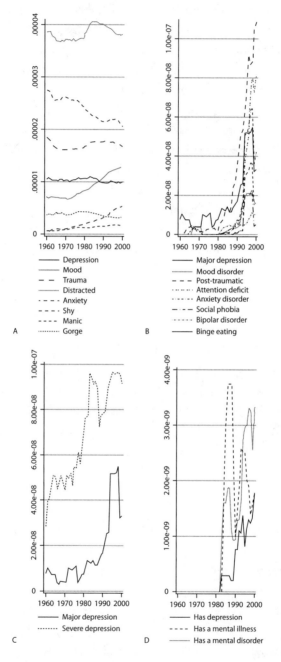

FIGURE 8.7 Google nGram frequency of psychiatric terms.

same time. The addition of "major" is not trivial, of course. In *DSM-III* "major" is used to indicate the severity of something that, in every language, exists on a spectrum. It is also used to distinguish the disorder from symptoms that are common and, therefore, could easily be regarded as "minor." "Major," then, is a crucial element of formal clinical parlance, and, for this reason, the choice of the word presents an interesting decision in the context of fiction. There are other ways an author could choose to modify "depression." An author could choose to describe a character's depression as "severe," which is, in fact, a popular choice. One way to think about the *DSM*'s influence would be to see the manual as promoting a greater appreciation of how significant depression can be. In this case, an author might be compelled to describe depression as "severe," perhaps so the character's misery is not dismissed by a reader, but not so compelled as to describe the depression strictly as "major." In fact, though, the frequency of both formulations has gone up over time, with references to "major depression" increasing quickly sometime in the mid-1980s.

The fourth panel turns to the verbs used in conjunction with mental illness. None of the nouns explored in this panel is entirely unfamiliar to English fiction. "Depression," "mental illness," and "mental disorder" have been used somewhat frequently since 1950. In fact, there are references to "mental disorder" as far back as the late eighteenth century (although they are not presented in the figure). Yet the verbs preceding these terms have changed. The fourth panel presents the frequency of three phrases: "has depression," "has a mental disorder," and "has a mental illness." There are virtually no references to these phrases from 1960 to 1980. In 1983, though, their use jumped, and this, too, likely represents how *DSM-III* has created a particular type of entity. Characters in fiction, just like people in general, are more likely to "have" mental disorders and to be described according to the more precise terms set by the *DSM*.

* * *

All this indicates that the *DSM* is influential and, if one chooses to interpret it in a certain way, perhaps a bit nefarious. But is the *DSM correct*? The foregoing has been about how the *DSM* is used. I have discussed the *DSM*'s power, its consequences, its values, and its limits. And I have discussed these things from the standpoint of different actors. This type of discussion prevents any simple answer to the question of the *DSM*'s usefulness. The value of the *DSM* to scientists, for example, is not the same as its value to clinicians. And clinicians, in turn, think about the *DSM* in a different way from patients. This suggests some built-in incompatibility among perspectives. It is difficult to imagine a revision of the *DSM* that would satisfy all the relevant interests, especially one that would not also induce at least some of the unintended consequences I have highlighted, especially in this chapter. It is possible, though, that science could eventually absolve psychiatry of the difficult task of finding an adequate compromise. If a single premise shared by all parties is that psychiatric disorders are *real* and that validity is important, it is possible that science, more so than any other sector, is in the best position to serve as the ultimate authority. The demands placed on a concept such as mental illness—not to mention its ability to absorb all sorts of external influences and its susceptibility to being stretched to serve other goals—might be greatly reduced if all parties could eventually concede that major depression, for instance, results from a predictable combination of stress and risky genes, or that generalized anxiety disorder resides in a dysfunctional amygdala, or that schizophrenia represents the accumulation of a set of specific genetic polymorphisms. The next chapter turns to this possibility.

9

THE CONTEMPORARY SCIENCE OF PSYCHIATRIC NOSOLOGY

Although the *DSM* succeeded in creating reliable diagnoses, it may have done so only by sacrificing any real discussion of validity. But what does the science of psychiatric disorders actually reveal? Increasingly there is evidence confirming at least some of the assumptions of the *DSM*. There is evidence, for example, regarding whether psychiatric disorders are categorical. In addition, there is evidence regarding how porous the boundaries are between different disorders. The *DSM* is presumed to "carve nature at its joints"—and it certainly carves—but has it done so precisely?

In this chapter, I will focus on the science of psychiatric nosology. I will focus on contemporary research, much of which was not possible when *DSM-III* was set in motion more than thirty years ago. It is important to keep in mind, however, that science has long played a role in the writing of the *DSM*. Even before the publication of *DSM-III* there were efforts to create a more scientifically defensible taxonomy using empirical methods.[1] This was especially the case, though, with *DSM-III*. Its authors used science when it was informative. The problem was the limited reach of the science available to them. At the time, scientific research did not speak directly to the issues that most concerned the task force. The contemporary science of psychiatric disorders, by contrast, is more directly relevant. And for this reason it has fueled a great deal of enthusiasm among those interested in creating more accurate criteria.

Yet contemporary science has also revealed a paradox. Even as science has provided clues about the nature of psychiatric disorders, it has also revealed that most disorders are probably not waiting to be uncovered by the right set of tools. Even as science has plumbed the depths of genes and neuroscience, it has not obviated the importance of clinical insight or experience. Nor has it unequivocally declared one particular set of scientific tools the winner. It has not diminished the importance of simply observing symptoms, for example, in favor of, say, testing for genes. To be sure, the contemporary science of psychiatric disorders has uncovered a great deal, but it has also laid bare the centrality of *judgment*, whose relevance goes deeper than expected. The more insights science provides, the more decision points it creates. It has discovered, for example, that psychiatric disorders are, indeed, genetic. Yet the degree of genetic influence must always be evaluated, as the genes behind psychiatric disorders are never strictly Mendelian. Science has also revealed that many psychiatric disorders overlap at a biological level. Yet the amount of overlap psychiatrists are willing to tolerate is a matter of choice. There are no external standards that permit a single answer to questions of degree or amount. The emergence of new forms of measurement—the measurement of brain activity, for example, as it relates to psychiatric symptoms—perhaps lends credibility to the pursuit of more "natural" classifications, but that credibility is based on a decision regarding what sort of evidence to admit as influential rather than on one kind of evidence obviously dominating another. In the end, the acceptance of new taxometric frameworks is not based on evaluating how well those frameworks correspond to the world—to what psychiatric disorders are in nature—but rather on valuing what aspects of validity those frameworks most represent.

ARE THERE GENES FOR MENTAL ILLNESS?

For many clinicians, the brightest star in the scientific sky is genetic research. Genetic research is promising for many people and for many reasons, but it is perhaps especially promising for those who want a cleaner nosology. In disease classification, the usual gold standard is etiological or pathophysiological information. A certain infectious agent, for example, gives rise to a certain infectious disease and, so, can lead to perfect identification. Although that disease might vary in its symptomatic presentation, it nonetheless reflects the same underlying pathology and can be identified accurately when antibodies for the pathogen or the pathogen itself have been identified. The basic idea of diagnosis through pathology informed the construction of the *DSM*, even if the underlying pathology of psychiatric disorders was not well established. Indeed, the idea was informative long before science understood much at all about psychiatric pathology. Almost a century before the development of *DSM-III*, Emil Kraepelin established the basic premise. He held that psychiatric disorders originating with the same pathology should present with approximately the same symptoms, and the authors of *DSM-III* used this idea as their guide.[2] For them, the idea was also aspirational in the sense that they not only thought the pathology existed; they also assumed it could be eventually identified, even if it was not obvious at the time. *DSM-III* was to be regarded as the interim authority— a placeholder for what psychiatric disorders should look like—but only until better pathological information was discovered.

The overlap between Kraepelin's idea and modern genetic research is obvious. If scientists could discover a gene (or genes) for, say, major depression, they would be able to define the disorder more crisply. The identification of a gene for depression would even aid those interested only in finding the correct symptoms. After identifying people who were positive for the genetic risk for depression, researchers could provide a more accurate and complete list of the true symptoms of the disorder.

Research has unequivocally shown that genes are important for psychiatric disorders, but this has not produced much insight relevant to diagnosis per se. One basic indicator of the role of genes in a phenotype is heritability. Heritability is the amount of variation in a phenotype that can be explained by genetic variation in a population. Heritability is usually estimated in samples of twins. Although heritability can also be calculated in samples consisting of other relatives having varying degrees of genetic similarity, including, for example, siblings and cousins, twins are especially useful because they have the right mix of influences. Identical twins share 100 percent of their genes at conception, whereas nonidentical (or fraternal twins) share 50 percent. Twins are also born at the same time, so we can assume they share similar experiences (though this also makes heritability calculations specific to a particular environment, and, as discussed shortly, heritability can change according to prevailing environmental conditions). Heritability is estimated based on these facts, along with information on differences between how similar identical and fraternal twins are. Consider, for purposes of illustration, the case of major depression. If both twins in a pair of identical twins are more likely to have major depression than twins in a pair of fraternal twins, this provides evidence that major depression is at least partly heritable. The greater similarity (or "concordance") among identical twins is presumed to derive from their greater genetic similarity, as little else would seem to explain it. Estimating in this way, heritability is a matter of degrees. For strongly heritable conditions, there will be almost perfect consistency among identical twins but considerably less among fraternal twins. For conditions that are not heritable, identical and fraternal twins should have the same level of similarity, whether high or low, because genes are irrelevant and other influences prevail. Studies based on this method reveal that the heritability of most psychiatric disorders is moderate to high. The heritability of psychiatric disorders ranges from around 35 percent for a major depressive disorder to around 75 to 80 percent for schizophrenia.[3]

Yet these studies also provide, at best, ambiguous information for crafting better criteria. There is no conventional psychiatric disorder for which identical twins are 100 percent concordant, as we would expect for a perfectly genetic disorder.[4] For example, among identical twin pairs where one sibling has schizophrenia—which is among the most heritable disorders—the lifetime risk for the other twin developing schizophrenia is only about 48 percent.[5] In other words, knowing that one sibling has a psychiatric disorder is informative, but it is not determinative of a disorder in the other.

INTERPRETING GENETIC INFLUENCES

Before we further discuss the implications of this research for psychiatric taxonomies, it is important to be clear about what we mean when we say there is "a gene for" a disorder. The optimism surrounding genetic research is often cast in such terms. What if we find the gene for schizophrenia? Or the gene for anxiety? When applied to psychiatric disorders, language of this sort implicitly aligns psychiatry with other areas of research where scientists have, in fact, discovered very strong genetic connections. There are, for example, genes for breast cancer. There are also genes for cystic fibrosis. And there are a number of conditions, such as sickle-cell anemia, for which the condition stems from a *single* mutated gene. In these cases, patients can be tested for the gene (or genes) and make informed decisions regarding prevention or treatment. Furthermore, testing can be done very early, even, in some cases, during gestation. In the case of sickle-cell anemia, for instance, testing can be done as early as eight to ten weeks into a pregnancy. Even short of accurate and early testing, genetic conditions lend themselves to a broader approach to prevention. The presence of a genetic condition in one family member alerts other family members that they, too, might be at risk.

Genetic research is not only compelling to clinicians or the families of those affected. The public, too, responds to research demonstrating genetic influences, interpreting such research to mean that a disease is real, that a diagnosis is uncomplicated, and that a cure is iminent.[6] And, in many cases, this optimism is warranted. Phenylketonuria is a genetic condition that prevents the body from converting one amino acid into another. The condition produces excess phenylalanine in the body, which poisons the brain and can eventually produce intellectual disability. Although the condition cannot be cured, it can be managed effectively by restricting dietary protein. In this case, then, the identification of a gene for the disease has, in fact, led to an effective treatment. Demonstrating genetic influences over psychiatric disorders could reverberate through all aspects of the diagnostic system described in this book.

But psychiatric disorders represent more complex phenotypes. Kenneth Kendler outlines the criteria necessary for claiming there is "a gene for" something and applies his framework to the case of psychiatric disorders.[7] First, he argues that the association between a gene and an outcome should be strong and substantial. If the gene increases your risk for major depression, it should increase your risk a great deal, not simply move a person somewhat closer to developing depression in a probabilistic sense. The benchmark for statements of this sort is a Mendelian relationship, which is purely deterministic: The presence of a certain gene always produces, for example, a purple flower. Few common illnesses have this character, but the idea is implied when we say there is "a gene for" something. Second, the gene should have a specific association. If there is a gene for major depression, for example, it should affect major depression and little else besides. Otherwise the gene might be "for" something else, either in addition to depression or anterior to depression. Its association with depression could be entirely incidental. Third, the effects of a gene should not be contingent on the presence of another risk factor. In this sense, saying there is a gene for depression is different from saying there is a gene that produces depression but only when combined with a traumatic life event. Contingency of this sort blunts the idea that the disorder is purely genetic, although it might very well be scientifically accurate. Fourth, the effects of the gene should be proximate to the outcome. If there is a gene for depression, the gene should affect depression in a direct way. If instead of a gene that produces depression, there is a gene that causes a person to ruminate over negative life events and in the process become depressed, we would not say the gene is for depression as much as it is for something related to depression through a chain of other influences. This example is straightforward. If there were even more steps between the gene and depression, we would have even less basis to claim it is the gene for depression.

If we employ Kendler's criteria, there is little evidence to support the idea that there is a gene for any psychiatric disorder. For one, the association between even the most well-established genetic markers and the most heritable psychiatric disorders is not terribly strong. The genetic markers for schizophrenia, for example, increase the odds of developing the disorder by only around 43 percent.[8] This is large, to be sure, but hardly deterministic. Furthermore, the genes associated with schizophrenia are located over a wide swath of the genome, suggesting little correspondence between a gene's actions and a specific disorder.[9] Bipolar disorder is likewise strongly heritable, but the actual genes associated with the disorder increase the risk by only around 18 percent. An especially large genome-wide association study of major depressive disorder was unable to identify any robust and replicable genetic effects, despite widespread acceptance of the idea that major depression is at least partly genetic.[10] If there are genes for depression, as revealed in twin studies, those genes are not visible in molecular research in any obvious way. To put these numbers in context, it is useful to compare the effects of genes with other well-known risk factors. Heavy smoking—thirty or more cigarettes per day—increases the risk of lung cancer by a factor of four to eighteen, with the risk growing even larger with more years of smoking.[11] To be sure, it is possible that science has yet to discover the most important genes for psychiatric disorders. It is also possible that interactions among genes are critical. Thus far, however, the evidence suggests that there are many genes for psychiatric disorders, that they are spread over various points in the human genome, and that each individual gene makes only a small contribution to the total risk.

Even this modest and circumspect conclusion can only be made in a general way. Genetic research on psychiatric disorders is, like genetic research on many other topics, plagued by problems in replication. If the effects of candidate genes are real, they should be found regardless of a study's sample or a scientist's technique. This is not the case, however. Studies routinely produce inconsistent findings. A failure to replicate can result from many things. And, indeed, in the case of psychiatric disorders it might be built into the phenotype itself: Complex genetic effects can mitigate against perfect replication. Yet replication is especially critical if science is to be used to craft better diagnostic criteria. Deciding there is a gene for a psychiatric disorder, and then using that gene for purposes of diagnosis, essentially reifies its influence. If the research is wrong, the diagnosis is wrong, too. By the same token, it is abundantly clear that there is a great deal of contingency in the relationship between genes and psychiatric disorders. Although research on gene-environment interactions also suffers from problems with replication, there is, at a minimum, a good deal of evidence indicating that genes and the environment work hand in hand. In the absence of significant environmental stress, the presence of risky genes alone is unlikely to produce depression, for example.[12]

The diagnostic value of genetic information is further diluted when considering the pathways connecting genes to psychiatric disorders. These pathways are usually not direct, and the distance is far from proximate. For many disorders, the pathway involves a long chain of events and steps. Furthermore, instead of a direct connection, the pathway likely involves a potentially large number of *endophenotypes*, lying somewhere between genes and psychiatric disorders.[13] An endophenotype refers to stable phenotypes that govern otherwise separate behavioral symptoms. Depression, for example, consists of a variety of different behaviors and symptoms, but the endophenotypes for major depression involve more abstract influences, such as a bias toward negative emotions, greater stress sensitivity, and dysfunctions in certain neurotransmitter systems.[14] Not only are these endophenotypes intermediate to the outcome of interest, but some are quite broad in their influence. In general, the genes related to psychiatric disorders probably pass through endophenotypes first and, at that, probably pass through several endophenotypes before landing on the symptoms of psychiatric disorders. They are likely related, first, to a variety of neurotransmitters, which, in turn, affect a variety of cognitive and affective processes, including learning, emotion regulation, and how individuals understand their social world. These psychological processes can, in turn, produce some of the symptoms of a psychiatric disorder, though only occasionally do they produce the entire syndrome—and they are often related to many psychiatric disorders at the same time.

Still, it is possible that endophenotypes provide a more promising avenue for creating credible diagnostic criteria, especially if we are willing to move well beyond the current parameters of the *DSM*. It is possible, for example, to regard a deficit in emotion regulation as, itself, a kind of psychiatric disorder. Furthermore, it is possible that at least some endophenotypes will satisfy aspects of Kendler's criteria better than conventional psychiatric disorders.

The relationship between genes and endophenotypes might be stronger, more direct, more specific, and less contingent than the relationship between genes and *DSM*-based psychiatric disorders. Yet in at least one important respect these endophenotypes are very different in their character from what is described in the *DSM*: They are not disorders per se. Virtually all the endophenotypes that scientists have discovered so far are apparent in those who have psychiatric disorders and those who do not. They are also apparent in those who experience significant impairment and those who do not. In the language of genetics, endophenotypes are state-independent, and, indeed, by the criteria scientists have used to study endophenotypes they *must* be state-independent if they are to be regarded as lying on the causal pathway between genes and disease.[15] This points to a another critical discontinuity: The interests of scientists studying endophenotypes and the interests of those focused on classifying psychiatric disorders are not in alignment, even when both have an avowed emphasis on genes.

ARE THE EFFECTS OF GENES SPECIFIC?

The specificity of the relationship between genes and psychiatric disorders deserves special emphasis. The concept of an endophenotype suggests that genes can affect multiple disorders simultaneously. Problems with working memory, for example, are not exclusive to schizophrenia. For this reason, any gene that affects working memory specifically will also affect several other psychiatric disorders. There is now more evidence bearing on the question of *diagnostic independence*, that is, the extent to which two or more disorders are distinct from the others at a genetic level. Evidence of this sort comes from two kinds of studies. The first is family and twin studies. Although early twin studies considered a single disorder at a time, recent studies have used the twin approach to study the contributions of genes to multiple disorders simultaneously. On this front, the evidence is clear. Studies find that the genetic contributions to a disorder are often not specific to that disorder and, instead, cut across many disorders simultaneously. Indeed, these studies find that the strong heritability found for many single disorders is artificial in the sense that it reflects the total contributions of genetic influences gathered from other disorders. The contribution of genes specific to a single disorder is generally very small, whereas the contributions to a broader set of disorders are much larger. Major depression, generalized anxiety, and phobia, for example, gain much of their apparent heritability from a set of strong and general genetic influences, but the genetic influences that affect major depression uniquely—and not anxiety or phobia—are quite small.[16]

Even for disorders that would seem to have distinctive symptoms, the case for diagnostic independence is complex.[17] Autism is a neurodevelopmental condition that involves three types of impairment: impaired social interaction, impaired communication, and rigid and repetitive interests and activities. According to the *DSM*, a diagnosis requires each of the three types of impairment. And because scientists use the *DSM* when identifying subjects, research on autism has followed suit: Studies have generally focused on the co-occurrence of all three types of impairments. Yet twin studies reveal that the three impairments are likely determined by different genes. To be sure, each type is highly heritable and, therefore, strongly genetic. But each type is shaped by genes different from those shaping the others. Even social and communication skills, which appear at least to resemble each other in that both involve communication, are separable at a genetic level. In short, there are no genes for autism per se, even if there are genes for its assorted elements.

Twin studies belong to an earlier era of science—indeed the intuition behind twin studies dates back centuries—but the insights of such studies are not so different from those of more cutting-edge research. Recent genome-wide association studies, for example, have reached essentially the same conclusions, albeit with different details. Linkage and association studies explore the role of specific genomic regions and polymorphisms in certain phenotypes. To date, studies of this sort have done more to bring psychiatric disorders together than to cleave them apart, albeit sometimes in unexpected ways. For instance, the specific genes for generalized anxiety disorder overlap with those for major depression.[18] In addition, there do not appear to be genes related only to schizophrenia.[19] On the contrary, certain regions of the genome are associated with both bipolar disorder and schizophrenia.[20] This overlap is especially provocative because it challenges one of the most longstanding distinctions in psychiatric nomenclature: the presumed division between mood disorders and psychotic disorders. To suggest that bipolar disorder, a mood disorder, shares some genetic antecedents with schizophrenia is to cast doubt over a premise many clinicians have accepted as fact. A recent study goes even further in this direction.[21] It identifies specific single-nucleotide polymorphisms (SNPs) at four loci that are associated with at least five disorders: attention deficit/hyperactivity disorder, autism-spectrum disorders, bipolar disorder, major depressive disorder, and schizophrenia. Although this genetic overlap does not cohere with the divisions of the *DSM*, it does point to some thematic commonalities. All the SNPs involved with these disorders are associated with calcium-channel activity, suggesting a shared neurochemical process.

THE NEUROSCIENCE OF PSYCHIATRIC DISORDERS

To date, genetic research has done little to validate the *DSM*, especially with respect to its organization and divisions. Yet this research at least points to a relationship between brain functioning and psychiatric disorders. The latest front in the science of psychiatric disorders is moving further in the direction of the brain. Research has sought to identify more precisely what neural abnormalities, whether in structure or function, produce psychiatric disorders. The appeal of neuroscience is, if anything, even greater than the appeal of genes, insofar as brain morphology is presumed to have a more direct correspondence to brain functioning. Perhaps there is no gene for psychiatric disorders, the reasoning goes, but there might still be a region of the brain that plays a critical role. In modern science, the brain is aligned closely with the mind, suggesting the sort of proximity that is preferred by those interested in psychiatric classification.

Neuroimaging is the best tool for the task. Neuroimaging involves a diverse set of technologies.[22] Functional magnetic resonance imaging (fMRI) uses blood flow to indicate brain activity, assuming that flow reflects an elevated neural response and, therefore, where different tasks are processed. fMRI data can be collected in an ongoing fashion, making it especially useful for tracking changes in a controlled setting. Positron-emission tomography (PET) is also a functional-imaging technique, but it tracks a different signal. PET detects gamma rays emitted following a collision of positrons and electrons. After the introduction of a radioactive agent to the body, the assumption is that areas of high radioactivity indicate heightened brain activity. In addition, a PET scan is unusually detailed in that it can yield a three-dimensional image of the brain, providing an improvement over cruder fMRI data, but at higher cost and lower safety.

Whatever their strengths and limitations, these tools are certainly useful when set in the context of observing patients and manipulating their experiences. Studies using PET scans, for example, are able to visualize and compare brain-region activity in revealing ways. Patients with major depression, for example, can be compared to those without major depression to check for chronic differences in neural activity. In addition, researchers can induce sadness in "normal" subjects in order to assess how brain activity changes in the presence of depression-like stimuli. The information derived from PET scans is especially useful in documenting differences between the brains of psychiatric patients and others. Studies of those suffering from schizophrenia, for example, find significant deficits in gray-matter material located in the prefrontal cortex.[23] These deficits are significant. They are correlated with symptom severity and with genetic risk factors for schizophrenia, suggesting potentially useful diagnostic information. Brain research on depression has, likewise, yielded significant insights. The symptoms of depression, including the full range of the disorder's emotional, cognitive, and psychomotor aspects, involve abnormalities in brain structure.[24] Among depressed patients, for example, activity in the prefrontal cortex tends to be lower than in nondepressed people. Much of the activity in this area of brain is related to the generation and regulation of emotions, suggesting a connection between depression and emotional control and, thereby, cementing an impression already alluded to by research on endophenotypes.[25]

Altogether, this research has successfully established a neurological substrate to many psychiatric disorders. The brains of those suffering from psychiatric disorders are, in ways that we can now identify, different. Yet the implications of this research for creating better diagnostic criteria are unclear. On one hand, neuroimaging can validate symptoms that might otherwise be neglected. Neuroimaging studies, for example, have illuminated some of the cognitive deficits associated with schizophrenia, ones, as discussed earlier, that have traditionally been neglected in the *DSM*. On the other hand, greater precision with respect to a specific class of symptoms does not, in itself, provide greater clarity with respect to the diagnosis of schizophrenia as a whole. Schizophrenia has a variety of symptoms, not all of which are located in a single part of the brain. Furthermore, it is unusual to regard the fate of "neglected" symptoms as hinging on the validation of neuroscience. Indeed, the status of cognitive symptoms in schizophrenia was elevated among clinicians long before PET scans came along. Clinicians appreciated the presence of cognitive deficits simply through the observation of patients. Other disorders suffer from similar problems in neuroanatomical specificity. White-matter hyperintensities are more common in people suffering from unipolar depression than among those who are not, suggesting, again, differences in brain functioning. Yet such hyperintensities also occur naturally with aging. Furthermore, they are found for a variety of other psychiatric disorders, not just unipolar depression.[26] Depression might produce white-matter hyperintensities, but the presence of hyperintensities does not reveal the presence of depression uniquely insofar as such hyperintensities have many other causes. This issue reflects a more general problem with fMRIs: They invite problems in causal inference. It is difficult to infer that activity in a specific region of the brain indicates a specific psychological state without explicitly testing that state against others that might also be associated with the same brain activity.[27] Psychiatric diagnoses thrive on distinctions; fMRIs elide them.

Even in the hands of the best scientists, neuroimaging does little to absolve psychiatry of the obligation to make decisions. Neuroimaging provides clues regarding the location of some moods, to be sure, but activity in a region alone cannot reveal whether the moods associated with that region are transitory or chronic.[28] From the standpoint of neuroimaging, chronic and transitory moods appear similar, even though from a clinical standpoint chronic depression is far more significant. Furthermore, neuroimaging alone cannot provide a general definition of mental disorder. To identify a relationship between depressed moods and specific neural activities says little about whether or when that mood ought to be regarded as dysfunctional or when sadness is appropriate (if one regards appropriateness as a useful consideration in the first place). Indeed, neuroimaging does just as well in identifying the location of joy as it does of misery.[29] In addition, neuroimaging is better at detection than falsification. It provides data on the location of an activity in the brain, but it does not provide information that can be used to discredit the existence of something. The failure to map some psychological state to an area of the brain does not, in itself, make that state artificial or warrant excluding it from consideration in formal diagnostic criteria. What we decide constitutes a symptom is based on additional considerations.

The more general problem with neuroscience is the lack of a *psychophysical identity*, the idea that the psychological can be derived from the physical. There is considerable philosophical and scientific debate regarding this issue, and, to be sure, not everyone agrees about whether there is a lack of identity.[30] But even those who try to elaborate some relationship between the brain and the mind appreciate the difficulty of translating between the two. For the purposes of illustrating the difficulty, a moderate standpoint is worth considering. Daniel Dennett provides a framework for thinking about how the psychological and the physical diverge, while still allowing for the fact that the mind depends entirely on the brain.[31] For Dennett, the mind and the brain operate in different ways, much like the difference between hardware and software in computers. Whereas the brain functions as a parallel processor, with neurons functioning in tandem, the mind functions as a serial processor, with psychological experiences flowing in a sequence from one event to another. This metaphor provides a way of thinking about the complex connection between mind and brain and especially for thinking about the mind as qualitatively different. Yet, if anything, the metaphor further undermines the promise of neuroimaging for psychiatry.

If the mind emerges in a way that is difficult to map onto how the brain functions, and if symptoms are experienced primarily as features of the mind rather than of the brain, the tools of neuroimaging can only take us so far in the task of diagnosis.

IS MENTAL ILLNESS CATEGORICAL?

At this point, the mind-brain connection is as much an issue of philosophy as it is of science, but there are other debates in psychiatric classification—ones nearly as abstract—to which science can speak with more clarity. In particular, science can now provide evidence regarding whether mental illness is categorical. A categorical approach implies a *natural kind*, which is a concept the most mature sciences have grappled with for a long time. A natural kind is any entity that has some essence—hidden or apparent—that defines it. That essence separates it from other entities and renders a definition of it a "natural" one rather than an "artificial" one, in the sense that it can be made in reference to some external standard. In addition, natural kinds have an identical character regardless of where they are found. Carbon is carbon regardless of where it is located. This idea is relevant to what science hopes to achieve with respect to classification. If something is a natural kind, science might eventually *discover* what the essence of that kind is, but science will not *invent* it; that is, the essence of natural kinds—whatever that essence happens to be—existed long before someone uncovered it. Perhaps the most well-known system of natural kinds is the periodic table of the elements, wherein each element is distinct and defined by its molecular properties. The periodic table is updated occasionally, but not frequently, and only in response to new discoveries. Although some psychiatrists look to the periodic table for inspiration, the *DSM* is far from it. At present, we do not have enough scientific evidence to say what the essence of a psychiatric disorder is, though at a minimum science can begin to test the idea that a disorder is categorical rather than dimensional and, therefore, that a disorder might be closer to a natural thing than an invented concept.

Evaluating whether a disorder is categorical is a statistical exercise. The idea of a categorical disorder implies what is referred to as a "zone of rarity," a point at which a disorder should be separable from a closely related but normal experience.[32] Even if we assume that virtually all *symptoms* exist on a spectrum—one can be more or less happy—the zone-of-rarity concept implies a point at which symptoms suddenly break from expected patterns, a threshold at which major depression, for example, is truly distinct from ordinary sadness. This idea leads to some testable statistical properties. For example, it implies some point on a spectrum at which symptoms become *rare*. Wherever that point happens to be, few people are likely to have symptom levels just below it because, at that point, all the symptoms of a disorder suddenly become more prominent, and the distribution of symptoms breaks from the continuous pattern that is apparent at lower levels. Another way to think about this idea is in terms of the set of symptoms that make up a major depressive episode. If major depression is truly categorical, the presence of high levels of some symptoms should be associated with high levels of virtually all the other symptoms as well. At a certain point, the other symptoms of depression come into play because some essence is apparent.

The empirical study of dimensionality and its counterparts is referred to as bootstrap taxometrics, in reference to the fact that no external information is used. Information on whether a disorder is categorical is derived only from the symptoms scientists observe. The technique makes no assumptions about what causes a disorder to be categorical. It only tests whether that disorder is likely to be categorical rather than dimensional.[33] In addition, bootstrap taxometrics does not require scientists to posit the precise level at which symptoms become a disorder. Although the *DSM* imposes thresholds using diagnostic cutpoints, bootstrap taxometrics can test whether a disorder is categorical without stipulating a priori exactly where that cutpoint should be drawn. The cutpoint will, instead, be estimated from the data.

Evidence from bootstrap taxometrics generally favors a dimensional approach. At this point, evidence for a categorical approach appears to be confined to schizotypy and substance use disorders. Some of the most prevalent psychiatric disorders, including mood and anxiety disorders, are likely dimensional.[34] Another interpretation of these findings is that some of the most *contested* disorders are likely dimensional. It is important to be clear about what this means. The idea, for example, that depression is dimensional still means that major depression is more severe than minor depression, but it also means that major depression is not qualitatively different from minor depression. The two differ in degree but not in kind. For this reason, any cutpoint assigned along a spectrum of depressive symptoms is likely to be arbitrary with respect to some essence, if not with respect to some spectrum. Even psychiatric disorders that would seem, on their face, quite severe are probably dimensional. Psychopathy, for example, is a personality disorder characterized by a combination of callousness, impulsivity, emotional detachment, and an extreme disregard of others. In everyday language a "psychopath" denotes an extremely manipulative and dangerous person, and, befitting this, the term is often associated with criminal behavior. Yet psychopathy, too, appears to reflect a dimension of personality rather than a category.[35] It manifests itself as a dimension among both criminal offenders and nonoffenders alike.

Other studies tackle the categorical-versus-dimensional issue in a different way but reach a similar conclusion. Kendler and Gardner, for example, focus on major depression.[36] They use identical twin pairs who vary along three dimensions of severity: in the number of symptoms of they have, in the amount of impairment caused by those symptoms, and in the duration of their symptoms. In the study, some twins were clearly above the threshold for a major depressive episode, but many more were below it. The design of Kendler and Gardner's study focuses on predicting the future, based on the symptoms of one twin or the other. Is there a point, they ask, based on current symptoms, at which a person becomes much more likely to experience an episode of depression in the future? Furthermore, is there a point at which the level of current symptomatology of one twin strongly increases the likelihood of a future episode of depression in the other twin? The zone-of-rarity concept informs their research design. If major depression is categorical, there should be a point at which the risk of a future episode of depression is much greater than the simple sum of current symptoms—that is, there should be a threshold that is discontinuous from the levels preceding it. Their results, however, provide little evidence for such a threshold, regardless of the criteria they use. They find that the number of symptoms is certainly related to the risk of depression in the future, but in a monotonic fashion: Each additional symptom increases the risk, but there is no point at which the risk is suddenly and decisively elevated. Similarly, the duration of symptoms has no consistent relationship with the risk of depression: Episodes of short duration are just as predictive of future depression as episodes of long duration. The same is true of impairment: Even episodes of depression that are only mildly impairing increase the risk of more severely impairing depression later on. In short, there is little evidence that major depression is more than the sum of its parts (although the sum itself is clearly still relevant). Nor is there evidence that minor depression is entirely distinct from its major counterpart.

ARE MAJOR AND MINOR DISORDERS CAUSED BY DIFFERENT THINGS?

This lack of an obvious distinction between minor and major depression can be pushed further. Even if we accept that the symptoms of depression are dimensional, we might still prefer a categorical approach if minor and major depression have different causes. As noted earlier, a longstanding (if still controversial) distinction is between depression with and without cause. The distinction is a misnomer in the sense that all forms of depression have causes, but the distinction is still useful insofar as it draws attention to how apparent causes are and, thus, how "deep" those causes might be. In this way, depression "without cause" might be regarded as genetic in the sense that it does not obviously reflect something apparent in the environment. And some regard depression caused in this fashion as "real," or as closer to a natural kind. Depression "with cause," by contrast, might be more superficial, in the sense that it reflects something in the environment and not an obvious genetic predisposition for the disorder. Depression of this sort is seen as "normal," in that it reflects what any person might experience after, for example, the death of a spouse. And the presumption is that such depression will remit once the individual has coped sufficiently. A general way to regard this distinction is to think about depression without cause as biological in origin and, therefore, obdurate, whereas depression with cause is social in origin and, therefore, fleeting. The former is closer to a natural kind than the latter.

Yet science has found little evidence for a clear distinction of this sort. If depression is divided into grades of severity, the causes of higher grades tend to be very similar to those of lower grades.[37] Social support, for example, promotes greater well-being generally, reducing the risk of both minor depression and major depression in near-equal measure. To be sure, some causes become more apparent at higher levels than lower levels, suggesting some important distinctions, but the causes that become more relevant are not biological in nature. Poverty, for example, is more strongly associated with major depression than minor depression (although it is significantly associated with both). Similarly, negative life events have a complex relationship with the severity of depression, belying a neat distinction. In general, there is a great deal of scientific evidence that negative life events cause major depression, especially when combined with risky genes. Yet the relationship between life events and depression is, if anything, *weaker* for more severe depression. One explanation for this is that those who suffer from "real" depression are more prone to a depressive response regardless of the stress that occurs in their lives.[38] For this reason, their depression tends to return whether or not they experienced a negative life event. Yet there is little evidence that social causes become entirely *irrelevant* when it comes to major depression. Major depression, too, is brought on by negative life events. For this reason, thinking about causes is not terribly useful as a framework for thinking about severity. Genetic influences suffer from a similar problem. There is a good deal of evidence, for example, that happiness is strongly shaped by genetic factors, just as major depression is.[39] Genes are not concerned with valence, though psychiatrists obviously are. In any case, a distinction premised on presumed pathologies, whether biological or social, is not especially useful for those interested in taxonomies. Deciding when depression is social and when it is biological is virtually impossible. There is no point at which the environment becomes less relevant and biology takes over. Depression is caused by a mix of causes, each of which varies across cases.

A version of the with-or-without-cause distinction is especially prominent in debates regarding bereavement. One proposed revision to the *DSM* is to expand the so-called bereavement exclusion, by applying it to more life events and perhaps also to more disorders. Critics argue that depression resulting from the death of a spouse (or, for that matter, any other major life event, especially involving loss) should not be regarded as "real" depression because it represents an expected response. If the response is proportional to the stressor, it represents a natural reaction and is, therefore, not a disorder. To be sure, the death of a spouse is a severe event and can plainly produce something like major depression, but because this response can be explained, it ought to be regarded as normal. By the same token, it is easy to imagine cases of anxiety that reflect a reasonable response to a threatening environment and so should not be regarded as a disorder per se.

Is bereavement really a different form of depression? This question lends itself to several testable ideas. One intuition anticipates that major depression that developed in light of the death of a loved one should be very different from major depression not developed in this fashion. For one, cases of depression following bereavement might have a different course, resolving more quickly than other cases of depression. In addition, such cases might respond differently to treatment, especially insofar as depression without cause is thought to reflect a different biological entity. Psychiatric medications, for instance, might not work as well for depression that is social in origin, like bereavement-related depression. Research has found little support for these ideas. Those who develop major depression in light of a significant life event like bereavement tend to resemble those who develop depression without such a precipitating event. They tend, for example, to have family members who also suffer from major depression and, therefore, presumably have a similar genetic profile. They also tend to have experienced more childhood adversity and, therefore, had similar social-risk profiles before they experienced the death of a spouse.[40] The idea of depression without cause anticipates the opposite: It anticipates that those suffering from depression in light of bereavement should have fewer preexisting risk factors than those suffering from depression without cause. Further suggesting little difference between the two, studies find that a major depressive episode beginning within the first two months of the death of a loved one is essentially indistinguishable from nonbereavement-related depression.[41] It has similar symptoms, including similar psychomotor disturbances. It also involves similar biological consequences, including increased adrenocortical activity and depressed immune function. And it tends to have the same degree of persistence, meaning bereavement-related depression is no more or less likely to remit and responds no better or worse to antidepressants. To be sure, bereavement-related depression is often quite mild, and many who are affected by it do not seek treatment. Furthermore, those who suffer from bereavement-related depression do differ on *some* demographic characteristics. They tend to be older, for example, and are disproportionately female.[42] Yet these are expected differences among those experiencing the death of a spouse, given the female advantage in life expectancy and the average age of death. Furthermore, most people with depression, irrespective of the cause, do not seek treatment. The fact that someone did not seek treatment does not mean he or she would not benefit from it. Bereavement-related depression might be considered normal from the standpoint of being *understandable*—and, to be sure, it is important for clinicians to comprehend a case as completely as possible—but it is probably not *distinct*. Like other forms of depression, bereavement-related depression is influenced by genes, causes significant impairment, and is responsive to treatment when and if that treatment is applied.

There is at least one major study, though, that points to some lingering differences between the two types of depression. This study is worth discussing in detail, because, as much as it illustrates the value of science, it also illustrates the limits of science in adjudicating matters of validity. In particular, it highlights the relevance of interpretation and how scientists differ in what they regard as valid. Ramin Mojtabai uses a large, nationally representative data set to compare the characteristics of those who experienced an episode of bereavement-related depression to those who experienced an episode of nonbereavement-related depression.[43] In both cases, the episode was brief, lasting under two months. He finds some differences between the

THE CONTEMPORARY SCIENCE OF PSYCHIATRIC NOSOLOGY

two, among the most important of which is a lower level of comorbidity among those with bereavement-related depression and a significantly lower risk of a new episode. In particular, the risk of a new episode in the two groups was 8.2 percent relative to 14.7 percent, which is not a small difference by conventional statistical standards. In addition, Mojtabai finds somewhat lower role impairment among those with bereavement-related depression. Altogether these differences suggest that bereavement-related depression is, indeed, milder and more self-limiting.

Yet another study, by Stephen Gillman and colleagues, uses the same data to reach seemingly the opposite conclusion: that bereavement-related depression is essentially identical to nonbereavement-related depression.[44] Although the reason for the different conclusions is not entirely clear, it likely reflects how the different authors chose to treat "complicated" bereavement and what comparisons they decided to emphasize.[45] When basic issues of taxonomy are always in play, precision in terminology is key. And in trying to resolve the differences, Gilman and colleagues focused on these issues, as they outlined in their subsequent reply. "Complicated" bereavement refers to a depressive episode occurring in the context of grieving that is, despite its relationship with bereavement, severe or prolonged. "Prolonged" is defined as lasting longer than two months, and "severe" is defined as involving suicidal thoughts, marked functional impairment, and certain symptoms like psychomotor retardation or feelings of worthlessness. Allowing for bereavement, so defined, it is possible to identify *three* different types of depression rather than just two (the conventional comparison): those who experience depression resulting from bereavement but do not qualify for a diagnosis because of the bereavement exclusion (group 1); those who suffer from complicated bereavement, formally defined by the *DSM* (group 2); and those who experience a major depressive episode that is unrelated to bereavement (group 3). The two studies are conflicting because they make different comparisons among the three groups. And, in this light, it becomes clear the two studies actually agree on some important points. Both studies, for example, find that group 1 suffers from milder depression than groups 2 or 3. The studies differ, however, in how they treat groups 2 and 3. Mojtabai combines groups 2 and 3 (except for a comparison with one outcome) and finds differences between that combined group and group 1. Gilman and colleagues do not combine groups 2 and 3 and find that group 2 is closer to group 1 than group 3. From this, Gilman and colleagues choose to emphasize the problems associated with excluding people based on poorly conceived criteria. At least according to their interpretation, the *DSM* criteria for complicated bereavement are inadequate for identifying differences, so it would be unwise and premature to extend the exclusion to other disorders or events. Mojtabai, meanwhile, uses the same evidence to support the inclusion and expansion of the bereavement exclusion. While focusing most of their comments on issues of statistical comparison, Gilman and colleagues summarize their concern by appealing to the issue of over- versus underdiagnosis: "Questions raised about diagnosing depression occurring in the context of bereavement are motivated by a concern for overdiagnosis; we think it is equally important to address the exception to the bereavement exclusion to guard against underdiagnosis."[46] They further note the importance of fine-tuning the criteria for complicated bereavement, which they find wanting, at least in *DSM-IV.*

This is more than a matter of semantics (although it might appear to be only that). And the issue of defining "uncomplicated" is more significant than it might initially seem. From evidence that uncomplicated bereavement is little different from no depression at all, some are willing to conclude that bereavement is normal. Citing Mojtabai, as well as his own work on the topic, Wakefield is direct on the point.[47] He argues that Mojtabai's research provides "powerful support for the hypothesis that such depressions are not pathological and are consistent with intense normal emotion."[48] Yet if the *DSM*'s diagnostic criteria for "uncomplicated" are essentially cast in terms of mild depression (albeit under a different guise), while the criteria for "complicated" bereavement resemble those for a major depressive episode, then the conclusion that uncomplicated bereavement is not as severe as major depression is a tautology, true virtually by definition.[49] In other words, the terms "complicated" and "uncomplicated" are defined ex ante in reference to severity. Studies that compare the two, then, are not terribly informative regarding the question of ultimate validity, although they can be used to test the adequacy of the devised diagnostic criteria for the purpose of distinguishing according to severity. Furthermore, if a scientist wished to advocate for diagnostic criteria premised on a more explicit concern with severity, they could do so, but demonstrating a relationship between the severity of a disorder and the risk of recurrence requires no consideration of the events that might precipitate depression. If severity is critical, there is no need to muddle things with a discussion of bereavement (or any other life event).

Another way of thinking about the bereavement exclusion, though, is to think about making exclusions on the basis of other losses as well. Critics argue that if discerning normal responses to the environment is the principal concern (of which bereavement is only an especially powerful example), there is no reason to limit the exclusion to bereavement. This idea, too, can be tested empirically, but here again it is critical to think through how researchers choose to interpret their comparisons. There is evidence that bereavement is, indeed, not unusual as a cause of major depression. Wakefield and colleagues find that a variety of losses, based on answers to the question "was there anything else going on in your life at that time which caused you to feel sad?" yield similar symptoms to those of bereavement.[50] Whether depression is brought on by the death of a loved one or something else, like the loss of a job, it tends to result in the same number of depressive symptoms, in episodes that last about the same amount of time, in episodes that have the same likelihood of recurrence, and in episodes that have about the same likelihood of being treated. Yet here, too, the issue of comparison is critical. Even if a depressive episode brought on by the loss of a job, for example, is similar to an episode brought on by bereavement, a comparison between the two episodes says nothing about whether those episodes are also similar to an episode brought on by no apparent cause. Advocates for the bereavement exclusion are certainly correct to point out that a focus on bereavement involves misplaced specificity if one is really interested in the idea of "normal" forms of stress. Under the rationale that was initially applied to bereavement, there are lots of other things that ought to be included as exclusions as well. Yet comparing depression with and without cause—the other dimension of the framework—is very difficult as an empirical matter, and for reasons that might undermine our enthusiasm for extending the bereavement exclusion. The best test of the with-versus-without-cause idea would be to compare those whose depression developed from an environmental trigger with those whose depression did not, but only about 3 percent of cases of a major depressive disorder involve no obvious trigger.[51] Even in that very small number of cases with no apparent trigger, it is unclear whether there was, in fact, no trigger or whether there was simply no trigger the person could remember (or feels sufficiently comfortable to report). Science knows a good deal about the causes of mental illness, more than it did in the past. And the work of both critics and advocates of the bereavement exclusion have advanced our understanding. Yet science does not have the tools to say with confidence that depression in one case was brought on by some dysfunction and in another by a normal response. Furthermore, much of the evidence cycles back to an issue that has been demonstrated in a variety of ways: Psychiatric disorders are dimensional, virtually to the core.

In the end, the bereavement exclusion is perhaps less consequential than all the debate surrounding it would suggest. One reason the issue attracts so much attention is the presumption that it is significant in ways that speak to the credibility of psychiatry. Some critics charge that eliminating the bereavement exclusion would further inflate the prevalence of major depression beyond its already dubious and artificial levels. If bereavement is common, the argument goes, allowing the *DSM*'s diagnostic criteria to admit bereavement as a major depressive episode would, perforce, increase the prevalence of depression. Yet research finds that the diagnostic implications of the bereavement exclusion are, in fact, quite limited. In the largest survey of its kind, 1,308 of the 8,098 people surveyed met the lifetime criteria for a major depressive disorder, but only sixty-five of those people—less than 5 percent—would not be counted as depressed using the bereavement exclusion.[52] If they live long enough, virtually everyone experiences the death of a loved one, but that experience alone does not and cannot elevate the prevalence of major depression by much. Most bereaved individuals do not experience all the symptoms necessary to meet the diagnostic criteria for a major depressive episode.[53] Among those who do, however, bereavement can be the trigger, setting in motion a disorder that can persist long after the loved one's death.

SCIENCE AND THE *DSM-5*

Much of the evidence discussed thus far was conducted using *DSM-III*, *III-R*, and *IV* diagnostic criteria. Another revision of the *DSM*, however, was published in 2013.[54] The timing is important. In contrast to earlier revisions of the *DSM*, *DSM-5* had, in principle, a much larger base of scientific evidence to draw from, especially from the natural sciences. The authors of *DSM-5* were well aware of this, noting "the last two decades . . . have seen real and durable progress in such areas as cognitive neuroscience, brain imaging, epidemiology, and genetics."[55] And the authors' apparent enthusiasm regarding the science of psychiatric disorders was matched by a sober sense of responsibility. Among other things, they recognized the great many people who could be affected by the revisions of the *DSM*, something they discussed extensively in *DSM-5*'s prefatory matter.[56] *DSM-5* gestated for a long time. Planning for *DSM-5* began in 1999, more than a decade before its publication. It began with a series of conferences, each involving a variety of stakeholders with different backgrounds and interests. The conferences included academic and clinical experts such as psychiatrists and psychologists, practicing mental health professionals, and researchers from a variety of disciplines, including the natural sciences, statistics, and public health.[57] The conferences also included people indirectly involved with mental health, such as lawyers, consumer organizations, and the families of patients. In perhaps the clearest acknowledgment of the very large number of stakeholders involved, a website was created to allow the public to comment on draft diagnostic criteria. Through this, the committee received more than 13,000 comments.[58]

Revisions were vetted through an integrated organizational structure, arranged by the task force. Working groups were established to explore specific diagnostic areas. Though they focused on different disorders, they shared common aims. For one, they were instructed to write diagnostic criteria that would avoid the widespread use of the "not otherwise specified" category. Recognizing the many problems associated with NOS, the APA noted that a "too-rigid categorical system does not capture clinical experience or important scientific observations."[59] In addition, the working groups were instructed to maintain as much continuity as possible between *DSM-5* and previous editions, although the task force also encouraged all types of proposals for revisions and updates. They would entertain proposals to change existing criteria, to add new disorders, to add new subtypes, or to delete disorders altogether. In a nod to some of the research discussed earlier in this chapter, the groups were also encouraged to include more dimensional elements to the diagnostic criteria, potentially allowing clinicians to employ *both* categorical diagnoses and graded assessments of severity. In addition, the groups were instructed to better align the *DSM* with international psychiatric nomenclature, especially the World Health Organization's International Classification of Disease. The revision effort was, indeed, international. Experts from thirty-nine countries were eventually involved in the process. Although no single working group was capable of revising the *DSM*'s overarching organizational structure, especially given their responsibilities for specific diagnostic areas, the task force recognized that the axial features of the *DSM* should be revised as well.

Despite a broad and ecumenical approach, the task force set some limits on the nature of the revisions. Above all they stipulated that all proposals required supporting scientific evidence. In their procedures, the task force mandated that any revision would need a "memorandum of evidence" prepared by the working group and including all the scientific evidence supporting the change, especially regarding issues of validity.[60] In addition, the proposals would be reviewed by the Scientific Review Committee, which was tasked with scoring each proposal according to the strength of its evidence. Another committee, the Clinical and Public Health Committee, would deal with proposals that were seen as potentially useful but scientifically premature. They too, however, would have a firm eye on issues of validity, despite a mandate that granted them some allowance for "extrascientific" revisions. Although the process was inclusive as an organizational matter, a final recommendation would come from the top. It would be provided by the APA Board of Trustees and the APA Assembly's Committee on *DSM-5*.

These procedures insured a wide-ranging and rigorous vetting process, but the goals set by the APA involved difficult tradeoffs. Some of the goals could easily conflict. For instance, the APA ceded that the "historical aspiration of achieving diagnostic homogeneity by progressive subtyping within disorder categories is no longer sensible."[61] Yet the APA still hoped for more homogenous diagnoses, even if under a very different taxometric framework. At the same time, the APA recognized that psychiatric symptoms crossed diagnostic boundaries, stating, "we have come to recognize that the boundaries between disorders are more porous than originally perceived."[62] Yet the revision process was organized around diagnostic categories, an organizational structure that virtually ensured artificial siloing. Tensions were produced in other ways as well. The APA encouraged the input of a variety of stakeholders, but they also elevated the authority of science. It is not hard to envision situations wherein the interests of patients could be in conflict with the insights of scientists.

In the end, the interface between science and *DSM-5* was incomplete. As a way to illustrate further the limits of science for questions of taxonomy, it is instructive to review in detail the conditions in which scientific evidence was and was not used. There are clearly places where evidence played a decisive role. Moreover, many of the revisions brought on by scientific research are consequential. For example, *DSM-5* created a single "autism-spectrum disorder," incorporating previous diagnoses such as autism, Asperger's, and pervasive developmental disorder not otherwise specified. This blending of disorders stemmed from scientific evidence indicating a shared genetic and neurological substrate. In addition, in other places, science played a role in either eliminating disorders or creating new subtypes. For example, various subtypes of schizophrenia that were included in *DSM-IV* were eliminated in *DSM-5* because of their poor apparent validity. In addition, science played a role in enhancing the diagnostic criteria for neurocognitive disorders, previously referred to as dementias. These disorders were unpacked into more specific subtypes, based on differences suggested by brain imaging and genetic research.

The organization of the *DSM* was revised as well, based in part on evidence regarding comorbidity. Recognizing the superficial boundaries between disorders, *DSM-5* revised the manual's axes. Axes I, II, and III were combined in order to avoid the implication that the disorders on different axes were different in any fundamental way. *DSM-5* still imposes some structure to the categories, albeit of a different type. Disorders occurring more frequently in childhood appear at the beginning of the manual, whereas disorders occurring more frequently in later life appear near the end. This, too, reflects a better scientific understanding of psychiatric disorders, especially regarding their age of onset.

In a few instances, new disorders were created in an attempt to stem the potential for overdiagnosis that was apparent in old disorders. One new diagnosis, disruptive mood dysregulation disorder, was created in order to provide an alternative to the diagnosis of bipolar disorder in children. The diagnostic criteria for the new disorder stipulate that the diagnosis is intended for children under the age of eighteen who are unable to control their behavior, thereby encouraging the diagnosis of disruptive mood dysregulation rather than bipolar disorder. Similarly, in the case of anxiety disorders, there was some fear of misclassifying "transient" fears as disorders.[63] To curtail this possibility, *DSM-5* includes a duration statement of "typically lasting for 6 months or more" for separation anxiety disorder and for specific phobias. A concern with overdiagnosis hardly pervades the entire *DSM-5*, though. On the contrary, in a few instances there was an interest in promoting greater sensitivity. In the case of PTSD, for example, the diagnostic threshold for children and adolescents was lowered.[64] Furthermore, separate criteria were added for children under the age of seven, a tacit acknowledgment that psychiatric disorders can, in fact, appear at a very young age. Similarly, the required minimum average frequency of binge eating for a diagnosis of bulimia was reduced from twice a week to once a week.[65]

Some long-simmering political controversies were also readdressed, especially surrounding how the *DSM* deals with sex and gender. *DSM-5* introduces gender dysphoria, for example, as a new diagnostic class. This class moves further in the direction of emphasizing gender *incongruence* as the diagnostically relevant issue rather than someone simply identifying as a member of the opposite gender. In addition, the word "sex" was replaced with the word "gender" in order to emphasize the social aspects of sex rather than its biology, as is conventional in the social sciences. Furthermore, the language of "some alternative gender" was used in tandem with "the other gender" in order to acknowledge transgender identification.[66] In the same vein, *DSM-5* acknowledges the complexities of gender identity, especially in social settings. For the child criteria for gender identity disorder, for instance, the phrase "repeatedly stated desire to be . . . the other sex" was replaced with the phrase "strong desire to be of the other gender," thereby acknowledging that "stating" a preference can be difficult, especially when doing so is stigmatized and the patient is young.[67]

In perhaps the most controversial revision, the bereavement exclusion was eliminated from the diagnostic criteria for a major depressive episode. The rationale for doing so drew on the research discussed earlier in this chapter, especially research showing that bereavement is a severe form of stress that can cause significant suffering lasting much longer than two months. The removal of the exclusion was not done lightly, nor was it done without any appreciation of a distinction. The introduction to the section on depressive disorders states that when bereavement and a major depressive disorder occur together, "the depressive symptoms and functional impairment tend to be more severe and the prognosis is worse compared with bereavement that is not accompanied by major depressive disorder" and, further, that depression related to bereavement "tends to occur in persons with other vulnerabilities to depressive disorders."[68] In addition, a footnote was added to help clinicians distinguish between bereavement and major depression. The footnote is not part of the formal diagnostic criteria, but it nonetheless provides considerable detail and specificity.[69] Recognizing the artificiality of much of the discussion surrounding the course of bereavement, the footnote states that grief "occurs in waves," whereas a major depressive episode is more persistent. It further specifies several significant differences in associated symptoms. Grief, for example, tends to be focused on thoughts regarding the decreased; depression is more self-focused. In addition, grief tends not to result in a loss of self-esteem, but depression almost always involves chronic feelings of worthlessness. In a nod to those who wished to expand the bereavement exclusion rather than contract it, a note in the diagnostic criteria lists bereavement as only one of several loss events that can produce symptoms resembling those of a depressive episode. This note also stipulates that clinical judgment regarding the appropriateness of the feelings of depression should consider the "individual's history" and "cultural norms" regarding the expression of distress.[70] This acknowledgment appears elsewhere as well. In an earlier section of the manual, the APA demurred that "normal life variation" and "transient responses to stress" make diagnosis difficult.[71]

Despite these caveats, however, the APA *did* eliminate the bereavement exclusion. Furthermore, in doing so it elevated the role of clinical judgment, even as it insisted on using the emerging insights of science. In particular, it put the onus of distinguishing between bereavement and depression on clinicians rather than the criteria themselves, noting that diagnosis requires clinical expertise and experience.[72] This emphasis is not incidental. It reflects a more general theme of the manual. Indeed, the *DSM-5* emphasizes clinical judgment even in its definition of a mental disorder, which is not a radical departure from earlier definitions provided when the science was not as strong:

A mental disorder is a syndrome characterized by clinically significant disturbance in an individual's cognition, emotion regulation, or behavior that reflects a dysfunction in the psychological, biological, or developmental processes underlying mental functioning. Mental disorders are usually associated with significant distress or disability in social, occupational, or other important activities. An expectable or culturally approved response to a common stressor or loss, such as the death of a loved one, is not a mental disorder. Socially deviant behavior (e.g., political, religious, or sexual) and conflicts that are primarily between the individual and society are not mental disorders unless the deviance or conflict results from a dysfunction in the individual, as described above.

(*DSM-5*, 20)

Repeated references to concepts that require clinical judgment, including dysfunction and cultural appropriateness, ultimately reveal the limited scope of the *DSM-5*'s revisions. Despite the ambitions of the task force, *DSM-5* is much like the editions before it. And it uses science in, at best, a halting way. In 2011, with the revision process well under way, David Kupfer and Darrell Regier admitted that, despite their earlier optimism regarding the potential role of science, they found the pace of impact much slower than anticipated.[73] This assessment is echoed throughout the final version of the manual. By the APA's own admission the revisions to *DSM-5* do not amount to a paradigm shift.[74] And, in many instances, the *DSM-5* falls back on the old theme of clinical utility, stating, for example, "until incontrovertible etiological or pathophysiological mechanisms are identified to fully validate specific disorders or disorder spectra, the most important standard for the *DSM-5* disorder criteria will be their clinical utility for the assessment of clinical course and treatment response of individuals grouped by a given set of diagnostic criteria."[75] At best, the task force found scientific validators "useful for suggesting large groups of disorders rather than for 'validating' individual disorder diagnostic criteria."[76]

Clinical utility and scientific validity are not the same, but they need not be in conflict. One place where science could have played more of a role in *DSM-5* is in assessing "clinically significant impairment." Like the editions before it, *DSM-5* specifies that the symptoms of the disorder must cause "clinically significant distress or impairment" in important areas of functioning. This is a critical aspect of assessing severity. Furthermore, the concept of impairment lends itself to scientific investigation. A variety of instruments have been developed to measure impairment. *DSM-5* notes that these instruments are useful but acknowledges, again, that there are limits to the role of science in the revision process, at least with respect to the science the task force most wants, noting that "in absence of clear biological markers or clinically useful measurements of severity for mental disorders, it has not been possible to completely separate normal and pathological symptom expressions."[77] A similar tone pervades *DSM-5*'s discussion of the categorical-versus-dimensional debate, in this case with the authors stating, "despite the problem posed by categorical diagnoses, the *DSM-5* Task Force recognized that it is premature scientifically to propose alternative definitions for most disorders."[78]

Yet the incomplete use of science in *DSM-5* likely reflects something more than prematurity. Indeed, it may be rooted in conflicting conceptions of validity itself. In the absence of a gold standard, validity is contentious.[79] And, in the presence of many different ideas about validity, along with many different proposed ways of assessing it, the difficulty in providing unequivocal evidence for validity is even greater. Having reviewed the science of psychiatric nosology, it is useful to circle back to the issue of validity. Behind all the disappointment surrounding *DSM-5* is an enduring problem, one that stretches beyond the kinds of evidence science is now capable of delivering. Even the most cutting-edge science will have a difficult time reconciling all the potential forms of validity that have been proposed. In the case of psychiatric disorders, validity is not a single target, no matter how much some advocates might like it to be.

10

THE ENDLESS SEARCH FOR VALIDITY

The integration of science in *DSM-5* was, at best, incomplete. Although many observers explained this lack of integration in terms of prematurity, perhaps an even bigger obstacle surrounded the concept of validity itself. In debates regarding the *DSM*, the term "validity" is used frequently, usually in critical ways. Critics charge that the *DSM* employs "invalid" criteria and that it creates "false positives," an assertion premised on a precise definition of validity. By the same token, the idea of "true positives" involves a clear idea about what that "truth" is. Critics charge, too, that reliability is counterpoised against validity, specifically that the *DSM* achieves reliability only by sacrificing validity, so that even this limited and generally accepted success of the manual is ultimately artificial vis-à-vis what should be its most important goal.

Yet for all of validity's rhetorical significance, it is rarely debated outright. Furthermore, alternative frameworks for assessing validity are seldom evaluated against one another. Instead, the concept is reduced to the choice of a right *validator*, or the specific criterion used to evaluate validity. Only after committing to a criterion do claims of invalidity gain resonance. A researcher might decide, for instance, that a psychiatric disorder is valid only insofar as it has genetic causes. A different researcher might replace an emphasis on genes with one on brain regions, to much the same effect. That researcher would insist that psychiatric disorders must involve neuroanatomical dysfunctions and would therefore trim from the *DSM* those disorders that do not involve such dysfunctions. Yet in debating between one type of validator and another researchers often leave unaddressed larger questions regarding the most appropriate way to think about validity, and many of these questions are philosophical as much as scientific. In the abstract, scientists certainly agree on the value of validity—after all, who would tolerate an "invalid" definition, or support the proliferation of "false" positives, or fail to appreciate the identification of "true" positives—but they disagree vociferously about what constitutes validity.

The issue of validity is even more complicated, though. It is possible to imagine diagnostic criteria that yield positive results on multiple kinds of validators. Psychiatric disorders might involve genes and brain abnormalities, for instance, and a scientist could produce evidence linking a psychiatric disorder to both. Yet different concepts of validity are often pitched in competition with one another. To the extent that one conception of validity is seen as correct, it is also seen as obviating the relevance of another.[1] If, for instance, a researcher insists that real disorders must be genetic in origin, disorders that are plainly caused by environmental influences are seen as invalid, unless those environmental influences can be traced through genetic mutations or if they reveal the influence of the more significant genes.[2] If, by the same token, a researcher insists that real disorders involve brain abnormalities, then genetic influences are regarded as, at best, subordinate to identifying those abnormalities. More generally, then, to the extent that one definition of validity prevails, no other diagnostic criteria are regarded as necessary or, in some cases, even admissible.

It is easy to see why the debate has calcified along these lines, even if it has some complicated implications. If we regard psychiatric disorders as somehow existing in nature, then the discovery of the correct classification means no other taxonomies are necessary. Indeed, the intuition of a natural kind implies the possibility of perfect classification. The periodic table, for example, has no competition because it perfectly classifies the elements. When it comes to psychiatric disorders, though, it is difficult to discern a concept of validity that would satisfy everyone, even if everyone agrees that psychiatric disorders are real. To date, the controversy surrounding psychiatric diagnoses has been cloaked in terms of a search for "better" criteria and for more accurate ways to measure disorders. In this vein, researchers have eagerly sought more "objective" criteria, ones that are removed from the otherwise subjective experiences that count as symptoms. By the same token, criticisms of the *DSM* have revolved around how its diagnostic criteria have been contaminated by a variety of "external" influences. This idea is found, for instance, in concerns about pathologizing social deviance, wherein the influence of culture becomes apparent in something that should be purely medical. The move toward "objectivity" is seen as a necessary step toward limiting these and other outside considerations.

What, though, do scientists mean by *validity*? In general, validity refers to verisimilitude with something existing in nature. In psychiatry, the concept usually has a less philosophical meaning: It refers to the *measurement* of a concept, and the term is often used in the context of psychological testing.[3] A measure is said to be valid if it measures the concept it was intended to measure. In some areas, this is not terribly difficult. Sonar, for instance, can be used to measure the size of a fetus or a submarine, and its accuracy can be assessed by comparing sonar with the actual thing. In psychology, though, validity is more difficult to ascertain and risks circularity. Edwin Boring famously argued that intelligence—which, like mental illness, is a difficult concept to define—is "the capacity to do well in an intelligence test" or, simply, that intelligence "is what the tests test."[4] For concepts that cannot be observed directly, validity must be assessed through indirect means. For example, validity can be assessed by looking at how strongly the measure is related to other things known to be associated with the concept; this is referred to as criterion validity. A measure of depression, for example, gains validity if it can be correlated with levels of certain neurotransmitters, for example serotonin, known to be associated with the symptoms of depression. The concept of validity is complicated by the fact that reliability and validity are logically distinct. A test can be reliable without being valid, meaning it can produce a consistent measure of a concept that has no validity. But a test cannot be valid unless it is reliable. This is the essence of the problem for the *DSM*. The underlying philosophy of the *DSM* has been that psychiatrists, using the same criteria in a uniform way, should be able to render the same diagnosis reliably. The *DSM* has been relatively silent, though, on the issue of validity.

The underlying theory of validity for psychiatric disorders is sometimes stated directly, but it is more often implied. Even when authors proffer a definition of validity, they often spend little time justifying the criterion by which they argue validity should be assessed. Instead, they presuppose the dominance of their conception, thereby claiming other criteria are invalid relative to the criteria they prefer. To take one example, Horwitz and Wakefield advocate for the expansion of the bereavement exclusion, arguing that bereavement, as well as other loss-related events, can produce the symptoms of depression even when a real disorder is not present.[5] Context, then, is important in their view and should be included in diagnostic criteria in order to distinguish the real from the illusive. Their proposal is an entirely reasonable one. There are good reasons to expand the bereavement exclusion, especially if we fear overdiagnosis, as discussed in the preceding chapter. Yet in making the case, they emphasize the importance of validity per se. They are not simply proposing a practical revision or a conservative adjustment. They are proposing a definition they regard as closer to the truth. For them, then, the issue is less that bereavement could be mistakenly regarded as depression than the putative fact that, without the bereavement exclusion, the *DSM*'s criteria are entirely invalid. They emphasize this in several ways and highlight how others appear to agree with their approach. They argue, for example, that the diagnostic criteria for a major depressive disorder are "obviously invalid," that they are invalid "because they misclassify intense but naturally selected loss responses as disorders," that they are "invalid and encompass some conditions that should not be diagnosed as disorders," that they are "known to be invalid," and that it is "obvious" the *DSM* should exclude other negative reactions to events beyond bereavement.[6] They further highlight the frequency of false positives using existing diagnostic criteria, noting that the potential for false positives increases "exponentially" as the number of required symptoms decreases and, similarly, that the *DSM* criteria create the potential for an "unprecedented" number of false positives.[7] Yet judgments regarding what is "false" imply knowing for sure what is "true." According to the diagnostic criteria Wakefield and Horwitz prefer, the *DSM* criteria do indeed produce false positives. But the

DSM's criteria are only obviously invalid when the alternative criteria you prefer are obviously preferred by everyone else. Recognizing this, a good deal of Horwitz and Wakefield's book *The Loss of Sadness* centers on showing how conceptions of depression have changed over time. They use a range of literary and historical examples to make the case that modern society has lost the ability to appreciate normal sadness. Perhaps befitting the cycles of doubt and retrospection endemic to the field of psychiatry, Robert Spitzer provides an approving foreword to the book. Yet the community of users currently involved with the *DSM* is hardly univocal on the matter of what validity looks like. And if validity itself is not something all parties can agree on, the existence of false positives relative to one standard does not in itself reveal an obviously better way to think about things.

This is not to say that there are never formal discussions of validity wherein competing conceptions are entertained and debated. Nonetheless, the contested nature of validity is often obscured. In many cases, for example, utility is seen as tantamount to validity (and not just something to maximize). Robert Spitzer, for example, equates the two when he states that a diagnostic concept has validity when it provides "useful information not contained in the definition of the disorder," in particular regarding features such as etiology, risk factors, and prognosis.[8] He further states that this sort of information is especially valuable when it helps with treatment-related decisions. The *DSM* returns repeatedly to the importance of clinical utility, stressing the role of the manual in clinical practice.

Some scientists proffer alternative definitions of validity. Kendell and Jablensky provide an especially sharp contrast between the utility and validity of diagnostic criteria.[9] They correctly note that the *DSM* has much in the way of utility, but they push explicitly for more validity. For them, a diagnosis is valid only insofar as it has been shown to be produced by "discrete entities with natural boundaries that separate [the disorder] from other disorders."[10] They argue that their conception of validity is appropriate given the implicit disease-entity assumptions already contained in the *DSM*. Yet their proposal represents only one of many. The persistence of debate regarding the *DSM* in part reflects the coexistence of many potential conceptions of validity as well as the many different validators available within any of those conceptions. The debate becomes even more insoluble once we recognize that not all validators—even those consistent with the idea that at least a general class of influences, like biology, ought to be important—will agree with one another. Even the idea that an emphasis on clinical utility is acceptable only in lieu of a more ambitious definition of validity is misleading in the sense that an entirely valid definition of a psychiatric disorder might have very little clinical utility. It is important, then, to understand the entire universe of validators in order to understand what science can and cannot achieve as well as what clinicians and the public do or do not want.

THE UNIVERSE OF VALIDATORS

When researchers discuss validity, it is often as a prelude to selecting validators. Validators indicate how good a proposed diagnostic criterion matches a certain conception of validity.[11] The identification of genes, for instance, can validate a disorder if one regards genetic causes as essential to the definition of a disorder: In order to have depression, one must have the genes for depression. But the validators are not, in and of themselves, an argument for validity. Furthermore, a single definition of disorder can imply several different validators, but these validators need not reach the same conclusion. In that case, scientists must weigh validators in order to reach a decision, and doing so requires even more of a rationale. The RDoC, for instance, discusses multiple validators but places more emphasis on neural mechanisms because it regards mental illnesses as diseases of the brain. It is important, though, to understand the long history of different validators, not just what has prevailed in the early twenty-first century, as a way to understand the ongoing debate surrounding diagnostic criteria.

Perhaps the most influential framework for assessing validity was articulated more than forty years ago. Eli Robins and Samuel Guze developed their framework with respect to schizophrenia, and subsequent research extended that framework (or a very similar one) to other disorders.[12] Robins and Guze envisioned five phases for establishing validity, all based on systematic study. The idea of *phases* was critically important; Robins and Guze were not proposing some ultimate arbiter of validity that could settle matters once and for all but were suggesting a strategic unfolding of empirical research that could eventually yield more valid diagnostic instruments. The process, then, is one of refinement and self-correction rather than ex ante assumption. In the absence of a solid framework for guiding the process, they feared there would be no possibility of iterating toward a better model, so their proposed phases were central to their approach.

The first phase was clinical description, consisting primarily of a detailed portrayal of the symptoms of a disorder but also its demographic correlates and precipitating factors. The second phase was referred to as "laboratory studies," in reference to the tools the natural sciences had available at the time. In this phase, researchers looked for relevant biomarkers of the disorder, including anatomical and physiological tests. The third phase involved separating a disorder from others, which might appear similar but reflect different underlying dysfunctions. The fourth phase involved follow-up study, in order to allow scientists to evaluate whether people initially diagnosed with the same disorder had similar experiences over time, consistent with the idea that disorders are "homogenous" in their character. The fifth phase was the use of family studies. In effect, this phase elevated the importance of genetic influences, as it was assumed that a valid diagnosis would be one that "ran in the family." Diagnostic criteria that did not produce family aggregation would be regarded as suspect. The Robins and Guze framework has been enormously influential. Among other things, it was cited as the spirit guiding *DSM-5*'s scientific-review committee.[13]

Since its articulation the Robins and Guze framework has evolved, and, in particular, the importance of genes has been elevated. A contemporary version of the framework was articulated in the mid-1990s by Nancy Andreasen.[14] She begins first by noting the general failure of the laboratory tests Robins and Guze referred to, but she sees a better corollary in contemporary organ-based tests, including tests of neural abnormalities and molecular mechanisms. For her, the criteria of family aggregation was merely a more primitive placeholder for emphasizing specific genetic and neuroanatomical abnormalities, which, she notes, can now be ascertained directly and with precision. With this in mind, she recommends amending the Robins and Guze criteria with validators at the level of neural substrates. She refers to the branches of science that can provide these validators, including molecular genetics, neurochemistry, neuroanatomy, and cognitive neuroscience.[15] She states her goal plainly and is optimistic that her framework is already in place, albeit not articulated in precisely the terms she employs. Her goal, then, is "to make conscious the largely unconscious fact that this second program for validation is vigorously in progress."[16] She states, too, that the evidence emerging from this program will give mental illness a "powerful credibility" that it lacked before.[17]

SCIENCE AND JUDGMENT

The elevation of genes can be regarded as a natural outgrowth of the development of genetic research in the era of the human genome. The twenty-first century has provided scientists with a better opportunity to identify the kinds of influences they have long suspected are relevant. There is another way to read this development, however, a way less focused on innovation as the driving force. The history of psychiatric diagnosis is largely one of wavering tension between essentialists and nominalists.[18] Essentialists argue that real disorders are waiting to be discovered and correspond to entities that exist in nature. Nominalists, however, argue that psychiatric disorders are created and that nature provides no clues regarding the appropriate boundaries of a disorder. Disorders, then, must be a matter of judgment rather than of science. Although nominalists once had a prominent voice in psychiatry, essentialists have slowly dominated the discussion, in part because of the ascendance of the natural sciences. This ascendance is frequently cast as a victory over the error of nominalism. Yet in assuming more control over the debate—and under more plausibly essentialist terms—scientists have largely jettisoned serious discussions of choice, culture, and discretion. In hoping for an answer in the natural sciences, essentialists have neglected the ways in which the science of psychiatric diagnosis is informed by values, scientific and otherwise. Empirical data can provide answers to specific questions, as those questions are posed, but sometimes there is little agreement over what exactly are the right questions to ask. Psychiatric nosology is bound up in questions of evaluation that can be obscured but never obviated.

Consider the case of genetic research. Although evidence that a disorder is at least partly genetic is often interpreted as evidence that the disorder must be real, the substantive significance of heritability—and, indeed, of genetic influence writ large—is a matter of interpretation. For one, there is no necessary connection between genes and dysfunction per se. Genetic research has, in fact, demonstrated heritability for a wide variety of phenotypes, including church attendance, abortion attitudes, patriotism, and occupational attainment.[19] All these behaviors, traits, attitudes, and experiences are at least partly genetic, too, but that fact alone does not mean that any one of them is a *dysfunction* in a meaningful sense. In addition, dysfunctions often have an implied threshold, whereas many strongly heritable phenotypes do not. Height, for example, has a heritability around 60 to 80 percent, but that range provides no guidance regarding what we ought to regard as "tall" or "short." Even if we stick to the area of health, where there is evidence that a wide variety of diseases are at least partly and occasionally entirely genetic, accepting the claim that a disease *must* be genetic significantly narrows the range of problems medicine can and should treat. The connection between smoking and lung cancer, for example, is very real, but no one would regard the lung cancer of a smoker as less real because it was brought on by a behavior. The same low relevance applies to less fatal conditions. Type 2 diabetes can be caused by genetic factors and/or excess weight (among other things), but it requires treatment irrespective of the cause.

A further complication stems from the fact that heritability is a population-level statistic. Heritability is in reference to explaining *variation in a population*. It only speaks indirectly to whether a phenotype is genetically caused for an individual. Indeed, if there is no variation in a phenotype, heritability will shrink to zero, even if that phenotype is entirely genetic. For example, the fact that humans possess two legs is driven by genes. And two legs provide a clear fitness advantage, consistent with evolutionary theory. In developing embryos, genes provide the instructions that produce two legs, no more and no less. But precisely because there is no variation in the number of legs (apart from variation produced by environmental accidents), the heritability of the number of legs in humans is zero. By the same token, if a phenotype unequivocally produces a fitness advantage, nature should select that phenotype and eliminate variants that produce less of an advantage. If depression always and everywhere reduced fitness, for example, it would be eliminated by natural selection. The fact that there is still variation in depression implies that depression does not yield a clear fitness disadvantage under all conditions.

Genetic research is much more useful in providing insights regarding whether two or more disorders are genetically distinct, but even here decisions about the strength and relevance of these revealed distinctions are subject to judgment.[20] Genetic relatedness exists on a continuum. It is unlikely that any pair of disorders will overlap perfectly, especially given polythetic criteria, meaning clinicians will still have to decide at what point two disorders should be regarded as sufficiently related to be considered the same disorder. Even if we have information about the specific genes that are involved, as is increasingly the case, it is unclear whether ten or one hundred genes is the point at which we should conclude that two disorders are identical. Both of these decisions presuppose that genes are an appropriate arbiter of diagnostic independence (albeit a complicated one), but even this premise can be questioned. Psychiatric disorders are caused by many factors, including but not limited to genes. Moreover, many of these causes, whether social or biological, are related to multiple disorders simultaneously. Stressful life events, for example, are related to many different disorders that are, in fact, highly comorbid, including anxiety and depression. Yet few scientists would regard information on social influences as diagnostically relevant in the same way as genetic influences. Genetic influences are seen as dominant. The same sort of complication pertains to neurotransmitters, which are blind to the distinctions drawn in the *DSM*. One could decide that disorders that co-occur *for any reason* ought to be regarded as nosologically identical, but this is not the sort of framework science has pursued. Science has decided, instead, to focus on genes.

A similar binding emphasis pervades the harmful-dysfunction perspective. Here, too, there is only so much that science will be able to accomplish, especially because there are limits to how well science can test the underlying theory. Evolution is a scientific fact and a key principle of biology. It is impossible to understand organisms without it. It is difficult, however, to discern what a normal response to stress is based on intuitions regarding what evolution has equipped the mind with. It is also difficult to evaluate what level of sadness might be appropriate from a fitness standpoint. Recall that Wakefield's harmful-dysfunction perspective stipulates two things: that a disorder must be harmful and that it must reflect a dysfunction. The idea of harm is not as controversial—even here, though, there are some very real controversies, as I will discuss shortly—but the notion of dysfunction has certainly proven much trickier. Wakefield would like the concept to be purely scientific, based on the theory of evolution. In this vein, Wakefield argues that dysfunction should be defined as the failure of a system to function in the fashion for which it was intended, according to evolution. Especially when it comes to psychological functions, though, it is difficult to assess functionality backward in time. In particular, it is difficult to discern the purposes of natural selection when functions are performed in current environments but were evolved in environments that prevailed millennia earlier. Some functions are seemingly straightforward, which is part of the appeal of evolution for those interested in articulating a more essentialist framework. Nature might have selected opposable thumbs, for example, because they permit gripping. But psychological functions are much more difficult to evaluate. It is difficult to see what *harm* could come from opposable thumbs, certainly, but many psychological functions involve complex and concatenated effects. One could even argue that, under some conditions, depression is a helpful response and is, therefore, functional. Depression diminishes motivation, which would seem to undermine fitness and produce real harm. Depression can also lead to suicide, which is a direct expression of fitness. These are real aspects of the disorder. But another interpretation of depression is that its symptoms provide a signal to the individual to stop engaging with the current environment and begin searching for alternatives, whether with respect to finding more fertile soil, avoiding predators, or, in a more modern vein, searching for a different job or spouse. In a similar but more abstract vein, Paul Andrews and Anderson Thomson focus on the role of depression in solving complex problems.[21] Depression has several "active ingredients" in this regard, all of which can be set in motion by challenging environments: Complex social problems trigger depression; rumination focuses attention on that problem, encouraging a slow and methodical approach to solving it; anhedonia reduces the desire to engage in other activities, which might ordinarily produce pleasure and divert attention from the difficult problem at hand; and a lack of energy prevents exposure to new stimuli that might also be distracting. To be sure, rumination is often painful and intrusive, and anhedonia is not pleasant by definition, but these experiences do not mean depression serves no positive function at all.

Further complicating matters is the fact that many features of the mind are unlikely to be a direct consequence of natural selection.[22] To the extent that the genes related to depression, for example, reside in close proximity to the genes related to more plainly adaptive traits, the genes for depression will persist despite affording no obvious fitness advantage with respect to that one phenotype. Research thus far suggests that even for a single psychiatric disorder the genes related to that disorder are usually spread widely over the genome. Similarly, some features of the mind might evolve for one function but serve another; this is termed exaptation. A variety of seemingly evolved physical functions can be more correctly characterized as co-opted exaptations. Bones, for example, might have initially evolved as a way to store minerals effectively when organisms moved to fresh water, but they later served as a means of body support when those organisms moved to land.[23] It is possible that mental functions even more than physical functions have this character. Indeed, at least one biologist characterized the vast majority of cognitive functions as exaptations rather than strict adaptations.[24] The brain is complex. Its large size provides humans with the capacity for a variety of complex skills, including speech, but the brain might have grown for an entirely different evolutionary reason. Still another possibility, one that implies even more difficulty in discerning evolutionary intent, is that the genes related to depression, for instance, might confer some advantage earlier in life, like sensitivity to the environment, even though they confer considerable risk later on. Evolution is based on the fitness value of genes during reproductive ages, but the average age of onset for major depression is in the late twenties and early thirties, beyond at least the first part of the human reproductive window.

There are even more difficulties in relying on evolution as a guide. Evolution does little to address dimensionality, at least in a clean way. Some evolved morphological features are either present or absent, but evolution is entirely comfortable with complexity. It can produce experiences that are adaptive at low levels but maladaptive at higher ones. Fear, for instance, might be selected in order to spark the flight response. When a mortal threat makes us anxious or fearful, we avoid it and, thereby, prevent injury or death. That avoidance is functional. But one could push the point, as Wakefield has. One could argue that such a response is functional *only to a point* and that evolution never intended the fear response to persist long after the situation that elicited it has passed. At that point, we might regard the fear response as dysfunctional, in the fashion Wakefield encourages. Yet this, too, reveals the importance of judgment more than the designs of nature. Nature does not provide us with answers regarding the appropriate duration of fear or anxiety. Sometimes the answer might be obvious, but that does not make the answer natural. Nor does nature provide us with answers regarding the appropriate length of, for example, mourning. Perhaps recognizing this, Wakefield frequently appeals to "common sense" as an appropriate framework for evaluating the functionality of disorders. In *The Loss of Sadness*, for instance, Horwitz and Wakefield point to some evidence regarding dysfunction and evolution but ultimately lean on "commonsense judgment" to distinguish real disorders from false ones.[25] Commonsense judgment and evolutionary intent are very different things. Returning to our earlier example, natural selection might have produced two legs in humans—as two legs provide more balance than one and also conserve more calories than four—but when it comes to mental functions, natural selection does not provide a uniform value for the optimal level of happiness, anxiety, and fear.[26] In fact, when presented with complex social and ecological environments, evolution might produce *variation* rather iterate toward a single value.[27] In many things, nature has left us to our own devices.

In this vein, Daniel Nettle outlines a framework in which natural selection yields heritable variation in personality as a tradeoff between different fitness costs and benefits when there is no perfect optimum across all environments and situations. Different dimensions of personality have complex relationships with fitness (and Nettle focuses only on the major dimensions of personality, though the logic could be applied to other psychological characteristics). Extraversion, for instance, is positively associated with fitness insofar as it is related to the number of sexual partners (among other things). Yet it also increases exposure to risk. Neuroticism is associated with many psychiatric disorders, as well as with impaired physical health, and, therefore, might reduce fitness. Yet neuroticism is also a form of psychological vigilance and sensitivity, which might help in avoiding predation in especially dangerous environments. Conscientiousness involves a high degree of self-control and is positively related to life expectancy (routine visits to the gym can be boring, but they are beneficial). Yet conscientiousness might also inhibit people from discovering new opportunities. If across these many different dimensions of personality there is no single optimal value, especially as a set of dimensions, nature might prefer variation. Under some conditions, neuroticism might be beneficial, but a short while later, it might lose that benefit. Under these conditions, natural selection might create or at least preserve variation in personality. In other words, natural selection will not winnow the dimensions of personality down to an optimum, as it might the number of legs. It is up to us, then, to decide where dysfunction lies in the sea of variation.

The harmful-dysfunction framework necessitates even more judgment insofar as it also invokes the concept of a "proportionate" response to an environmental stressor. A proportionate response necessarily involves considering the person's particular situation and what a normal response to that situation should be. Here, too, natural selection does not provide an answer regarding what to expect. In fact, natural selection might (again) favor a wide variety of responses. In this case, though, Wakefield has a clear sense of what a proportionate response is. His view is reasonable. Minor setbacks should not be disturbing, he argues. They might lead to disappointment, sure, but they should not lead to outright despondency. He provides other examples, all in the same vein. And while these examples are all sensible, his interpretation of the concept of proportionality is less scientific than normative. Rendering a decision about whether a person is responding in an appropriate fashion is, in the end, a judgment. Furthermore, the concept of proportionality ultimately requires the input of a clinician, since it is articulated with respect to a person and not, at least easily, in a set of uniform diagnostic criteria.

It is also difficult to discern from a scientific perspective when a disorder is with or without cause. I discussed this difficulty earlier, but it is instructive to revisit this discussion in reference to what science has discovered with respect to the actual causes of depression. Much of the "with cause" discussion centers on bereavement. This is an understandable focus given the severity of the event, but it is also a bit too easy, given other characteristics of the experience. The death of a loved one is easy to demarcate. The event happens at a specific time to a person with whom one had a specific relationship. Lots of events, though, are not so easy to recall, define, or date. And even bereavement can be complicated, in the sense that the death of a spouse, for example, is often preceded by a long period of deteriorating health. In the same vein, chronic stress—as opposed to eventful stress—has a very strong relationship with the symptoms of depression, but it is generally impossible to demarcate, even as a span of time. Further complicating matters is the nature of depression as a cognitive phenomenon. Among its other aspects, depression distorts memory, leading depressed persons to recall different life events than nondepressed persons. Yet scientific research on depression depends to some degree on the accuracy of self-reports. Precisely because depression shapes perceptions and retrospection it is often difficult to discern the degree to which depression is brought on by stressful life events or reflects cognitive phenomena moving in the other direction. In one study, for example, students induced to feel mild depression reported more negative life events and lower social support than did students made to feel happy.[28] This makes the measurement of stress difficult, at a minimum, but it actually has deeper implications. Real depression can conjure its own causes, disguised as aspects of the external environment.

A different sort of problem stems from having multiple potential validators. Even if scientists agree on what the appropriate set of validators is, there is no guarantee that all the elements they select will yield the same result.[29] For instance, scientists might decide that valid psychiatric disorders involve a family history and have a poor prognosis, assuming, then, that psychiatric disorders are genetic and chronic. Yet there are many instances in which these two validators will not align. Schizophrenia is a strongly heritable disorder, for example, but there are different subtypes of the disorder, some of which have a good prognosis and others of which do not.[30] Of course, a researcher might then conclude that only one type of schizophrenia is real, but that revised definition will exclude many cases of schizophrenia that are at least strongly genetic (not to mention disabling). Similarly, major depression can emerge even in individuals who lack the most significant risk alleles. Yet regardless of the genetic profile of those suffering from it, major depression is strongly related to disability. In fact, the heritability of major depression is lower than that of many other psychiatric disorders, even though it is among the most disabling.[31] ADHD presents a different problem. It is nearly as heritable as schizophrenia, but it is also highly sensitive to developmental influences and will often remit.[32] In these cases, what should researchers do? Should they regard one validator as more important? Should they seek other validators instead?

Even assessing harm can be difficult. Although there is still a great deal of scientific controversy regarding the causes of psychiatric disorders, the harm associated with them would seem to be indisputable. Psychiatric disorders cost jobs, productivity, relationships, and sometimes lives. Furthermore, some disorders are more harmful than others, suggesting places where the *DSM* could be trimmed. And there is a good deal of granular scientific information when it comes to harm, which is precisely the sort of data those interested in taxonomic improvements look for. There are numerous complications, however. For one, the harm associated with psychiatric disorders does not always stem purely from the disorder itself. Because those who suffer from psychiatric disorders also tend to suffer from physical disorders, allocating what part of their disability comes from the psychiatric side is often very difficult.[33] Furthermore, the harm caused by a psychiatric disorder depends a great deal on the environment the person finds herself in. Depending on the type of job someone has, for instance, major depression may be more or less detrimental to productivity. This complexity might be regarded as an acceptable form of inconsistency, and it might also be something worth specifying in the diagnostic criteria themselves. Yet it also introduces a paradox for those interested in identifying natural kinds: Emphasizing the harm caused by a disorder and setting its parameters in a more specific and contingent way will necessarily move diagnostic criteria away from the characteristics of the disorder to the characteristics of the person, something that is not consistent with thinking about disorders as natural kinds.

An even more elementary concern pertains to the *object* of harm. Using the concept of harm requires judgments not only about whether the psychiatric disorder impairs some ability, which is at least partly an empirical question, but also what abilities we value. Sigmund Freud emphasized the role of psychoanalysis in allowing the person to engage better in the essential tasks of life, which he regarded as work and love.[34] Although Freud's version of psychoanalysis is less influential today than it was during his lifetime, his framing of the goals of treatment remains close to the modern approach. In fact, science has adopted a definition of harm that is not at all inconsistent with his formulation. When scientists study disability, for example, they do so in terms of a set of specific capacities that are potentially affected by health. One popular instrument for measuring disability is the World Health Organization Disability Adjustment Schedule (WHO-DAS).[35] The instrument asks questions regarding the amount of difficulty a person experiences in six different domains: understanding and communicating; getting around, including basic mobility and endurance; self-care, such as bathing, eating, and getting dressed; getting along with other people; performance in various activities and settings, including at work, home, and school; and participation in society, including joining community activities. Other disability instruments are more narrowly focused but still involve performance in specific domains rather than general capacities. Another popular way to measure disability, for example, is simply in terms of the number of days in the last month in which the person's health problem impaired his ability to work, either reducing his productivity or forcing him to forgo work altogether. Psychiatric disorders have been shown to affect all of these things, often quite strongly. Indeed, the effect of psychiatric disorders on disability often exceeds that of physical disorders.[36] From this finding, some scientists have concluded that psychiatric disorders are, indeed, harmful and, therefore, must be valid. But accepting this interpretation—based on a fact—requires accepting that there are certain things individuals ought to be able to do. This, again, makes psychiatric disorders different. A shellfish allergy, for example, is a real condition—it can be accurately characterized at the level of biochemical reactions to a certain protein found in shellfish—but most of us would not regard the condition as "disabling" insofar as consuming shellfish is not essential to a well-lived life. In the case of psychiatric disorders, though, science has stipulated certain values regarding what it means to be an active and well-functioning person. It has concluded that harm involves impairment in routine daily activities and productive endeavors, and it has elevated certain values with respect to those activities. Science, for example, has elevated the importance of *social* experiences insofar as most dimensions of the WHO-DAS involve activities at the intersection of the person and his or her social world. Science has also elevated the importance of *external* evaluations above *internal* ones. It is possible to evaluate disability in terms of what each individual values and thus to ask people, for example, whether their depression impairs their ability to engage in a hobby they love rather than a job they might not. Yet the WHO-DAS conventionally assigns the same weight to each domain across all individuals. The merits of this practice are debatable—some scientists prefer a bit more relativity, and the WHO-DAS can, in principle, accommodate that preference—but at a minimum the conventional practice reveals the implied relevance of values. Facts are ordinarily held to exist independent of values, but in providing facts about the harm caused by psychiatric disorders—for example, major depression leads to about half a day of work loss per month—scientists necessarily reveal something about values, too.[37]

COMPETITION AMONG SCIENTIFIC FRAMEWORKS

Another way to think about different validators is to think about competition among scientific frameworks. Psychiatric disorders are complex phenotypes. It is difficult to argue that they are *entirely* biological or *entirely* social. But if we accept, for the moment, that a more valid diagnostic system will ultimately be one informed by innovations in genetics and neuroscience, perhaps in tandem with the social sciences, it is still worth considering what a more "essentialist" framework of this sort might cost us. Moving toward more biologically informed diagnostic criteria can be misleading if the character of the object being studied is not well established in the first place. And the same is true, it should be said, of more *socially* informed diagnostic criteria. Biological reductionism can be problematic, but it is the *reduction* that matters more than the biology per se.

A biological view is perhaps especially misleading, though, from the standpoint of symptoms. Scientists addressing the question of validity often take the symptoms of a disorder as given. The problem in doing this is that any explanation that might be consistent at the level of the entire syndrome need not be consistent at the level of discrete symptoms. Genetic research, for example, often focuses on discerning genetic influences related to a major depressive episode *as a diagnostic category*. Yet the genes related to a major depressive episode need not be the same as the genes related to that episode's individual symptoms, including depressed mood, fatigue, weight loss, insomnia, and so on. This partly reflects the fact that the diagnostic criteria for a major depressive episode do not, in fact, *require* insomnia or weight loss, so scientists studying major depression are, in effect, forced to uncover genes that will lead to weight loss in some people but not in others. A moving target is hard to hit. Yet the problem is much bigger. There are, in fact, very few genetic mechanisms capable of explaining *all* the symptoms that compose a syndrome. Moreover, the symptoms that make up a syndrome are probably connected to one another through pathways that stretch well beyond the influence of genes. There are many real causes of psychiatric disorders that cross different levels of explanation, from the genetic, to the neurological, to the psychological, to the behavioral, to the environmental.[38] In considering the significance of this problem, it is instructive to consider, again, the case of a major depressive episode, which can involve a variety of things, including fatigue, diminished ability to concentrate, changes in weight, and feelings of worthlessness. It is easy to imagine a biological substrate governing either fatigue, impaired cognition, or diet (in fact, all these things can be studied independent of a psychiatric disorder). Yet it is also easy to imagine processes that connect these psychological symptoms, as when feelings of worthlessness lead to undereating and, in turn, to weight loss and an inability to concentrate. The many plausible connections between cognition, behavior, and physiology render it difficult to envision an explanation that resides *entirely* at one level, whether genetic, neuroanatomical, or social.

The current focus on endophenotypes is, in part, an attempt to circumvent this issue. The idea of an endophenotype directs researchers to look for more abstract phenotypes that span many systems and symptoms. In the context of major depression, for example, some endophenotypes that have been proposed include a cognitive bias toward negative moods, a diminished ability to derive pleasure and reward, impaired learning and memory, and increased stress sensitivity.[39] All of these endophenotypes are thought to be related to numerous symptoms of depression at the same time. A bias toward negative moods, for instance, might be related to depressed mood, diminished interest or pleasure, and feelings of worthlessness. An even cleaner set of endophenotypes has been proposed with respect to obsessive-compulsive disorder. At least according to some frameworks, the disorder might simply reflect the failure of certain cognitive systems that ordinarily inhibit impulsive behavior.[40]

All these efforts are promising, especially for being synthetic. Yet for those interested in crafting better diagnostic criteria, they still present problems. Although the heritability of many of these endophenotypes is quite high, their actual genetic architecture is nearly as complex as that of traditionally defined psychiatric disorders.[41] In fact, the effects of specific genes on endophenotypes are generally no bigger than that of specific genes on psychiatric disorders. At the same time, endophenotypes generally have effects that cut across disorders. Of course, this might be regarded as a *strength* of endophenotypes rather than a limitation, especially from the standpoint of those who advocate for a radical pruning of the *DSM*, one that moves toward more elemental deficits in functioning. To this end, endophenotypes could help in efforts to create a manual with far fewer disorders. One could imagine, for instance, a new disorder being developed around the idea of a bias toward negative moods, obviating the need for a whole host of mood disorders and perhaps many anxiety disorders as well. Nevertheless, there are still many disorders that do not have an obvious endophenotype associated with them that clinicians would be loath to discard. The strongest evidence for an underlying endophenotype is limited to ADHD, alcoholism, anxiety, autism, bipolar disorder, depression, and schizophrenia.[42]

There are other ways scientists have considered the issue of validity. One way to think about disorders that are essential rather than nominal is in terms of evolutionary counterfactuals. In this case, the question to ask is: If evolution could be restarted and run again multiple times, what sorts of disorders would appear consistently?[43] According to this idea, we should only consider those disorders that reappear every time. Repeated disorders are real—in effect, part of human nature—whereas the rest are merely artifacts of random fluctuations, something that could be eliminated under different environmental conditions. This approach would, thus, eliminate what have been called *conditionalities*.[44] If fear, for example, is an evolved response that promotes fitness in hostile environments, anxiety disorders might emerge repeatedly because the environment of a hospitable planet is consistently threatening. On the other hand, if the nature of gender identity fluctuates over time, space, and geography, gender identity disorders might be discarded. For some critics, this framework would rightly deflate considerations of culture and social deviance in favor of an emphasis on evolved dispositions and natural kinds.

Although the logic of this thought experiment is compelling, there are still reasons we might want to retain conditionalities, even *deeply* conditional disorders. And on this point, too, science provides compelling evidence. Some very serious and uncontroversial disorders are, in fact, highly conditional, both in when they are recognized and how they present. At this point in time virtually everyone agrees, for example, that post–traumatic stress disorder (PTSD) is a potentially devastating disorder. The controversy surrounding PTSD, such as it is, is nowhere near as piqued as the controversy surrounding the bereavement exclusion, and it rarely centers on the question of whether the disorder is real. But it has not always been this way. The acceptance of PTSD was conditioned by history. It was largely with the emergence of PTSD-like symptoms in veterans of foreign wars that the condition became widely recognized as a disorder. The disorder was first codified in *DSM-III*, shortly after the Vietnam War, although clinicians apprehended the basic elements of the disorder much earlier in the century, especially following World War I. In the experiences of returning veterans, clinicians witnessed the symptoms necessary to appreciate the experience as a sickness. "Shell shock" and "battle fatigue," as they were then known, were eventually transformed into the formal nomenclature of PTSD. The putative reality of the disorder was supported by widespread agreement that the underlying stressor was severe. And it was further supported by being evident in a sympathetic group. Veterans exposed themselves to trauma in defense of the country, and some suffered as a result. For this group at least, clinicians saw little reason to debate whether the response to combat was proportionate.

Subsequent research has complicated matters. For example, the symptoms of PTSD do not require *direct* exposure to trauma, nor do they require exposure to especially severe and unusual experiences like combat. The terrorist attacks on Manhattan on September 11, 2001, for example, greatly affected those in and near the Twin Towers, as expected given the nature of the event. Yet they also affected those who had no direct experience with the attacks and were not living in close proximity. About 4 percent of those with no direct exposure to the attacks nonetheless developed PTSD.[45] Research further demonstrated how even indirect effects had a deep reach. The frequency of exposure to 9/11 images, for example, was positively associated with the symptoms of PTSD two to three years after the event.[46] These effects occurred even after controlling for the presence of psychiatric disorders prior to 9/11, suggesting that the effects of image exposure were not driven by the possibility that those who already suffered from a psychiatric disorder were merely responding to the new traumas they were seeing on television. Findings of this sort can be extended in provocative ways. The proliferation of handheld devices suggests the symptoms of PTSD can now spread even faster than they did in 2001, as there are more opportunities for seeing traumatic images frequently and, if one is so inclined, seeking them out.

PTSD is even more conditional, though. The presentation of PTSD symptoms has varied greatly over time. Studies have gone back into historical records to explore the manifestation of PTSD in different eras, assuming that if PTSD is a natural kind it should manifest in a similar way.[47] In testing this idea, studies have explored the case files of UK servicemen. These files, available from the 1850s onward, provide an unusually long window of high-quality data. The time period covers a number of foreign conflicts, and because servicemen were awarded pensions for postcombat disorders, the records contain detailed information for adjudicating the merits of their claims, including comprehensive records of their symptoms. Little of this evidence, however, suggests that PTSD is a timeless natural kind with an ordered and regular presentation. The symptoms of PTSD vary a great deal, for instance, depending on the war. Although flashbacks were common among Gulf War veterans, they were rare among World War I and II veterans. In addition, the ability of clinicians to detect PTSD has varied over time. The case files suggest that some World War I and II veterans were clearly suffering from *something*, but they also indicate that many of these veterans would probably not meet the contemporary diagnostic criteria for PTSD because they rarely experienced the disorder's primary symptoms: exaggerated startle response and social avoidance. In this light, some scientists have provocatively concluded that PTSD is—despite all claims and assumptions to the contrary— a "culture-bound syndrome" that reflects the "continually evolving picture of human reaction" to trauma and adversity.[48]

The *DSM* criteria for PTSD have been revised in ways that reflect some of these research findings, but at the same time they have been revised in ways that will increase the prevalence of the disorder. Indeed, for critics of the *DSM*, the revision of the criteria for PTSD provides an especially vivid example of "conceptual bracket creep," defined as broadening some aspect of the diagnostic criteria so as to admit more disorders.[49] It is not at all clear, however, that revisions of this sort are inappropriate or that they would not pass a scientific review. In *DSM-III*, the diagnostic criteria for PTSD stipulated that the disorder could only result from direct exposure to a relatively small set of events, ones that are "generally outside the range of usual human experience."[50] To illustrate the point, *DSM-III* listed specific examples, including military combat, death camps, torture, rape, and airplane crashes. Subsequent editions of the manual, however, expanded the criteria considerably, including direct experiences with a broader set of traumas, witnessing trauma experienced by someone else, and being exposed to information related to trauma that was experienced by someone else.[51] These revisions were not made lightly. They were made in light of evidence much like that regarding 9/11. Nevertheless, these revisions have strong implications. The revised criteria imply that virtually everyone has experienced some sort of traumatic event in their lifetime. One study, for example, estimated that about 90 percent of adults had experienced at least one trauma in their lifetime as defined by the *DSM*.[52] The same study found that the effects of traumatic events on PTSD were not equivalent. The effects were smaller when traumatic events included witnessing trauma relative to when traumatic events were restricted to direct exposure. But "made smaller" does not mean "eliminated altogether." Even when traumatic events were defined as merely learning about an event, the risk of subsequently developing PTSD was not zero. In fact, just under 40 percent of PTSD cases diagnosed under the expanded criteria were brought on by the set of events added to the original criteria.[53]

A similar contingency applies to bulimia and anorexia. Although bulimia is strongly shaped by biological factors, it is also influenced by cultural considerations. The rise of thin as the ideal body type, for example, led to an increase in bulimia in the United States.[54] In the absence of such an ideal, the prevalence of bulimia would almost certainly be lower than it is now, although perhaps not zero. Furthermore, anorexia has crossed cultural borders as the thin ideal has migrated.[55] The prevalence of anorexia has increased sharply in Hong Kong, for example, which some attribute to the Westernization of the region, including the ascendance of a Western ideal body type. These contingencies are difficult to ignore. If evolution could be replayed, anorexia might recur in every instance, at least to some degree. Indeed, some argue that anorexia evolved as an adaptive mechanism to facilitate migration in response to famine.[56] The same perspective, though, notes that the *decision to diet* is different from the evolved dimensions of anorexia. The decision to diet is determined by social and psychological factors. For this reason, it is doubtful anorexia, even if evolutionary in origin, would appear in precisely the same place at precisely the same time in every run of evolution. Evolution establishes the risk but not the actuality. Complex evolutionary frameworks of this sort complicate how we evaluate disorders. At a minimum, evaluating whether we prefer essential disorders (that will consistently recur over multiple iterations of evolution) to contingent ones (that will vary greatly depending on cultural considerations) requires debate about what degree of contingency we are willing to tolerate (or even embrace), not just whether it is apparent at all.

Culture is relevant in another way. In some eras, culture can produce symptoms that have at least some precedent in other disorders but assume such an unusual form that they would be difficult to identify without allowing for conditionalities. In this vein, Joel Gold and Ian Gold describe the emergence of a new form of psychosis, referred to as the "Truman Show delusion," wherein the person believes he is being filmed and that others are watching the footage for their own entertainment.[57] The name of the delusion is in reference to the 1998 film of the same name, in which the character Truman Burbank is unaware he is living in a reality-television show. The idea, however, is more general and does not depend on the movie itself. The idea is that modern culture has produced technologies that create a form of delusion that is entirely contingent on those technologies. In the case of the Truman Show delusion, the delusion is a product of low-cost home-video recording that can be easily broadcast and consumed. In this vein, research has found that watching a large amount of reality television, especially when coupled with a desire to feel self-important, increases the risk of the disorder. Associated characteristics include other fears, such as living in an artificial environment wherein other people are playing a role and not acting as themselves. The emergence of this delusion challenges the ability of scientists to identify the core features of psychosis. To be sure, delusions of persecution, a sense of grandiosity, and a fear of a lack of privacy are not unique to the twenty-first century (or to television viewers, for that matter). And, in principle, it is possible to craft *DSM* criteria that are sufficiently abstract to capture accurately the *form* of the delusion if not always the *content*. Yet relaxing the diagnostic criteria in this fashion reintroduces a different problem: It reduces the clinical utility of the *DSM* and invites more diagnoses insofar as the criteria would necessarily rely on more abstract concepts, as discussed earlier. If clinicians are instructed only to evaluate "delusions," they might have a more difficult time doing so than if instructed on the specific potential content of those delusions. Those interested in adapting the *DSM* to the times argue that, in order to be maximally useful, the *DSM*'s criteria should reflect the content of delusions that prevail at a particular cultural moment. Of course, however, those who wish to purge the *DSM* of conditionalities resist precisely these sorts of recommendations.

As this discussion implies, there are strong and weak arguments regarding the influence of culture. The case of psychosis could be interpreted as a sort of middle ground insofar as it suggests culture provides the veneer through which the underlying psychosis is made legible. If so, culture is powerful, to be sure, but under the right conditions the entity of psychosis would perhaps be apparent without having to detail the content of the delusions of those who suffer from it. There are, however, stronger cultural arguments that render the task of adequate description even more difficult. Some argue that culture is so powerful as to produce disorders that have no natural counterpart in history, that emerge entirely de novo at a particular point in time. Ian Hacking recounts episodes of what he calls "transient mental illness," including epidemics of hysteria and fugue in late nineteenth-century France.[58] Both historical episodes can be considered epidemics in the sense that they affected a large number of people (in this case, mostly men). Yet both also quickly faded from view. The *fugueur* (or "mad traveler") experienced a compulsion to travel, with seemingly no motivation or destination. The wandering itself was often harmful, in that the person wandered through inclement weather and other environmental hazards, often to the point of physical exhaustion. In addition, the fugueur was not conscious in the usual sense and later awoke with little sense of how he got to where he was. With this as an illustration, Hacking argues for strong conditionalities. He argues that the fugueur emerged and was sustained by a confluence of factors that were only apparent at the time. Fugueurs first appeared as the possibility of travel grew, and it was coupled with an idea about what travel meant. At the time, to wander was regarded as a way to discover one's identity. As Hacking emphasizes, these were novel cultural developments, and they were abetted by a medical system that was increasingly inclined to name and diagnose symptoms. In addition, the men who suffered from the compulsion often fit a certain psychodemographic profile, lending itself to a seemingly coherent interpretation of the disease. The men were of high income but felt trapped by work or family and, thus, wandered as means of release from their normal obligations. Providing further support for Hacking's argument, the disorder was more prevalent in places where these social and historical influences were stronger, thus affecting men in France but not in the United States. Although it is possible to regard the fugueur through a contemporary lens—to see it as a form of epilepsy, for instance, or as an aspect of multiple personality, or as a type of dissociation—the appearance of this precise disorder, with its specific symptoms, was, in fact, unique to the time.

One risk of seeking only disorders that will withstand multiple runs of evolution is that highly conditional disorders of this type will be overlooked. To be sure, with the benefit of hindsight, we do regard some old psychiatric disorders as errors, as artifacts of a mistaken, superstitious, or bigoted set of beliefs or as misapprehensions of the real problem. And we might regard fugueurs in this fashion. Certainly there is no reason to include "mad travelers" in *DSM-5*. But a fear of repeating past mistakes should not encourage us to discard all disorders that might appear grounded in historical or cultural contingencies. Some disorders are, in fact, entirely modern. They emerge only in certain cultures and at certain times. Other disorders are more biological but, even so, only become legible through the idioms a culture provides. To the extent that the scientific project of biological essentialism is accepted under strictly reductionist terms, psychiatry forsakes the possibility of identifying transient disorders that nonetheless cause real suffering.

THE PROBLEM OF CONSCIOUSNESS

One roadblock to developing completely satisfying diagnostic criteria is more elementary: The core symptoms of many psychiatric disorders are *subjective*. Consider the case of depression. Sadness is a central feature of depression, but it resides in the mind of the individual. It is something the person experiences, and it reflects beliefs about who he or she is. Sadness, of course, is something the individual can report to a clinician, but there is very little to corroborate those reports. Depression, then, is irreducibly a disease of consciousness. This distinguishes psychiatric disorders from many other forms of illness. Blood pressure, for example, can be measured, and, in fact, high blood pressure is generally symptomless. For this reason, individuals cannot apprehend hypertension without some tool that provides them with objective measurements. Diagnosis requires some form of technological mediation. Treatment is the same. The treatment of hypertension requires no subjective awareness of its efficacy. It can be successful regardless of whether the individual experiences any reduction in his or her symptoms. The experience, identification, and treatment of depression, though, begins and ends in the mind. The treatment of depression cannot be regarded as completely successful if the individual is still sad.

From the standpoint of science and medicine, the problem with human consciousness is twofold. First, it is difficult for researchers to study depression as a pure experience without also studying all the other things associated with depression.[59] In other areas of behavioral research, animal models have been a highly productive research strategy because they permit an unusual degree of control. Studying depression in humans demands more. To be sure, scientists can study some aspects of depression in animals, especially mice, but these are not perfect analogues to depression in humans.[60] It is possible, for example, to induce learned helplessness in mice through difficult obstacles or by forcing them to swim. In addition, mice can be made to fear certain stimuli, as when scientists shock a mouse following an auditory tone.[61] In addition, mice can be put in unfamiliar environments to explore responses to novelty, and bonds between parents and offspring can be severed to explore responses to stress.[62] All these research strategies can inform our understanding of depression, but it is unclear whether the psychological experience of mice is truly the same as the human experience of depression. At best these studies explore concepts related to depression, such as stress reactivity and uncertainty, but their ability to speak to the entire syndrome of depression is limited.

The second problem with consciousness pertains to the credibility of self-reports and, relatedly, to whom or what we grant the authority of insight. Patient reports of symptoms are an inescapable feature of psychiatric diagnosis. And, to be sure, many of the symptoms of psychiatric disorders are reportable experiences. With little psychological acumen, a person can report sadness, anxiety, and the content of delusions because they are eminently available to awareness. Yet there are circumstances under which we might doubt the veracity of such reports, and, in any case, consciousness is internal and private. At times, for instance, individuals might be loath to admit sadness, especially given the stigma surrounding psychiatric disorders. For some people, depression is a sign of weakness. Furthermore, some people, especially children, might lack the ability to articulate their symptoms verbally. The *DSM* explicitly allows for this possibility by noting that certain symptoms have behavioral corollaries, thereby allowing other people to report symptoms on a patient's behalf. In this sense, the *DSM* expands the range of admissible symptoms beyond that of verbal self-reports. Yet for some symptoms the *experience* of the symptom is the symptom itself.[63] And, for this reason, the authority of others to report on a symptom is unclear. If a parent reports depression in a child but a child denies that depression, the clinician must weigh the credibility of both sides of the testimony. Similarly, the behavioral aspects of a psychiatric disorder will usually be secondary to its psychological aspects, even if the *DSM* puts both on the same plain. If other people infer sadness by virtue of someone's behavior but the person does not in fact experience any sadness, we ought to disregard those behaviors as relevant. Behaviors have many causes. Weight loss and insomnia, for example, are behavioral aspects of depression by definition but can occur for many reasons apart from depression. Bizarre delusions are the most heavily weighted symptom of schizophrenia, and, even if delusions motivate behavior, schizophrenia is impossible to diagnose without assessing the logic and plausibility of a person's stated beliefs.[64] At this point there is no technology that provides an impartial intermediary. Neuroimaging provides information on the location of certain functions of the mind, but many psychiatric disorders likely exist as higher-order functions, cutting across regions of the brain. Even if neuroimaging demonstrates some apparent location of sadness—something current technology in fact permits—this location is unlikely to be determinative of the experience of depression. To be sure, brain scans are important for some clinical questions, especially those for which local traces of activity are relevant. They are useful, for example, in detecting signs of consciousness in nonresponsive patients.[65] But determining whether an otherwise unresponsive person is conscious is a simpler assessment than evaluating whether someone is depressed. If a brain scan reveals activity in the area corresponding to sadness but the individual credibly does not report any sadness, we might not regard that person as sad.

The third problem with consciousness is related but might be even more intractable. In addition to being problems of the brain, psychiatric disorders are problems of experience. Consciousness is a complex phenomenon. It entails the full stream of intertwined moment-to-moment events. Sadness, for instance, is not experienced as a single object that might be part of one's awareness at any one time.[66] Consciousness involves many other experiences and is set in narrative form, so sadness is not experienced apart from something else. Philosophers of science point to the difficulty of explaining consciousness in terms of the brain, as discussed in the preceding chapter.[67] Some philosophers go further, though, and assert that consciousness is an explanandum of its own.[68] If this is correct, it is unclear what a reductive explanation should reduce to.[69] In the standard disease framework, reductionism is useful and has an endpoint. To the extent that the explanation of tuberculosis, for instance, is reduced to the identification of a bacillus, science has condensed the explanation of that disease to that pathogen. We need no longer talk about the symptoms of tuberculosis as a way to identify the problem. We need only test for the bacillus. It is unlikely that aspects of consciousness can be reduced in the same way. Even if we accept the idea that the mind derives entirely from the brain, it will be difficult to reduce aspects of consciousness to, say, the firing of certain neurons in a certain sequence. Consciousness refers to ontologically subjective experiences, so to reduce it to neurons is, in effect, to describe it as something else.[70] Contemporary neuroscience has largely operated in a reductionist vein, in that it has tried to reduce psychological experiences, like emotions, to activation in certain brain regions. This can be a very useful scientific enterprise. Indeed, with this information we might choose to define psychiatric disorders entirely in terms of brain function. But in doing so we would be implying that psychiatric disorders are not disorders of consciousness, and, at least in terms of current science, we would be employing a more impoverished view of psychological experience.

The problem with reductive explanations complicates the task of psychiatric taxonomy in several ways. The *DSM* creates apparent simplicity from real complexity. For instance, it attempts to impose equivalence between symptoms. According to the *DSM*'s criteria, a particular set of symptoms indicates a disorder when experienced in combination during a defined period of time. In principle, some of these symptoms could be mapped to brain regions, but at the level of consciousness there is a pervasive incompatibility between symptoms and the goal of reduction. Symptoms are a product of experiences, beliefs, intentions, biography, and personality. They cannot be isolated from other experiences, as if they were things in and of themselves. Social phobia, for example, can be interpreted in many ways: as an emotion, a belief, or a feature of personality. Each of these explanations implies a different experience and also implies a different *thing* to explain. Alva Noe draws a parallel between consciousness and visual perception.[71] Perception is not a passive experience wherein the individual takes in information through the eyes and recognizes objects based on the information she receives. The brain, instead, actively interprets the information and does a good deal of condensing it based on past experience (among other things). For this reason, two people can look at exactly the same object and see very different things. Consciousness, too, is more complex than the sum of its functions. There is, in short, an "explanatory gap" between what neuroscience studies, such as the firing of neurons, and what the individual consciously experiences.[72]

There are related risks to disregarding the psychological aspects of mental disorders. Some have proposed bundling the assorted obsessive-compulsive disorders into a single broader spectrum disorder related to obsession. Disorders on this spectrum would share the core feature of repetitive thoughts and behaviors. This proposal makes sense from the standpoint of symptoms that are currently shared by a variety of different disorders as well as from the standpoint of the genetic influences that appear to be common to these disorders. At both of these levels there is considerable scientific evidence to support the bundling of heretofore discrete disorders. Yet it is still problematic to regard all compulsions as sharing the same underlying etiology, especially at the level of psychological experience. Many psychiatric disorders are characterized by repetitive and compulsive behavior, but from the standpoint of the individual, the functions of these behaviors vary enormously, and not just in terms of the object of the obsession.[73] Those who suffer from a social phobia, for example, will obsessively avoid social situations, whereas those who suffer from a drug addiction will obsessively seek a fix. In addition to the object of obsession, the motivations behind these two behaviors are very different: One person seeks to avoid discomfort; the other seeks pleasure. There might be common neurological features to both activities—addictions of all kinds can appear very similar in a brain scan, which is, in fact, the finding that sparked enthusiasm for a common neurological substrate to obsession—but the reasons for the behavior are still very different. Similarly, many disorders involve fear, but an unreasonable fear of flying is likely to appear identical on an fMRI as a more reasonable fear of parachuting. An analysis of the neurological aspects of fear, then, is unlikely to say much about how that fear is appraised or certainly how rational that fear is, despite the fact that many other critics of the *DSM* have elevated the importance of commonsense adjudication. Insofar as all these disorders are forced to reside on the same spectrum, clinicians risk mixing very different motivations and experiences, from harm avoidance, to anxiety reduction, to pleasure seeking. More generally, attempts to rewrite the *DSM* based on a single perspective, including brain activity, would superimpose a particular standpoint regarding the ultimate cause. Those who emphasize neurological causes would favor one framework, whereas those who favor psychological causes would favor another. This, too, might be something psychiatry would prefer to do, but, if so, it is a choice regarding what evidence the discipline finds compelling rather than something that emerges from the evidence itself.

THE APPEAL OF THE NATURAL SCIENCES

Despite some ambiguity surrounding neurological causes—which, to be sure, is a relatively new entrant to the field—the enduring appeal of the natural sciences writ large is clear. The natural sciences are role models in at least one important respect: Whatever they might have to say about psychiatric disorders, the natural sciences have certainly produced other classification systems that are considered ideal. The periodic table of elements is perhaps the most well known. The periodic table provides a taxonomy for perfectly and uniquely identifying elements. Having twenty-six protons in the nucleus, for example, is the essence of iron. There is no other way to think about iron. Closer to psychiatric disorders is the biological classification of organisms, where the natural sciences have been successful as well. The classification of organisms is often done on the basis of shared evolution, yielding species as the basic unit of classification, followed by larger hierarchical ranks, including genus, family, order, class, and so on. Species have the appearance of being "natural" categories because they share certain identifiable characteristics and are capable of reproducing with others within that species. Psychiatry would like to classify psychiatric disorders in the same fashion, and, indeed, some psychiatrists turn to evolution for answers to the discipline's most vexing questions, as discussed earlier.

Yet a closer look at some of these seemingly clear and natural taxonomies reveals considerable complexity as well as perhaps greater tolerance on the part of natural scientists than is appreciated by psychiatrists. Indeed, the complexities behind these other taxonomies are not unlike the complexities we have discussed thus far with respect to psychiatric disorders. For this reason, scientists holding up the classification of species as a role model for psychiatry might be revealing more than they intend. The underlying process that produces species is referred to as speciation, which is premised on evolution. Speciation would appear to be perfect. It seems to yield entirely different groups who are genetically isolated from one another and, thus, are reproductively unrelated.[74] Humans and chimpanzees, for example, share common ancestors, but they evolved independently and cannot reproduce with each other. This clear differentiation is the key to producing a clean taxonomy. Yet it does not, in fact, apply neatly to all organisms. Reproductive barriers are occasionally weaker than supposed, and genetic material can move from organism to organism. Hull puts the matter directly: "One can rarely discover a set of traits which is possessed by all members of a species and by no members of some other species."[75] The centrality of reproduction is also debatable. Genetic interchange is not necessary for the maintenance of the characteristics of a species. Some species are so geographically removed from one another that reproduction is impossible, but they still maintain morphological similarity.[76] To be sure, the standard understanding of speciation might apply very well to some animals, including animals we care greatly about, such as mammals, but it does not work equally well for all organisms, including microorganisms and plants and, thus, cannot be applied to all forms of life that evolve, which is, after all, the putative universe of the phylogenetic tree.

Although some psychiatrists envision taxonomies of psychiatric disorders that would lead to something like species, it is notable that some natural scientists have already accepted taxonomies of species based on concepts other than evolution.[77] Different definitions of a species can produce very different classifications, but rather than regard these classifications as more or less correct—or more or less valid—scientists accept them as more or less useful for different purposes.[78] For instance, those interested in evolution have different ideas about the best classification from those interested in ecology (although those interested in ecology plainly recognize the truth of evolution). If there is general agreement on a certain taxonomy, it is only of a tentative kind. As Dupré puts it, a taxonomy of species should be considered "no more than the currently best (and minimally revised) general purpose reference system for the cataloguing of biological diversity," one that provides a "lingua franca" for the parties involved.[79] By this standard, the *DSM* might very well be acceptable to some natural scientists insofar as it already serves science well. Furthermore, the idea of a lingua franca is precisely the thing many psychiatrists have emphasized all along. In encouraging conservative revisions to the *DSM*, Allen Frances treads this ground. He emphasizes that the *DSM* is "more an exercise in forging common language than in finding a truth" and that we need a "strong reason to change the syntax."[80] The tentative satisfaction of scientists has another dimension as well. One reason scientists might accept classifications as more or less useful is simply that there might be little to be gained from trying to derive the single best classification system (even presuming such a thing were possible). Those interested in ecology and those interested in evolution are ultimately pursuing different goals. And in neither scientific enterprise is the incentive to derive a perfect classification system all that strong. What works in ecology works in *ecology*. What works in evolution works in *evolution*. In that context, few scientists are tempted to focus their careers on taxonomies per se. They would much rather study what interests them, including one organism or another.

THE INESCAPABLE IMPORTANCE OF VALUES

One way to read the trajectory of the science of psychiatric classification is in terms of progression toward at least identifying more *objective* disorders. When prior attempts failed, or when they provided ambiguous information, researchers pursued alternative strategies. In this way, a new scientific horizon always fed new hope, if not necessarily a new outcome. In recent years, there has been a good deal of enthusiasm surrounding genes, especially in terms of thinking about how evolution produced psychiatric disorders. The parallel between these efforts and speciation is obvious. Furthermore, evolution implies an especially obdurate kind of objectivity: What is given in nature is not invented by man. Yet here, as elsewhere, the importance of values is inescapable. For one, evolution seeks something very simple: the maximization of fitness and the production of offspring. It is possible to evaluate psychiatric disorders in this light and regard only those disorders that impair fitness as reflecting dysfunction. Earlier I reviewed the complexity of assessing current functions in light of earlier evolution, but setting that issue aside, there remains the more elementary distinction between *function* and *purpose*. Humans have many purposes apart from fitness, so deciding which functions to value involves thinking about the existential dimensions of life and not just the evolutionary aspects of psychology.[81] Some definitions of disorder turn on this distinction, as when we elevate the importance of social participation in measures of disability. In addition, the symptoms of psychiatric disorders often reflect experiences around which individual preferences will vary. Some people, for example, might accept sadness as a fact of life, whereas others might demand greater emotional well-being. Virtually everyone, though, is likely to agree that heart disease is something worth treating because the purpose of the heart is easy to deduce. In this way, evaluating the "function" of mental processes is far more difficult than evaluating the function of simpler organs.

There is a tendency to view values as competing with objectivity. By the same token, there is a tendency to view science as emancipatory, as freeing society from the misconceptions of the past. Given some prominent controversies in its history, psychiatry has understandably shied away from explicitly discussing values. Among these controversies is the classification of homosexuality as a psychiatric disorder, which still looms large in historical memory. Other examples are much older, but they are no less cautionary. In the mid–nineteenth century, the physician Samuel Cartwright proposed a mental illness known as drapetomania, characterized by a slave's compulsion to run away.[82] Neither drapetomania nor homosexuality is considered a disorder today, but they weren't eliminated by better science. Drapetomania was eliminated from consideration when the country began to employ a different moral framework for thinking about slavery. Homosexuality was eliminated through the efforts of gay rights advocates and because of changing public views of homosexuality. To be sure, science played some role in the process insofar as homosexuality was increasingly seen as a biological disposition rather than a choice, but the role of science was largely secondary to the role of activism. The facts of science required an interpretation, and advocates provided one. Although in the scientific literature values are often cast in contrast with empirical insight, it is notable that in both of these examples values served a progressive and emancipatory function.

Thinking about psychiatric disorders in terms of evolution and genes introduces a number of problems, but the importance of values is apparent even for less scientifically ambitious validators. One way to think about valid psychiatric disorders is in terms of disorders that can be treated, especially through pharmaceuticals. In this case, disorders that we might regard as real are those that reflect the actions of neurotransmitters—change the neurotransmitters and change the disorder. Yet here, too, values are inescapable. Advocates for eliminating the bereavement exclusion, for example, have emphasized that psychiatric medications are effective regardless of the precipitating cause: Patients whose depression was caused by the death of a spouse respond just as well to antidepressants as those whose depression was caused by something else. The more general logic behind this idea is that if a newly proposed disorder responds to the same medication that treats an already accepted disorder, the new disorder must have a pathology similar to the old one. Although recognizing the appeal of this essentially Kraepelin-based approach, some critics reject this transitivity. They note—correctly—that even nondisordered people respond to medication. Wakefield asks rhetorically: "Do college students whose examination performances benefit from psychostimulants therefore have a mild form of ADHD?"[83] For critics, the fear is one of "pharmacological assimilation," whereby the universe of accepted disorders expands merely from the presumption that *any* effective treatment reveals the presence of a pathology. Again, though, this criticism sits uncomfortably at the nexus between facts and values. Psychiatric disorders are complex. They are caused by many things. Furthermore, many disorders are naturally dimensional. For these disorders, treatments will move individuals along that dimension, starting from the point at which they began. Both sides of the debate are in some sense correct. We should fear growth by assimilation. But when the debate is framed in terms of *science*—in terms of which side has the facts on its side or what study provides the most compelling evidence for or against a testable proposition—neither side appears willing to take the next step and argue for or against including that "mild form of ADHD" in the *DSM*, for example, or whether "assimilating" more disorders into the *DSM* might promote better mental health care if it alerts clinicians to a wider variety of treatable problems.

This issue of treatment response is particularly complex. A well-known finding in the pharmaceutical literature is that people respond positively to placebos. In controlled experiments, subjects given inert pills show improvements in their symptoms relative to those given nothing at all. In clinical trials, this finding is used knowingly and strategically: Placebos are used to identify more precisely the effects of a pharmaceutical agent. In particular, they are used to simulate a so-called therapeutic context, like taking a pill prescribed by a physician in the context of a doctor-patient interaction. This context might itself affect a patient's behavior or physiology, but it is not, of course, the result of an active pharmaceutical agent and therefore should be eliminated from consideration. To identify the effects of an active agent, then, the placebo effect is subtracted from the total. This is no small matter. Studies that look at major depression provide an especially clear picture of the placebo effect's significance. In such studies, about 30 percent of people respond to a placebo, whereas about 50 percent respond to the medication.[84] Furthermore, the significance of the placebo effect is growing. In the early 1980s, the placebo effect was a little more than 20 percent. In the late 1990s, however, it started to exceed 30 percent and in some studies reached as high as 50 percent. A similar increase has been found for antipsychotic medications, suggesting a general psychological process related to receptivity to psychiatric medication.[85] Although scientists have yet to establish the precise reasons for this increase, a plausible explanation is that the public is increasingly convinced about the efficacy of psychiatric medications: The public expects more from such medications and so responds in a more positive way, even to placebos. Recent studies point to other cultural influences as well.[86] Like the placebo effect for drugs used in the treatment of depression, the placebo effect for drugs used in the treatment of chronic pain increased between 1990 and 2013. In the case of pain, however, the increase was limited to studies conducted in the United States. An increase was not found in trials conducted in Europe and Asia, where, among other things, direct-to-consumer advertising of pharmaceuticals is not allowed.

One interpretation of results of this sort is that they highlight the superficial nature of psychiatric disorders. If major depression can be treated effectively with a sugar pill, perhaps the disorder was superficial to begin with or at least something the *DSM* failed to identify properly. These results probably reveal something else, though. What they reveal is the inability of pharmaceutical evidence to address questions related to the accuracy of diagnostic criteria. In fact, the placebo effect is found for a variety of diseases and physiological systems whose ontological status is not in doubt, including Parkinson's disease,[87] the cardiovascular system,[88] and the endocrine system.[89] Furthermore, the fact that an effective treatment for a disease can be internally generated need not imply the disease was superficial to begin with. The immune system effectively eliminates many bacteria and viruses, but no one regards a viral infection as insignificant. In this vein, some scientists are loath to equate placebo with "useless," characterizing the placebo effects as a real psychobiological event and asking clinicians to reconsider its meaning accordingly.[90] An endogenous psychological immune system may be just as real as a viral immune system, and our failure to acknowledge it as such might simply reflect a lingering prejudice against the psychological.

There is another way to think about the reality of the placebo effect, which also speaks to the classification of disorders. The act of diagnosis can itself change the nature of the disease. Consider the case of "primary orgasmic dysfunction," discussed by Richard McNally.[91] Primary orgasmic dysfunction did not appear in *DSM-III* but was widely recognized and studied at the time of its development, especially in the influential work of Masters and Johnson. The dysfunction was characterized by never having experienced an orgasm.[92] At the time, studies indicated that the problem was quite prevalent, with an incidence somewhere between 7 and 15 percent.[93] Studies also suggested that psychotherapy was generally ineffective in treating the problem. Yet research had identified a potential cure: Professionally guided masturbation was shown to be highly effective.[94] For some, the superficiality of the treatment revealed the superficiality of the condition.

Wakefield, for instance, regards the disorder as yet another unjustified expansion of the diagnostic enterprise, arguing for the need to distinguish those who fail to have an orgasm because of a dysfunction and those who fail for other reasons.[95] He further asserts that codifying the disorder without appreciating this distinction "could easily blind us to the diagnostic practices which enforce our values but go beyond the demands of evidence and logic."[96] With this in mind, one could eliminate disorders concerned with "normal" sexual arousal, presuming such disorders reflect values rather than science. *DSM-III* included, for example, a disorder referred to as "inhibited female orgasm," characterized by a delay in or absence of orgasm following "normal sexual excitement."[97] No doubt disorders of this sort invite controversy, as there is a good deal of moralizing surrounding sexual behavior. Yet it is hard to discover a "cure" without some way of formally acknowledging a problem. The fact that inhibited female orgasm was a product of cultural forces—at the time, masturbation was highly stigmatized, and female sexuality was still met with considerable fear—does not mean the disorder was not real. This is especially so if we are willing to acknowledge that cultural forces can be powerful. By naming the problem—even on a dubious basis or on patently nonscientific grounds—scientists developed a more accurate understanding of female sexuality. Interpreting the end result critically, in terms of scientists identifying a "cure" for a disorder it invented whole cloth, is only one possible interpretation. One could even argue that the stigma surrounding masturbation declined in no small part because aligning it with health moved it further away from the area of morality. In this sense, a more progressive approach to female sexuality went hand in hand with a more clinical mindset and, indeed, the instinct to create a diagnosis.

SUMMARY

The intersection of science and psychiatric diagnosis is awkward. Psychiatry's occasional aversion to grappling with the complex ontology of psychiatric disorders would seem to be self-defeating. Psychiatry demands accurate diagnostic criteria. And psychiatry is clearly not unaware of the difficulty of reconciling science and values. In the build-up to *DSM-5*, Kenneth Kendler and others called for a working group devoted to conceptual issues, something that could address many of the issues discussed in this chapter.[98] In their proposal, Kendler and colleagues highlighted the difference between questions that are "fundamentally empirical" and those that are "conceptual or philosophical."[99] They further emphasized that conceptual questions should be central to *DSM-5*, even as Kendler and others appreciated the rich body of empirical findings that were now available to them. They appreciated that among the questions a robust conceptual debate could answer was: What validators, among many, should be given priority?

Yet these discussions ultimately had little influence. *DSM-5*'s conceptual definition of mental disorder is little different from the definition used in earlier editions. This is hardly the fault of any working group—the nature of psychiatric disorders belies easy classification. When revising a whole universe of diagnostic criteria in anticipation of producing a new manual, it is difficult to discuss overarching values. Furthermore, at many levels a discussion of values is dissonant. A focus on values, for example, draws attention to the nominal nature of psychiatric disorders. A focus on values also makes many people uncomfortable, given psychiatry's history. Altogether there is little in the entire ecology of diagnosis that welcomes a thoroughgoing review of values. The demands of that ecology go elsewhere. When the larger culture demands a more essentialist understanding, when clinical medicine demands crisp diagnostic categories, and when science has shifted to a focus on genetic and neurological markers, a discussion of values seems out of touch with the evolving conversation.

The task of writing better diagnostic criteria has been made even more difficult by an insistence on a *unified* view of psychiatric disorders. The *DSM* demands some harmony among its disorders. One implication of this view is that the validators that work well for one disorder—whatever they happen to be—ought to work for any other disorder. The idea of a *DSM* that would permit disorders with mixed ontological characteristics—some reflecting values, others reflecting science, some that are particular to a specific time period, others that reflect the failure of evolved psychological functions—risks the appearance of an ad hoc approach. To be sure, some scientists are entirely comfortable with uncertainty. In his discussion of scientific taxonomies, John Dupré advocates for a "promiscuous" view of classification, and, indeed, he sees no inherent weakness in nominalism.[100] His premise is that no single classification system is better than another *on a priori grounds* and, therefore, that we should not insist on one sort of classification over another. The grounds for assessing the best classification are likely to change, he argues, and classification systems ought to be able to adapt. As appealing as this idea is, a more flexible *DSM* would still have to contend with the many contradictions inherent in the field of psychiatry specifically. If useful criteria are always welcome, but promiscuity is something to be avoided, the most relevant question becomes, *useful for whom*? And that, too, has no easy answer. At this point we should return to our earlier discussion.

11

THE ENDURANCE OF THE
DIAGNOSTIC SYSTEM

In the preceding chapter I argued that science on its own is unable to arbitrate questions of psychiatric taxonomy. The creation of better diagnostic criteria requires judgment. It requires serious wrangling over values. And it requires actively choosing some forms of validity over others. Although science provides useful information—and science now provides more information than it has in the past—judgment is a scientific responsibility that cannot be abdicated in the name of objectivity. With this in mind, it is instructive to return our discussion to an earlier theme: how different constituencies use the *DSM*. Although current controversies in psychiatric taxonomy have a scientific sheen, at a deeper level they continue to reflect conflict regarding how different actors use the *DSM*. We can interpret the controversies of the past—and anticipate where controversies are likely to go in the future—by focusing on the standpoints of different actors and how those actors use the *DSM* for their own purposes. In this chapter I consider the contradictions of the diagnostic system in a more synthetic fashion than I have done to this point. I do so in terms of the intersections between three groups: science, clinicians, and the public. Although each of these groups might think in terms of more or less validity—and certainly some invoke the concept regularly—the real conflict is over what they regard as the proper goal of psychiatric classification. Furthermore, solutions to one set of problems can reverberate in ways that create new problems somewhere else. In light of the contradictions of the diagnostic system, I end with some principles for moving forward.

CONFLICT AMONG SCIENCE, CLINICIANS, AND THE PUBLIC

One reason the *DSM* remains so controversial is that it is difficult to envision criteria that would satisfy every stakeholder. Different parties have different interests and needs. Scientists seek an accurate description of psychiatric disorders. For them, dissatisfaction with the *DSM* stems from evidence that the *DSM* does not, in fact, provide criteria that precisely characterize all the dimensions of psychological functioning that scientists care about. The *DSM* overlooks, for instance, symptoms that are present in some patients; it separates disorders that, in fact, overlap with others; and it imposes artificial decision rules regarding when symptoms reflect a disorder, even though many psychological functions exist on a continuum. The frustration of scientists is made even more acute by the forces that compel them to use the *DSM* faithfully. The *DSM* sets the foundation for research on psychiatric disorders. The process of peer review demands fidelity to formal psychiatric nomenclature. Pharmaceuticals are tested and approved only for indications pertaining to *DSM*-classified disorders. Social, genetic, and neuroanatomical causes are tested for disorders as they are presented in the *DSM*. Furthermore, the *DSM* fosters little in the way of alternatives. Usually scientists test hypotheses that can be falsified—science proceeds best when deciding what is incorrect. Although it is possible to compare the *DSM* with other diagnostic criteria, the *DSM* prevents the development of alternatives.

The public is not seeking a scientific tool of the same kind, but people are looking for insights to shed light on their experiences. For them, the *DSM* provides a framework for thinking about mental distress as *illness*. For scientists, a diagnosis is merely descriptive—it only labels what is—but for patients a diagnosis connotes something deeper. A diagnosis helps explain why, for example, patients are sad or why their anxiety is extreme (even though the *DSM* provides nothing with respect to explanation per se). In many cases, patients actively distance themselves from a diagnosis, as discussed earlier, but people tend to seek clinical expertise in order to adjudicate whether they have a disorder, and they recognize the role of the *DSM* in this task. For the public, then, a diagnosis is closer to an explanation than a label.

Clinicians, too, recognize the value of a diagnosis for more than descriptive reasons. For them, the *DSM* provides a lingua franca for communicating with other clinicians and for representing their work to outside parties. Insurance companies, for instance, demand information about the disorder for which they are being billed, and, at least at this point, the *DSM* satisfies their demands. Like scientists, clinicians might regard the *DSM's* diagnostic criteria as superficial. Indeed, there is abundant evidence that clinicians distort the criteria on a case-by-case basis to serve interests they regard as paramount. Yet clinicians also appreciate how the *DSM* criteria at least provide a quick and easy summary, a kind of shorthand that allows them to move quickly to, as they see it, the more important task. Furthermore, clinicians appreciate that the *DSM* has done much to improve the professional standing of psychiatry. The *DSM* has produced an equivalence between what physicians do in diagnosing a physical illness and what mental health professionals do in diagnosing a psychiatric disorder. Even if this amounts to little more than borrowing the form of modern medicine without the content, the transposition has increased the reliability of diagnosis. This, too, helps clinicians. With all of these competing interests and needs in mind, it is possible to see ongoing controversies in light of incommensurability. Writing criteria that will better satisfy one party is difficult to do without frustrating another. The diagnostic system is a stubborn synthesis, if it is a synthesis at all.

CLINICIANS AND THE PUBLIC

One of the most prominent intersections in the diagnostic system is, of course, between clinicians and the public. A lingering source of apprehension among professionals pertains to how the *DSM* allows the public to appropriate some of the authority that should rightly be held by mental health professionals. This apprehension is longstanding. In 1983 Robert Spitzer wondered whether clinicians would really be necessary if the APA succeeded in writing especially translucent diagnostic criteria.[1] The dilemma he identified was even more acute, though, because of his avowed interest in fostering reliability. Insuring reliability requires writing clear and unambiguous diagnostic criteria, with few references to concepts that require interpretation or expertise, "identity," for example. The more the criteria reduce the need for interpretation, the more likely they are to promote consistent diagnostic decisions from clinician to clinician. At the same time, however, the less the criteria require inference, the more they can used by the public in almost exactly the same way as they are employed by professionals. Armed with the *DSM* clinicians will know exactly what other clinicians are referring to when they talk about a major depressive episode, but so too will anyone else who reads the manual. If the *DSM* puts clinicians on a stronger professional footing, it also makes the task of diagnosis more transparent and, indeed, launches disorders into the public sphere.

To the extent that the *DSM* remains tightly focused on the surface manifestations of psychiatric disorders, this tension will remain. To be sure, the *DSM* could be revised in ways that identify deeper and less apparent causes, including genes and neuroanatomical dysfunctions. Identifying these signs would require a technological intermediary and, therefore, would build a barrier—and potentially a safeguard—between the public and professionals. Yet a more biological *DSM* would also introduce a different set of tensions. Among other things the *DSM* provides a dictionary for interpreting the lay idiom of distress. The idea of an "idiom" is used by researchers to describe how patients talk about and articulate their suffering.[2] And for patients the language of mental illness is fundamentally a language of surface manifestations. It pertains to emotions, behaviors, and experiences. The symptoms cataloged in the *DSM* are evocative of mental illness because people generally share the same idiom of distress, and the authors of the *DSM* have historically felt compelled to be sensitive to the most important elements of that idiom. The symptoms of a major depressive episode, for instance, have not changed much between versions of the *DSM* because they appear to capture adequately the core symptoms of depression, as people experience it. If the *DSM* were redrafted so that disorders were defined according to more deep-seated biological pathologies, the subjective experience of mental illness would not suddenly change. Diagnosis would still require some correspondence between what a patient reports and how a clinician interprets it.

For their part, patients would still present their illness using the symptoms they regard as significant. And clinicians would still communicate with
their patients, at least in part, using that language. The lingering tension,
then, would be in squaring the newly created biological criteria with the
enduring cultural lexicon for presenting complaints. This issue is not limited
to psychiatric disorders. The lay public recognizes the distinct ontology of
heart disease, cancer, and infectious disease—these are not controversial illnesses—but when presenting their symptoms to a physician, even for what
they suspect are well-known physical disorders, patients routinely describe a
mix of experiences, not all of which can plainly be associated with a disease.[3]
Rather patients present those things that bother them most, including, quite
often, general signs of emotional suffering. The problem this introduces is
deeper than one of mere interpretation. Laurence Kirmayer and others elevate the significance of idioms of distress in arguing that the fit between such
idioms and formal diagnostic criteria is the essence of treating illness.[4] A
lack of correspondence between the two—even one based on formal diagnostic criteria rooted in neuroanatomical abnormalities—would undermine
the very things patients seek to alleviate.

SCIENCE AND THE PUBLIC

A related source of tension lies at the intersection of science and the public.
The contemporary science of psychiatric disorders has produced findings that
do not comport well with public conceptions of those disorders. For instance,
science has shown that many disorders exist on a spectrum rather than as a
category. Depression, for instance, is largely a matter of degrees, and even
mild forms of depression carry considerably more risk than no depression at
all. For the public, though, the instinct to categorize is very strong, and this
is indeed a consequence of the *DSM*, as shown in an earlier chapter. For the
public, *major* depression *is* different and perhaps the *only* form of depression
worth treating. Certainly the public thinks a lot about discerning when
depression is or is not an illness. Although the public might be willing to
accept some medical conditions as spectrums—in the case of, for example,

blood pressure or cholesterol—moving the *DSM* further in the direction of spectrums will be difficult to square with the public's current mindset regarding psychiatric disorders and other diseases. Indeed, moving in the direction of spectrums, although scientifically credible, might paradoxically induce a problem that critics of the *DSM* have long sought to correct: It might accelerate the problem of overdiagnosis.

In order to understand this possibility it is important to situate the concept of "risk" within a larger cultural backdrop. A variety of forces have converged to change how clinicians and patients respond to risk. Risk is probabilistic. High blood pressure is not a disease per se, but it is strongly associated with other problems, such as heart attacks, strokes, and organ failure, and is, therefore, treated. By the same token, physicians treat high cholesterol in order to lower the risk of a blocked artery. Risk and disease are, therefore, distinct. Yet from the standpoint of both patients and physicians, risk and disease have converged. An elevated risk for something is now itself a target of treatment, aligning those "at risk" for a disease and those who already have it.[5] Much like those who actually have a disease, those who are at risk monitor their condition, track progress toward improvement, and worry when they show signs of deterioration. Similarly, the idea of "watchful waiting," especially with respect to cancer, has created a new class of health care consumers who, like those who actually have cancer, see themselves as ill and experience much of the same uncertainty and fear that comes from actually testing positive for the presence of cancer cells.

The convergence of risk and disease, in part, reflects the spread of technologies that have made such a convergence possible. Clinical testing is far more common today than it was in the past, and, in general, Americans are very enthusiastic about testing.[6] For example, the vast majority of adults, 87 percent, believe that routine cancer screening is almost always appropriate. As much as this enthusiasm is based on a rational appreciation of what screening provides—who could quarrel with the virtue of being more informed?—it is also a *moral* issue, based on the public's emphasis on personal responsibility for maintaining good health. For instance, about 41 percent of adults believe that it would be "irresponsible" for an eighty-year-old woman not to avail herself of mammography. For a fifty-five-year-old woman, this percentage increases to more than 70. Even the possibility of false positives—which is hardly unusual—does little to dent this enthusiasm. Of those patients who experienced a false-positive cancer screening, for example, virtually all, 98 percent, expressed no regrets about seeking the initial test. From the standpoint of clinicians, this unwavering enthusiasm presents a problem. Clinicians want diagnostic tests that can accurately detect conditions, with no false positives or negatives. Especially if a condition is rare, even a small false positive rate can produce an enormous amount of misinformation. Yet from the standpoint of the public, even a small risk of disease is worth testing for, and the many downsides of misinformation occasion very little fear.

The risk is similar in the case of psychiatric disorders. Allowing for a graded assessment of psychiatric risk could create an even broader class of patients. To be sure, the public's enthusiasm for testing is likely stronger for mortal conditions than for nonfatal chronic conditions. Robert Aronowitz, for instance, explains the enthusiasm for aggressive cancer screening in terms of an "anticipated regret" heuristic: When thinking about the future, patients fear not having done everything possible to prevent death, even if it means testing for rare diseases or using unproven treatments.[7] Psychiatric disorders are different, both in profile and treatment. They are not mortal in the same way as cancer (although they are related to suicide). Furthermore, there are no prophylactic cures for psychiatric disorders in the same way that there are procedures that can eliminate the risk for cancer in some sites. Nevertheless, the class of people "at risk for a psychiatric disorder" is very large. Indeed, the evidence discussed earlier suggests that the risk of developing a psychiatric disorder almost never shrinks to zero for any population group. Once the public starts thinking about the risks for developing a psychiatric disorder, the leap to thinking in terms of actually having a disorder is very short.

SCIENCE AND CLINICIANS

The interface between science and clinicians also produces its own kind of tension. Science prefers diagnoses that are stable with respect to some underlying entity. Clinicians, however, prefer diagnoses that are sensitive to all the different kinds of patients they are likely to treat. Clinicians also prefer diagnostic criteria that will reflect how patients' fears might shift over time, while scientists prefer concepts that are sufficiently abstract to cover as many cases as possible, such as generalized anxiety rather than a fear of, say, electronic surveillance specifically. If anything, the tension between science and clinicians has grown sharper as the tools of science have progressed. Scientists now use instruments that allow them to identify neurological traces of fear, for example, even if those traces reveal nothing about the specific content of those fears. Likewise, genetic research supports the existence of broad categories of internalizing and externalizing disorders, but for clinicians these categories are not terribly meaningful. Clinicians would like, instead, to uncover the specific nature of a patient's moods or the specific targets of his aggression.

Science investigates other topics, of course, and not all of these topics are irrelevant to the concerns of clinicians. Science examines the causes of psychiatric disorders, for instance, and surely clinicians will benefit from better information along these lines. Yet here, too, the discoveries of science cannot be applied seamlessly to the work of clinicians. Much of the work of scientists is probabilistic and frequential, whereas the work of clinicians is concrete and unique. When scientists study the causes of major depression, for example, they typically base their research on samples of individuals, and from these samples estimate statistical models that allow them to infer probabilistic causes. This process can yield important insights. For example, research on the effects of stressful life events has provided insights into how the environment shapes psychological distress, showing that traumatic life events do, in fact, increase the risk of developing a psychiatric disorder. Yet the statistical models upon which these insights are based are set at the level of populations rather than individuals. For this reason, scientists are better at predicting how many people will experience major depression following a divorce, for example, than they are at identifying who exactly will experience major depression. At best, statistical models provide only probabilistic information, and, at that, they usually only demonstrate causes that are well outside the parameters of what a clinician might regard as a law. This dilutes the clinical relevance of science. To return to our earlier example, the relationship between stressful life events and psychiatric disorders is well known and widely regarded as "significant." Usually claims of significance are made in reference to statistical significance and occasionally relative to the effects of other established risk factors. Yet in terms of change in the probability of developing a disorder, the effects of stressful life events are often quite small. Stressful life events, for example, are often found to double the odds of major depression, but this increase in the relative odds amounts to only a small increase in the probability of depression. In addition, stressful life events are much more common than major depression, meaning that events provide information of limited relevance for clinicians. Although most cases of major depression are preceded by a negative life event, most people who experience a negative life event will not develop depression.[8] Also, when applied to individual cases, the meaning of "probability" changes. In statistics, a probability refers to the frequency of something happening over the long run, but in the minds of clinicians, a probability usually refers to their confidence surrounding an outcome.[9] This difference in semantics reflects the more fundamental problem that what can be demonstrated in science is often difficult to apply in clinical practice.

In the same vein, the science of psychiatric disorders sits at the intersection of a distinction between *understanding* and *explanation*.[10] As the term is often used, *explanation* refers to causal accounts, or how one event leads to another. Causal processes can be observed and tested empirically, and the subject matters of the natural sciences lend themselves to explanations of this kind, as when a physicist using classical mechanics studies the effects of a force acting on a body. In this case, the scientist is armed with the right theory, and a cause can be delimited and the parameters of its effect deduced. The subject matter of the behavioral sciences, however, lends itself to *understanding* more than explanation. Understanding is a more modest and particular endeavor, even though it is still science. In the case of mental illness, the goal of understanding is to comprehend the significance or meaning of behavior in reference to psychological states, motivations, social relationships, background, and so on. The conclusions, too, are different. Although it is difficult to anticipate who will get depressed—that is, to explain depression—once someone is depressed a scientist can provide a plausible account for the particular case. Any understanding of this sort, though, has limited application to other individuals. In short, science has not derived a full explanation for depression, even if it has developed a valuable understanding.

The interests of clinicians and scientists diverge in another way as well. Insofar as the *DSM* criteria are revised in ways that fail to reduce heterogeneity within disorders, the work of scientists grows more difficult. Consider, again, the case of PTSD. Over time the diagnostic criteria for the disorder have admitted an ever larger number of potential causes. In effect, this change in what counts as a traumatic event has increased the sensitivity of the diagnostic criteria and, thereby, reduced the number of false negatives. Yet increasing the sensitivity of the criteria has also introduced more heterogeneity into the diagnosis. People who meet the current diagnostic criteria for PTSD might share symptoms, but the social and psychological contexts surrounding those symptoms will vary greatly. Even if we accept this as an appropriate way to revise PTSD's diagnostic criteria, and even if we grant that the symptoms of the disorder can, in fact, stem from a wide variety of events, the use of expanded diagnostic criteria will necessarily dilute the ability of scientists to draw firm conclusions. In bundling together many different people, the *DSM* risks bundling different epidemiological contexts and maybe even different disorders. This can distort the conclusions of research studies, and it can do so in ways that will not always be obvious or correctable. For example, someone who survived the collapse of the Twin Towers on September 11 might resemble symptomatically someone who witnessed the towers falling on television, and we might properly diagnose both as suffering from PTSD, but in all likelihood these two people had very different personalities prior to the attacks. Neuroticism, for instance, is strongly associated with psychiatric disorders *and* with a preoccupation with stress. Those people most at risk for developing PTSD, then, might also be those people most likely to seek out traumatic television coverage and ruminate about it. In effect, the premorbid risks of the two people are different, and, indeed, their environments are different as well because they are construed in different ways. The problem is not with how these two people differ, though; it is with drawing inaccurate scientific inferences. Some of these preexisting risk factors are well known to scientists and could presumably be considered when designing a study. But unless scientists have a good understanding of these factors—and, in any case, these factors usually lie outside the existing diagnostic criteria themselves—they risk drawing misleading conclusions about the causes of PTSD.

In general there remains a remarkable deference to science in psychiatry, despite some incompatibility between what science provides and what clinicians need. Yet in the context of revising the *DSM* there has been a resurgent emphasis on empowering the public. In this vein, some clinicians explicitly cast the public as a credible judge of severity. Appeals to "common sense" move in this direction. Wakefield, for instance, interprets the low rates of help seeking among those with a psychiatric disorder as evidence that the public is capable of making reasonable decisions about when a disorder is truly significant.[11] To Wakefield, the fact that most people who meet the diagnostic criteria for a psychiatric disorder do not seek treatment only means the public has a different—and, in his mind, more appropriate—model of what constitutes a psychiatric disorder. Among other things, Wakefield is arguing that the public deserves a place at the table, especially when the *DSM* is, to him, so faulty. Another way to put this idea is that the public suffers from psychiatric disorders and, for this reason alone, has some bona fide expertise.

Wakefield is not alone in emphasizing a potential interface between science and the public. Others have more explicitly advocated for the inclusion of patient perspectives in the *DSM* and, under some conditions, for the dominance of patient perspectives. In the past, the relevance of the public for issues of psychiatric classification was cast in much more limited terms. The authors of the *DSM* recognized, for instance, that the manual should avoid any stigmatizing language, out of respect for those suffering from psychiatric disorders. And public input was used in revising the *DSM* along these lines. The authors of the *DSM* noted that the phrase "people suffering from schizophrenia" should replace the noun "schizophrenics." But recent calls for patient input have pushed for a more fundamental role, including a role in determining the symptoms of disorders and specifying the difference between disordered and normal. In this vein, Douglas Porter advocates for what he calls *normative validity*, premised on the idea that there are a variety of frameworks for evaluating the "good life" and that, in the presence of plurality, the moral imperative should be to respect each individual's capacity to develop his or her own views and, in turn, to use these views for evaluating some of the *DSM*'s core concepts, including clinically significant impairment.[12] This, of course, stands in sharp contrast with efforts to craft a more monolithic view of the concept. In a similar vein, Elizabeth Flanagan and colleagues focus on the concept of subjectivity, favoring criteria that not only emphasize subjectively experienced symptoms, as the *DSM*'s diagnostic criteria already do, but criteria that respect the significance patients may or may not grant to the different symptoms within a set of criteria. This proposal amounts to considerably more than just representing patient interests and showing respect for personal integrity. This proposal would, in effect, allow patients to shape their diagnoses through their own understandings of the disorder.[13] To emphasize her point, Flanagan proposes including subjective considerations in the diagnostic criteria and not shunting them to an addendum. Her proposal has important implications. Under it, diagnostic criteria would not be limited to a predetermined and fixed set of symptoms but rather would allow—even encourage—patients to nominate other symptoms they regarded as indicative of the problem. Of course this sort of revision would change the character of many disorders. Schizophrenia, for example, might still be characterized by many of the symptoms already included in the *DSM*—patients suffering from the disorder do, in fact, emphasize the symptoms that psychiatry regards as significant—but would probably also include reports of loss and loneliness, which are frequently mentioned by patients suffering from the disorder but are not part of the *DSM*.[14] Other patients suffering from schizophrenia, likewise, mention a loss of self, even though this idea has not appeared in the *DSM* since its third revision.[15]

Such proposals stand in sharp contrast to both what the profession of psychiatry has tried to accomplish with the *DSM* and what science intends to pursue in the future. Bruce Cuthbert and Thomas Insel—the architects of RDoC—published a response to Flanagan's specific proposal, although they used the occasion mostly to speak to the more general role of subjectivity in diagnostic criteria.[16] In this regard, their emphasis is clear: They regard diagnoses as *data*. And their different interests are clear. They note that the experiential dimensions discussed by Flanagan are "hypothetical constructs best studied by measurement in various response systems, including behavior, genetics, and activity in physiological systems, in addition to patients' reports."[17] They further imply discontinuities between Flanagan's proposal and the current scientific interest in reducing some unwanted features of the *DSM*'s criteria, including heterogeneity within disorders, comorbidity between disorders, and the frequent use of "not otherwise specified" designations.[18]

Although not explicitly included in Cuthbert and Insel's discussion, there are additional complications to proposals like Flanagan's. Proposals focused on respecting the phenomenology of psychiatric disorders usually depart from the scientific pursuit of causal explanations. For instance, well before Flanagan's proposal, science had rejected the theory that schizophrenia was caused by a loss of self. Indeed, this scientific consensus was the reason such symptoms were removed from *DSM-III*. Flanagan and others are still correct to note that symptoms of this type remain important to patients, but if science increasingly regards the symptoms of disorders in terms of underlying *causes* (rather than as any and all *signs* of the disorder), a "loss of self" per se no longer fits its diagnostic framework. Cuthbert and Insel have no problem with proposals that might enhance the therapeutic alliance between clinicians and patients, as they make clear, but they resist the idea that these proposals enhance diagnostic accuracy.[19] Accuracy is overwhelmingly their primary concern.

MOVING FORWARD

In this book I have adopted a "meta" approach to the debate regarding the *DSM*. I have sought to describe ongoing debates in ways that highlight how their details might evolve but showcase how their form rests on longstanding concerns. To this end, I have presented what might appear like a litany of controversies. A reader might want something else. Appreciating that the

DSM is one element of a larger diagnostic system is one thing, but what might a better *DSM* look like if one recognizes that larger setting? My analysis does not provide answers for improvements, though it does provide principles for moving forward.

Recognize that reification is virtually impossible to avoid. Concerns over the reification of psychiatric disorders are entirely warranted. The reification of psychiatric disorders has a number of consequences, which I traced in earlier chapters. Yet reification is virtually impossible to avoid. So long as there is *something* like the *DSM*, reification will occur because the social environment is poised to foment it. The public hungers for explanations for suffering. Scientists seek rules for moving forward with their research projects. And clinicians render diagnoses as part of their everyday practices. Any document from an authoritative body—whether or not it has authoritative scientific underpinnings—will be received in ways that promote reification. The only safeguard against the most adverse consequences of reification is a more self-critical approach. This is especially true in the case of science, which has perhaps suffered the most from reification. But as the ascendance of RDoC has shown, science is prepared to move in an independent direction, and at least one authoritative body, the National Institute of Mental Health, has given scientists permission to do so. Other parties, too, might benefit from a more self-critical approach, though this book has shown that clinicians and the public are less tied to the *DSM* than scientists. If neither is entirely *critical* of the *DSM*, they at least adapt the manual to their needs.

Realize that much of the cultural work of the DSM is already in effect. There is no doubt that the *DSM* influences the larger culture. The terms used in the *DSM* quickly seep into public culture, and old terms are extinguished much more slowly than new terms are adopted. One implication of the arguments made in this book, though, is that the most significant cultural work of the *DSM* has probably already occurred. The idea that psychiatric disorders are things—things with crisp boundaries and ontological features that resemble those of more traditional physical diseases—was accomplished with *DSM-III*. Following the publication of that edition of the *DSM*, how we talk about mental illness shifted dramatically and in ways that have not and likely will not recede. These cultural effects reflect how well the

DSM-III supplied people with the language they needed to talk about psychiatric disorders and aligned that language with ideas about disease generally. The authors of the *DSM* are correct to worry. They should write diagnostic criteria with care and precision; no change, no matter how small, is entirely inconsequential. Yet some of the most important cultural changes have already occurred: The public already talks about anxiety as a disorder, about major depression as distinct from sadness, about symptoms as signs, and about having a disorder rather than simply being depressed. Changing what symptoms constitute generalized anxiety, for example, will not change how the public already instinctively regards severe anxiety as a disorder.

Make normative discussions a central feature of classification. Modern science has illuminated the puzzle of psychiatric disorders in an unprecedented way. Perhaps one unfortunate side effect of this progress, however, is that the rise of a scientific approach has largely pushed normative discussions to the side. Yet normative considerations are no less relevant today than they were in the past. They continue to inform, for instance, what we regard as a significant disorder and continue to shape what we are prepared to admit as a major life event. They lie behind discussions of proportionate responses to stress, and they form the basis for what symptoms we regard as abnormal. Many scientific debates have persisted not only because parties differ in the evidence they bring to the table but also because they differ in their fundamental precepts. A better *DSM* would not only involve the use of better scientific evidence but also contain a full-throated defense of and wrangling with underlying concepts and principles.

Grapple with the deep dimensionality of psychiatric disorders. The importance of basic concepts becomes even more important in light of the dimensionality of psychiatric disorders. An especially illuminating finding of contemporary research is to lay bare the deep dimensionality of psychiatric disorders. The most common psychiatric disorders likely reflect dimensions rather than categories, and, with each additional step, further dimensionality is revealed. Disorders are themselves dimensional, as are the symptoms that compose the disorders, as are the endophenotypes that lie behind those symptoms, as are the genetic influences that move one along these endophenotypes. This deep dimensionality has a number of implications, but among the most important is that it necessitates *choosing* when something constitutes a disorder. The diagnostic system demands distinctions, but those distinctions will be a matter of discretion rather than fact. Major depression requires an understanding of what "major" is. Generalized anxiety requires agreement regarding how abstract anxiety ought to be. Although the *DSM-5* task force was well aware of these issues, the definition of a mental disorder they supplied in the manual poses questions more than it provides answers, perhaps because the task force also had an avowed commitment to scientific evidence. The definition of mental disorder continues to rely on the concept of "clinically significant disturbance." Moreover, it continues to rely on an ostensive definition of disorder, positioning mental disorder against an "expectable or culturally approved response to a common stressor or loss" and contrasting dysfunction with "conflicts that are primarily between the individual and society."[20] This definition is perhaps an implied admission of the difficulty of defining mental disorder directly. Nonetheless, the elements it contains are not especially directive. Adverbs and adjectives like "primarily," "significant," and "expectable" are where the rubber meets the road, but they hardly amount to a full-fledged theory.

Distinguish between the "right" way and the "only" way. The chapters in this book were organized according to the different parties vested in the diagnostic system. Across the chapters a key point was to illustrate how these parties use the *DSM* and the many ways in which these various uses are incompatible. Despite these incompatibilities, however, most revisions to the *DSM* are undertaken in the spirit that there is a right way to classify psychiatric disorders and that the *DSM*—along with certain other diagnostic frameworks, including the ICD, with which the *DSM* has increasingly tried to harmonize—is the only way. At a minimum the APA does not produce different manuals for different audiences. It might be useful, though, to allow scientists and clinicians to use different frameworks. The RDoC is already attempting to do this, of course, but the controversy surrounding that taxonomy reveals all too well how difficult it is to imagine different classification systems coexisting peacefully. At this point, science has a firm foundation of facts to stand on. Allowing science more flexibility with respect to taxometric issues is unlikely to demolish the scientific literature or to revert it back to the haphazard situation that prevailed prior to the publication of *DSM-III.*

Another general principle is to recognize that the meaning and significance of the *DSM* is determined by forces quite apart from its text. The reception of the *DSM* cannot be governed by its authors. There are a variety of ways to illustrate the implications of this idea, though perhaps the best way is to show how the diagnostic system maintains a state of equilibrium. No matter how radical a change we might envision in one aspect of the diagnostic system—in the diagnostic criteria proposed by the APA, in the research strategies adopted by scientists, or in the clinical practices of mental health professionals—there are forces that compel only incremental change in the system as a whole. It is important, then, to be clear about the power and limits of the *DSM.*

THE DIAGNOSTIC SYSTEM IN EQUILIBRIUM

Whatever it looks like in the future, the *DSM* is unlikely to satisfy all the constituencies who use it. The needs, interests, and tools of these constituencies are too often incommensurate, and controversy is, therefore, built in. Yet the idea of incommensurability has another implication: It implies that the *DSM* has less power than critics fear (or that advocates want). Some critics of the *DSM,* for instance, point to the role of the manual in encouraging medicalization, defined as the process of defining nonmedical problems as medical ones and using a medical framework to treat them.[21] For these critics, the *DSM* is an especially effective instrument for expanding medical authority, and it is easy to see their point. The number of diagnoses contained in the *DSM* has grown over time. Furthermore, the diagnostic thresholds for some disorders have fallen in ways that make it easier for individuals to be categorized as mentally ill. This expansion both within and between disorders is consistent with an expanding view of illness, and it is an expansion we might want to resist. Edward Shorter argues that the public is more inclined to see illness today than it was in the past, even in the same symptoms.[22] Although people have long suffered from pain, fatigue, and other psychosomatic complaints, how people interpret these symptoms has changed. In the 1920s, these complaints might have been disregarded or interpreted as inevitable, whereas today they are seen as symptoms of disease and worthy of treatment.[23]

Yet when it comes to psychiatric disorders there are reasons to question whether the *DSM* has produced a cultural effect of this sort. For one, it is unclear whether the high prevalence of psychiatric disorders is entirely *artificial*—whether it is driven by how we choose to categorize psychiatric disorders or by a truly high prevalence of psychiatric disorders. Furthermore, it is unclear whether the promulgation of the *DSM*'s criteria has produced an increase in the prevalence of disorders, consistent with the idea that labels create disorders. Both of these ideas involve long-term processes. The *DSM* is a modern invention, so it is difficult to assess what psychiatric symptoms looked like before science developed the formal taxonomies to study them. Some studies have, however, tried to use uniform diagnostic standards applied to different eras in order to test whether depression has truly increased over time. The best evidence suggests that it has. Since World War II there has been an increase in the prevalence of depression between birth cohorts, along with a decrease in the initial age of onset.[24] Each successive cohort—divided into approximately decade-long intervals, such as 1945 to 1955—has experienced an increased lifetime risk of depression. It is difficult to determine precisely why this is occurring, but scientists have ruled out some possibilities. One possibility is that younger cohorts are simply more willing to report depression. Another is that they are better able to remember depression. And still another is that they live longer and, therefore, are more likely to experience depression at some point in their lifetime. None of these explanations, however, is entirely adequate, and the increase in depression appears instead to be real. Other evidence supports this interpretation. For one, the increase in depression corresponds to a parallel increase in some known risk factors for depression, like social isolation. In addition, the increase is not unique to depression, as might be the case if we believed that people are only becoming more sensitive to symptoms that are especially resonant, like unhappiness. Anxiety symptoms, too, are increasing.[25] Between the 1950s and the 1990s reports of anxiety increased by about a standard deviation. In the United States, the average *child psychiatric patient* in the 1950s reported the same levels of anxiety as the average *child* in the 1980s. There is no doubt that what we regard as "normal" has shifted over time, too, but it also seems clear that a current lifetime prevalence of psychiatric disorders around 50 percent might not be so unexpected as to cast doubt over the entire enterprise of psychiatric classification or to support unequivocally the argument that the *DSM* is implicated in the creation of an epidemic.

Even if we accept that the prevalence of psychiatric disorders is too high by some standards, it is difficult to argue that the *DSM* alone is responsible. The *DSM*'s influence is ultimately facilitated or diminished by other factors, including other institutions. In other words, the influence of the *DSM* is shaped by things that have an obdurate reality, one that cannot be revised as readily as a text. Nor can we regard the *DSM* more narrowly as a powerful handmaiden to psychiatrists, to whom we might then assign more blame. One example is the diagnosis of psychiatric disorders in children. Formal diagnostic criteria for children are especially controversial. There have been frequent calls to revise the *DSM*'s criteria in ways that better tolerate normal misbehavior in people who have yet to mature. Yet identifying instances of overdiagnosis in children is complicated. Overdiagnosis is not a reflection of the *DSM* alone, and, indeed, it is unclear whether any revisions to the *DSM* would reduce the problem, however one defines it. One question pertains to what purpose a diagnosis serves. There is evidence, for example, that students—often in collaboration with their parents and clearly with input from their physicians—take stimulants to enhance test performance. For this reason, the diagnosed prevalence of disorders like ADHD will likely increase the more schools are required to emphasize tests. Sharpening the *DSM*'s diagnostic criteria for ADHD might encourage clinicians to think twice about prescribing medications, but there is also evidence that clinicians adapt the *DSM* to serve the goals of treatment, as clinicians envision those goals. This behavior is relevant to how we consider ADHD. If ADHD is regarded as detrimental to performance on tests that do, in fact, have significant consequences for children, clinicians are likely to weigh test performance heavily in their assessments, even if not explicitly asked to do so. Both critics and advocates of the *DSM*'s current diagnostic criteria agree that requiring symptoms to cause "clinically significant impairment" is critical to creating more accurate diagnoses. High-stakes testing is surely "significant."

PTSD presents a similar case. There is evidence that PTSD might be increasingly overdiagnosed relative to its naturally occurring prevalence. But the clearest evidence for such an increase applies to somewhat unusual conditions, as discussed earlier. Those people pursuing a diagnosis of PTSD were, in effect, seeking disability benefits rather than a diagnosis per se. Furthermore, there is little evidence that those seeking such benefits did not suffer from anything at all. The pressure to seek a diagnosis might have been considerably weaker if they had more attractive employment alternatives or if they had other ways to secure income while unemployed. It is difficult to imagine any revisions to the *DSM* that would blunt these external influences or even to imagine some sort of coordination between psychiatrists and administrators that might mitigate them. Although the diagnostic criteria for PTSD have certainly expanded to admit more sources of trauma, this expansion is not the explanation for the increase in diagnosed cases of PTSD. Indeed, an increase occurred even among those with combat experience, who would be considered eligible for the diagnosis even under the strictest version of the *DSM*'s diagnostic criteria for the disorder. In the case of both ADHD and PTSD, the underlying issue is less about the diagnostic criteria—how high or low the threshold is, how sensitive or specific the criteria should be, what does or does not count as a trauma—than about the incentives of those seeking a diagnosis and how those incentives are shaped by other institutions.

A more general concern with the *DSM* is with limiting the influence of "external" factors writ large. Virtually everyone agrees the *DSM* should be crafted on the basis of credible and disinterested insights regarding the nature of psychiatric disorders. Perhaps the most prominent external influence that concerns critics is, of course, the pharmaceutical industry. The authors of *DSM-5* were concerned about this as well. They invested considerable effort in trying to limit the influence of pharmaceutical companies or at least to make their influence more transparent. It is debatable whether they succeeded. There is little doubt that pharmaceutical companies fund a great

deal of research on psychiatric disorders and that their funding is consequential. Clinical trials sponsored by pharmaceutical companies are more
likely to report favorable outcomes than those funded by other sources.[26]
Yet despite the growing recognition of the industry's influence, its power is
increasingly difficult to constrain. As federal funding for mental health research has declined, the influence of pharmaceutical companies has likely
increased. Yet here, too, there are other factors to consider, and pharmaceutical companies share at least some of the same concerns about the *DSM*
that scientists do. In recent years, pharmaceutical companies have moved
away from developing new psychiatric medications in part because the *DSM*
does not provide them with clean clinical targets. The sort of diagnostic
instrument the pharmaceutical industry might favor—criteria that lend
themselves to identifying molecular mechanisms, for example—would look
very different from what ultimately became *DSM-5*.

Critics of the *DSM* also point to the influence of the manual on the public. In this case, the claim is less that the public uses the *DSM* than that the
DSM can create psychiatric disorders. In particular, some critics charge that
the *DSM* can generate "diagnostic panics" or "fads" that artificially inflate
the prevalence of disorders. Several aspects of this idea are certainly correct.
Critics are correct to highlight the fact that labels are stigmatized. The
stigma surrounding psychiatric disorders inheres around labels as much as
symptoms, as discussed earlier. Furthermore, the stigma surrounding most
psychiatric disorders has not diminished over time. In some instances, it has
grown worse. There is also evidence that the *DSM* has reified cultural conceptions of psychiatric disorders. There are risks, then, to describing someone as suffering from "major depression" relative to recognizing simply that
the person is sad. But the idea that the *DSM* creates disorders whole cloth
can only take us so far. This is also evidence that the public endorses a complex view of psychiatric disorders and approaches the *DSM*—if it approaches
it at all—with specific goals in mind. The public, for instance, accepts the
genetic and biological causes of mental illness more than it did in the past,
but its growing appreciation of a biomedical approach has not supplanted its
recognition of environmental causes. The public continues to regard stress
and family upbringing, for example, as important determinants of mental

illness. By the same token, when asked what people suffering from psychiatric disorders should do, the public recommends medical treatment to some degree, as expected given the rise in medicalization and pharmaceutical treatments in particular, but the public also still encourages more informal treatment, like talking to friends and family. If the process of medicalization is seen in terms of adopting a strictly *medical* approach to treating psychological problems, the public is not entirely on board.

When thinking about how the public interfaces with the *DSM*, it is perhaps more appropriate to think of the *DSM* as a lexicon of symptoms, as a method of talking about disorders in a way that will compel clinicians and others to act. Patients want to communicate the severity of their symptoms, and the *DSM* provides them with the means to do that. This represents a weaker strain of influence than claiming that the *DSM creates* disorders, but it is not inconsistent with the history of other kinds of symptoms. In his history of psychosomatic illness, Edward Shorter presents a theory for why certain symptoms tend to be present during specific historical periods.[27] In Shorter's framework, medical nomenclature provides the terms for what is to be regarded as the most credible signs of illness. As he puts it, "as the culture changes its mind about what is legitimate disease and what is not, the pattern of psychosomatic illness changes."[28] In the same vein, the *DSM* might not have created disorders that the public suddenly recognizes in its experience so much as it allowed those who are suffering to express their distress in ways that compel clinicians. Further evidence that the public uses the *DSM* as much as the *DSM* uses the public is apparent in how patients talk about their diagnoses. Patients talk about symptoms far more than disorders. Indeed, they actively distance themselves from diagnoses whenever possible. One interpretation of this behavior is that it reveals a rather sophisticated resolution to a sociomedical dilemma: Patients recognize that treatment is beneficial, but they also recognize that the stigma of a psychiatric diagnosis is severe. Presented with this problem, patients talk about *symptoms* and, therefore, behave in a way that ensures treatment, but this also allows them to distance themselves from a label and perhaps some of that label's negative connotations. This symptom-disorder discontinuity works in another way as well: When patients evaluate how well their treatment is working, they do so on the basis of how well it alleviates specific symptoms and not whether it cures the disorder altogether. When taking a prescription medication, for example, patients ask how it will reduce their fear or improve their appetite, something all people experience more or less of. Illness is sometimes regarded as a distant land, but psychiatric disorders are often closer than people think, and this characteristic of psychiatric disorders allows patients to migrate to and fro in ways that serve their needs.

Even if we accept that the public turns to the *DSM* only as a way to frame its symptoms, the influence of the *DSM* faces yet another filter. The credibility of the *DSM* is also mediated through clinicians. The *DSM* is clearly the central authoritative document for purposes of diagnosis, but a diagnosis is ultimately rendered by a clinician, and patients often accept what a clinician decides. In many cases, the diagnosing clinician is in fact their physician, who has much broader diagnostic authority. And some evidence suggests that physicians are the ultimate arbiters of the entire concept of disease, no matter how contested a disease might be. In a classic study, Campbell and colleagues asked a group of medical students and other adults about their concept of disease.[29] They asked participants to indicate whether some common diagnostic terms referred to actual diseases or not. They then compared the characteristics of those terms that were viewed as diseases with those that were not. Some differences between the two were obvious. The cause of the problem, for example, was very important to how it was categorized. Infectious diseases were classified as diseases by virtually everyone in the study. Yet apart from these obvious influences, the most important characteristic was whether a doctor was necessary for a diagnosis. In short, when thinking about whether a disease was real, the public asked, simply, do I need a doctor to diagnose it?

THE LAST *DSM*

One way to resolve some of the tensions in the diagnostic system is to accept different interests as a fact of life and craft suitable diagnostic criteria for different audiences. Some recent efforts can be interpreted along these lines. In effect, these efforts are attempts cleave the *DSM* according to its audience, to think, for example, about diagnostic criteria that are useful for clinicians and about different diagnostic criteria that are useful for researchers. The RDoC is the strongest statement in this regard. Its authors are affiliated with the NIMH, primarily a research organization, and want to create diagnostic criteria that are maximally useful for scientists. Indeed, the creators of the RDoC have essentially disavowed any clinical value for the criteria, at least in the short term. They also frame their effort as an attempt to circumvent some of the problems they see with subjectively reported symptoms. They cast the RDoC as a scientific workaround to the problem of self-reports, emphasizing the hard data of biological samples collected in labs over the soft data of symptoms reported in surveys. They also emphasize the importance of dimensions of functioning, rather than categories of disorder.

These differences are not slight. The RDoC is very different from *DSM-5* in intention and in reality. To be sure, *DSM-5* was written with many of the same concerns in mind—and the RDoC has been endorsed by the authors of *DSM-5*—but the *DSM* ended up in a very different place.[30] Despite a declared interest in producing more scientifically defensible criteria, the authors of *DSM-5* ultimately fell back on the relevance of clinical utility. In a statement that would not be out of place in *DSM-I*, the first paragraph of *DSM-5*'s preface states this directly: "*DSM* is intended to serve as a practical, functional, and flexible guide for organizing information that can aid in the accurate diagnosis and treatment of mental disorders," and, later, "this edition of *DSM* was designed first and foremost to be a useful guide to clinical practice."[31] These statements can be read as a plea for tolerance as much as a mission statement. The word "accurate" is smuggled into the passage, to be sure, but it carries no more significance than the word "flexible."

For all the controversy surrounding the *DSM*, its influence is remarkably constrained. It sometimes forestalls skepticism, and it often demands assent, but it does not do so through its own autotelic force. The meaning and significance of the *DSM* is filtered through many constituencies, each with its own set of interests and values. This distorts the *DSM*—few deploy the diagnostic criteria entirely faithfully—and it occasions a lot of fear and concern regarding the stewardship of the diagnostic enterprise. Professionals ought to be in charge of making accurate diagnoses. Yet this filtering also serves as a system of checks and balances. It might be difficult to extract the *DSM* from all forms of external influence—to, in effect, set it on the highest perch of objectivity—but it might also be undesirable. There is unlikely to be any one best classification system that adequately suits all purposes. Nor is there likely to be any one version of the *DSM* that stands the test of time, cataloging only eternal disorders and refusing to codify "problems in living" unique to a specific time or place. This situation has left many people uneasy, and it leaves people especially apprehensive when so many other areas of medicine have benefited from high-tech diagnostic tools. These tools allow physicians to apprehend deep causes when in the past they only saw surface clues. Yet, in the end, psychiatric disorders can only fit imperfectly into this emerging medical framework. Like some physical disorders, some psychiatric disorders lead to suffering and even death. But the only way to treat psychiatric disorders seriously is to grant them an ontological flexibility that we are no longer willing to grant other diseases.

It is useful to return to where we began. As a provocation, this book began by posing questions about the ontological status of psychiatric disorders. Yet it is important to draw a distinction between questions of *ontology* and questions of *epistemology*.[32] When it comes to psychiatric disorders, the two are often conflated. *Ontology* refers to whether disorders do in fact exist as some kind of abstract entity; *epistemology* refers to our ability to know anything about those disorders. Much of the discussion surrounding the *DSM* pertains to the latter. Most scientists are committed to the ontological reality of disorders and critique only whether one approach or another does a better job of approximating that reality. The RDoC, for instance, is cast in this vein. It might assert that it does a better job than the *DSM* in describing psychiatric disorders as they exist in nature, but the *DSM* and RDoC fundamentally agree that psychiatric disorders are real. One interpretation of the failure of contemporary science to say much about the accuracy of diagnostic classification is that psychiatric disorders are enormously complex in their etiology and presentation, far more complex than many other things science has studied and classified successfully. Science simply cannot do as well in describing psychiatric disorders as it can in describing, say, natural elements. Some critics go further, though. In reviewing all the controversy surrounding the science of psychiatric disorders, as I have done here, they conclude that disorders have no ontological reality, that they are entirely and only social constructs. In its strongest form this idea has faded from view, but elements of it remain.

Perhaps, though, ontological questions are irrelevant. Psychiatric disorders may be real when they are manifest in any one person—and maybe everyone involved in the debate can eventually agree on the nature of a particular case—but disorders are unlikely to manifest in exactly the same way in all people. If so, the "failures" of modern science are deep seated, in the sense that it is hard to imagine a time when better science will be able finally to deliver the best criteria for characterizing a deeply complex target. Yet it is also hard to imagine a time when society suddenly decides to disregard the idea of mental illness altogether or to abandon completely the tools it has at its disposal. Diagnostic *criteria* may be provisional, as most people agree with respect to the current *DSM*, but the idea of "mental illness" is not. Indeed, the idea of mental illness could be cemented even further as we develop better means of remediating suffering, whether those means are pharmaceutical, neurological, psychological, cognitive, or social. Even a fundamental paradigm shift in psychiatric classification—something many scientists aspire to—will only change the paradigm of *diagnostic classification*, not the commitment of clinicians, scientists, or cultures to the ontological reality of mental illness. That commitment is longstanding and was, if anything, solidified by the *DSM*. And it was solidified despite the *DSM*'s superficiality, its incomplete use of science, its latent judgments, its political controversies, its sometimes ad hoc definition of mental disorder, and the ways in which the authors of its prior editions seemed routinely to disavow its current editions. The *DSM* is a remarkable accomplishment. The last *DSM* will never be the final *DSM*, but mental illness is here to stay.

NOTES

1. THE CONTESTED ONTOLOGY OF PSYCHIATRIC DISORDERS

1. John W. Barnhill, ed., *DSM-5 Clinical Cases* (Washington, D.C.: American Psychiatric Association, 2014).
2. Katharina Meyerbröker, "Case 5.4: Flying Fears," in *DSM-5 Clinical Cases*, ed. John W. Barnhill (Washington, D.C.: American Psychiatric Association, 2014).
3. Richard A. Friedman, "Case 4.3: Grief and Depression," in *DSM-5 Clinical Cases*, ed. John W. Barnhill (Washington, D.C.: American Psychiatric Association, 2014).
4. Ibid., 80.
5. Jonna K. Vuoskoski et al., "Who Enjoys Listening to Sad Music and Why?," *Music Perception: An Interdisciplinary Journal* 29, no. 3 (2012): 311–17.
6. Maurice M. Ohayon, "Prevalence of Hallucinations and Their Pathological Associations in the General Population," *Psychiatry Research* 97, no. 2–3 (2000): 153–64.
7. Jerome C. Wakefield, "High Mental Disorder Rates Are Based on Invalid Measures: Questions About the Claimed Ubiquity of Mutation-Induced Dysfunction," *Behavioral and Brain Sciences* 29, no. 4 (2006): 425.
8. Allen J. Frances, *Saving Normal: An Insider's Revolt Against Out-of-Control Psychiatric Diagnosis, "DSM-5," Big Pharma, and the Medicalization of Ordinary Life* (New York: William Morrow, 2014).
9. Thomas Insel et al., "Research Domain Criteria (RDoC): Toward a New Classification Framework for Research on Mental Disorders," *American Journal of Psychiatry* 167, no. 7 (2010): 748–51.
10. Nick Craddock and Michael J. Owen, "The Kraepelinian Dichotomy—Going, Going . . . but Still Not Gone," *British Journal of Psychiatry* 196, no. 2 (2010): 92–95.
11. Michel Foucault, *Madness and Civilization* (1965; New York: Vintage, 1988).
12. Ian Hacking, *Mad Travelers: Reflections on the Reality of Transient Mental Illnesses* (Cambridge, Mass.: Harvard University Press, 1998). Hacking uses the concept of an ecological niche in a similar fashion to explain the emergence of transient illnesses.
13. Charles E. Rosenberg, "The Tyranny of Diagnosis: Specific Entities and Individual Experience," *Milbank Quarterly* 80, no. 2 (2002): 237–60.
14. Theodore Millon, "Classification in Psychopathology: Rationale, Alternatives, and Standards," *Journal of Abnormal Psychology* 100, no. 3 (1991): 245–61.
15. Ibid., 246.

2. WHAT DIAGNOSES ARE: *DSM-III* AND THE FORM OF CONTEMPORARY PSYCHIATRIC DIAGNOSES

1. The International Classification of Disease (ICD) also provides diagnostic criteria and is widely used. The ICD and the *DSM* share a similar spirit, though, and there have been efforts to make them more consistent with each other over time.

2. Roger K. Blashfield et al., "The Cycle of Classification: *DSM-I* through *DSM-5*," *Annual Review of Clinical Psychology* 10, no. 1 (2014): 25–51, provides an overview of the *DSM* revisions.

3. Steven E. Hyman, "Can Neuroscience Be Integrated Into the DSM-V?," *National Review of Neuroscience* 8, no. 9 (2007): 725–32.

4. American Psychiatric Association, *Diagnostic and Statistical Manual of Mental Disorders*, 2nd ed. (Washington, D.C.: American Psychiatric Association, 1968), 36–37.

5. Ibid., 36.

6. Ibid., 35–37.

7. L. N. Robins and J. E. Helzer, "Diagnosis and Clinical Assessment: The Current State of Psychiatric Diagnosis," *Annual Review of Psychology* 37, no. 1 (1986): 409–32.

8. Charles Brenner, "A Psychoanalytic Perspective on Depression," *Journal of the American Psychoanalytic Association* 39, no. 1 (1991): 25–43.

9. Ibid., 37.

10. Gerald N. Grob, "Origins of DSM-I: A Study in Appearance and Reality," *American Journal of Psychiatry* 148, no. 4 (1991): 421–31.

11. American Psychiatric Association, *Diagnostic and Statistical Manual of Mental Disorders* (Washington, D.C.: American Psychiatric Association, 1952), 5.

12. Ibid., 31.

13. Gerald N. Grob, "The Forging of Mental Health Policy in America: World War II to New Frontier," *Journal of the History of Medicine and Allied Sciences* 42 (1987): 410–46.

14. D. L. Rosenhan, "On Being Sane in Insane Places," *Science* 179, no. 4070 (1973): 250–58.

15. Philip Ash, "The Reliability of Psychiatric Diagnoses," *Journal of Abnormal and Social Psychology* 44, no. 2 (1949): 272–76.

16. R. E. Kendell et al., "Diagnostic Criteria of American and British Psychiatrists," *Archives of General Psychiatry* 25, no. 2 (1971): 123–30.

17. Thomas Szasz, "The Myth of Mental Illness," *American Psychologist* 15 (1960): 113–18.

18. Thomas J. Scheff, *Being Mentally Ill: A Sociological Theory* (London: Weidenfield and Nicolson, 1966).

19. APA, *DSM-II*, 44.

20. A. McDowall, S. Owen, and A. A. Robin, "A Controlled Comparison of Diazepam and Amylobarbitone in Anxiety States," *British Journal of Psychiatry* 112, no. 487 (1966): 629–31, 629; N. S. Capstick et al., "A Comparative Trial of Diazepam (Valium) and Amylobarbitone," *British Journal of Psychiatry* 111 (1965): 517–19, 517.

21. H. Keith H. Brodie and Melvin Sabshin, "An Overview of Trends in Psychiatric Research: 1963–1972," *American Journal of Psychiatry* 130, no. 12 (1973): 1309–18.

22. Charles E. Rosenberg, *Our Present Complaint: American Medicine, Then and Now* (Baltimore, Md.: Johns Hopkins University Press, 2007).

23. Grob, "Origins of DSM-I: A Study in Appearance and Reality."

24. D. Mechanic, "Emerging Trends in Mental Health Policy and Practice," *Health Affairs* 17, no. 6 (1998): 82–98.

25. Richard G. Frank, Howard H. Goldman, and Thomas G. McGuire, "Trends in Mental Health Cost Growth: An Expanded Role for Management?," *Health Affairs* 28, no. 3 (2009): 649–59.

26. Rick Mayes and Allan V. Horwitz, "DSM-III and the Revolution in the Classification of Mental Illness," *Journal of the History of the Behavioral Sciences* 41, no. 3 (2005): 249–67.

27. Roderick D. Buchanan, "Legislative Warriors: American Psychiatrists, Psychologists, and Competing Claims Over Psychotherapy in the 1950s," *Journal of the History of the Behavioral Sciences* 39, no. 3 (2003): 225–49.

28. Ibid.

29. Mayes and Horwitz, "DSM-III and the Revolution in the Classification of Mental Illness."

30. Theodore Millon, "The DSM-III: An Insider's Perspective," *American Psychologist* 38, no. 7 (1983): 804–14.

31. Roger K. Blashfield, "Feighner et al., Invisible Colleges, and the Matthew Effect," *Schizophrenia Bulletin* 8, no. 1 (1982): 1–6, 4.

32. Mitchell Wilson, "DSM-III and the Transformation of American Psychiatry: A History," *American Journal of Psychiatry* 150, no. 3 (1993): 399–410.

33. The *DSM-III* did not, however, adopt all of Kraepelin's foci. For instance, Kraepelin emphasized the prognosis of symptoms, too, though prognosis was largely ignored in *DSM-III*.

34. American Psychiatric Association, *Diagnostic and Statistical Manual of Mental Disorders*, 4th ed. (Washington, D.C.: American Psychiatric Association, 1994), 427–28.

35. Isaac R. Galatzer-Levy and Richard A. Bryant, "636,120 Ways to Have Posttraumatic Stress Disorder," *Perspectives on Psychological Science* 8, no. 6 (2013): 651–62.

36. Nancy Cantor et al., "Psychiatric Diagnosis as Prototype Categorization," *Journal of Abnormal Psychology* 89, no. 2 (1980): 181–93.

37. American Psychiatric Association, *Diagnostic and Statistical Manual of Mental Disorders*, 3rd ed. (Washington, D.C.: American Psychiatric Association, 1980), 6.

38. Ibid.

39. Ibid.; Eli Robins and Samuel B. Guze, "Establishment of Diagnostic Validity in Psychiatric Illness: Its Application to Schizophrenia," *American Journal of Psychiatry* 126, no. 7 (1970): 983–87.

40. APA, *DSM*, 44–45, 46.

41. APA, *DSM-II*, 2.

42. Ibid.

43. Ibid.

44. Robins and Helzer, "Diagnosis and Clinical Assessment: The Current State of Psychiatric Diagnosis."

45. APA, *DSM-III*, 24.

46. Lee N. Robins, "How Recognizing 'Comorbidities' in Psychopathology May Lead to an Improved Research Nosology," *Clinical Psychology: Science and Practice* 1, no. 1 (1994): 93–95.

47. Wilson, "DSM-III and the Transformation of American Psychiatry: A History," 407.

48. Robert L. Spitzer and Joseph L. Fleiss, "A Reanalysis of the Reliability of Psychiatric Diagnosis," *British Journal of Psychiatry* 125, no. 587 (1974): 341–47.

49. Robert L. Spitzer, "Values and Assumptions in the Development of DSM-III and DSM-III-R: An Insider's Perspective and a Belated Response to Sadler, Hulgus, and Agich's 'on Values in Recent American Psychiatric Classification,'" *Journal of Nervous and Mental Disease* 189 (2001): 351–59, 354.

50. Ibid.

51. APA, *DSM-III*, 26.

52. American Psychiatric Association, *Diagnostic and Statistical Manual of Mental Disorders*, 3rd. ed., rev. (Washington, D.C.: American Psychiatric Association, 1987), 32.

53. APA, *DSM-IV*, 4.

54. APA, *DSM*, 33.

55. Ibid., 41.

56. Ibid., 31, 41.

57. Ibid., 29, 31, 32.

58. Mayes and Horwitz, "DSM-III and the Revolution in the Classification of Mental Illness."

59. APA, *DSM-II*, 39.

60. Millon, "The DSM-III: An Insider's Perspective."

61. Ibid., 806.

62. J. P. Feighner et al., "Diagnostic Criteria for Use in Psychiatric Research," *Archives of General Psychiatry* 26, no. 1 (1972): 57–63.

63. W. L. Cassidy et al., "Clinical Observations in Manic-Depressive Disease: A Quantitative Study of One Hundred Manic-Depressive Patients and Fifty Medically Sick Controls," *Journal of the American Medical Association* 164, no. 14 (1957): 1535–46; Kenneth S. Kendler, Rodrigo A. Muñoz, and George Murphy, "The Development of the Feighner Criteria: A Historical Perspective," *American Journal of Psychiatry* 167, no. 2 (2010): 134–42, 136.

64. Robert L. Spitzer, Jean Endicott, and Eli Robins, "Clinical Criteria for Psychiatric Diagnosis and DSM-III," *American Journal of Psychiatry* 132, no. 11 (1975): 1187–92.

65. APA, *DSM-III*, 6.

66. Josef Parnas and Pierre Bovet, "Psychiatry Made Easy: Operationalism and Some of Its Consequences," in *Philosophical Issues in Psychiatry III*, ed. Kenneth S. Kendler and Josef Parnas (New York: Oxford, 2014). Parnas and Bovet provide a general discussion of this issue.

67. APA, *DSM-III*, 65, 66.

68. Julie Nordgaard, Louis Sass, and Josef Parnas, "The Psychiatric Interview: Validity, Structure, and Subjectivity," *European Archives of Psychiatry & Clinical Neuroscience* 263, no. 4 (2013): 353–64.

69. Robert L. Spitzer, Janet B. Forman, and John Nee, "DSM-III Field Trials: I. Initial Interrater Diagnostic Reliability," *American Journal of Psychiatry* 136, no. 6 (1979): 815–17.

70. Spitzer and Fleiss, "A Reanalysis of the Reliability of Psychiatric Diagnosis," 344.

71. The claim that *DSM-III* produced greater reliability is not entirely uncontroversial. Kirk and Kutchins provided a thorough critique of the kappa statistic and its interpretation in the *DSM-III* field trials, highlighting in particular that claims for greater reliability were "premature" and very difficult to generalize from given the centrality of the base rate of a disorder in determining a high or low reliability. Stuart A. Kirk and Herb Kutchins, *The Selling of DSM: The Rhetoric of Science in Psychiatry* (New York: A. De Gruyter, 1992), 158.

72. Buchanan, "Legislative Warriors: American Psychiatrists, Psychologists, and Competing Claims Over Psychotherapy in the 1950s," 232.

73. Ibid., 234.

74. Gerald L. Klerman, "A Debate on DSM-III: The Advantages of DSM-III," *American Journal of Psychiatry* 141, no. 4 (1984): 539–42.

75. Melvin Sabshin, "Turning Points in Twentieth-Century American Psychiatry," *American Journal of Psychiatry* 147, no. 10 (1990): 1267–74.

76. Robert L. Spitzer et al., *Structured Clinical Interview for DSM-III-R, Patient Edition* (Washington, D.C.: American Psychiatric Association, 1990).

77. Millon, "The DSM-III: An Insider's Perspective."

78. Blashfield et al., "The Cycle of Classification: DSM-I through DSM-5."

79. Wilson, "DSM-III and the Transformation of American Psychiatry."

80. Millon, "The DSM-III: An Insider's Perspective."

81. Ibid., 804.

82. Spitzer and Fleiss, "A Reanalysis of the Reliability of Psychiatric Diagnosis."

83. Spitzer, "Values and Assumptions in the Development of DSM-III and DSM-III-R," 353.

84. Ibid., 354.

85. Wilson, "DSM-III and the Transformation of American Psychiatry."

3. *DSM-III* AND THE DESCRIPTIVE SCIENCE OF PSYCHIATRIC DISORDERS

1. Leo Srole, "Measurement and Classification in Socio-Psychiatric Epidemiology: Midtown Manhattan Study (1954) and Midtown Manhattan Restudy (1974)," *Journal of Health and Social Behavior* 16, no. 4 (1975): 347–64.

2. Gerald N. Grob, "Public Policy and Mental Illnesses: Jimmy Carter's Presidential Commission on Mental Health," *Milbank Quarterly* 83, no. 3 (2005): 425–56.

3. Darrel A. Regier et al., "Limitations of Diagnostic Criteria and Assessment Instruments for Mental Disorders: Implications for Research and Policy," *Archives of General Psychiatry* 55, no. 2 (1998): 109–15.

4. Lee N. Robins and Darrel A. Regier, eds., *Psychiatric Disorders in America: The Epidemiological Area Study* (New York: Free Press, 1991).

5. R. C. Kessler et al., "Lifetime and Twelve-Month Prevalence of DSM-III-R Psychiatric Disorders in the United States: Results from the National Comorbidity Survey," *Archives of General Psychiatry* 51, no. 1 (1994): 8–19.

6. Estimates of the prevalence of psychiatric disorders are also sensitive to how people respond to surveys—and how they seek to *avoid* responding to surveys. The prevalence estimate in the NCS was much higher than in the ECA in part because of differences in the structure of their survey instruments. In the NCS, respondents were given screener or "stem" questions up front, whereas in the ECA each set of diagnostic criteria was conveyed sequentially, including their stem questions. Because of this, the NCS in effect locked respondents with qualifying symptoms into further questions later on, whereas respondents in the ECA eventually learned that by saying no to certain symptoms presented in a stem, they could avoid answering many more questions later on. For this reason, the prevalence of psychiatric disorders initially appeared much higher in the NCS

and the ECA, though attempts to standardize the two surveys' estimates, including on the basis of how they administered their questions, found that the differences between the two were probably smaller than they appeared at first. The lingering issue, as Regier and colleagues put it, was more fundamentally related to the *DSM* itself: whether either survey could "adequately differentiate between diagnosis and treatment need." Regier et al., "Limitations of Diagnostic Criteria and Assessment Instruments for Mental Disorders," 115.

7. Kessler et al., "Lifetime and Twelve-Month Prevalence of DSM-III-R Psychiatric Disorders."

8. Ibid.

9. R. C. Kessler et al., "Prevalence, Severity, and Comorbidity of Twelve-Month DSM-IV Disorders in the National Comorbidity Survey Replication," *Archives of General Psychiatry* 62, no. 6 (2005): 617–27.

10. Ibid.

11. Ibid.

12. Ronald C. Kessler et al., "Prevalence and Treatment of Mental Disorders, 1990 to 2003," *New England Journal of Medicine* 352 (2005): 2515–23.

13. Ronald C. Kessler et al., "Lifetime Prevalence and Age-of-Onset Distributions of DSM-IV Disorders in the National Comorbidity Survey Replication," *Archives of General Psychiatry* 62, no. 6 (2005): 593–602.

14. Ibid.

15. Josep Maria Haro et al., "Concordance of the Composite International Diagnostic Interview Version 3.0 (CIDI 3.0) with Standardized Clinical Assessments in the WHO World Mental Health Surveys," *International Journal of Methods in Psychiatric Research* 15, no. 4 (2006): 167–80.

16. The WHO World Mental Health Survey Consortium, "Prevalence, Severity, and Unmet Need for Treatment of Mental Disorders in the World Health Organization World Mental Health Surveys," *Journal of the American Medical Association* 291, no. 21 (2004): 2581–90.

17. Evelyn Bromet et al., "Cross-National Epidemiology of DSM-IV Major Depressive Episode," *BMC Medicine* 9, no. 1 (2011): 90–105.

18. Ronald C. Kessler and Evelyn J. Bromet, "The Epidemiology of Depression Across Cultures," *Annual Review of Public Health* 34, no. 1 (2013): 119–38.

19. G. E. Simon et al., "Understanding Cross-National Differences in Depression Prevalence," *Psychological Medicine* 32(2002): 585–94.

20. Kessler and Bromet, "The Epidemiology of Depression Across Cultures."

21. Ronny Bruffaerts et al., "Proportion of Patients Without Mental Disorders Being Treated in Mental Health Services Worldwide," *British Journal of Psychiatry* 206, no. 2 (2014): 101–09.

22. Simon et al., "Understanding Cross-National Differences in Depression Prevalence."

23. T. E. Moffitt et al., "How Common Are Common Mental Disorders? Evidence That Lifetime Prevalence Rates Are Doubled by Prospective Versus Retrospective Ascertainment," *Psychological Medicine* 40, no. 06 (2010): 899–909.

24. G. Andrews et al., "Recall of Depressive Episode 25 Years Previously," *Psychological Medicine* 29, no. 04 (1999): 787–91.

25. A. Frances, "Problems in Defining Clinical Significance in Epidemiological Studies," *Archives of General Psychiatry* 55, no. 2 (1998): 119–19.

26. In an interview with the *New York Times*, Kessler pushes the point in noting that some mental illnesses are little more than "psychiatric hangnails." Benedict Carye, "Most Will

Be Mentally Ill at Some Point, Study Says," *New York Times*, June 7, 2005, http://www.ny times.com/2005/06/07/health/most-will-be-mentally-ill-at-some-point-study-says.html.

4. RETHINKING THE *DSM*

1. Gary Greenberg, *The Book of Woe: The DSM and the Unmaking of Psychiatry* (New York: Blue Rider, 2013), 23.

2. I am here using the idea of a "conservative approach" as a catchall. Those behind the proposals I review do not necessarily regard their proposals as "conservative" or align themselves with others within this approach as I describe it. In fact, given the consequences of even slight revisions to the *DSM*, even seemingly "conservative" approaches can yield very different kinds of disorders.

3. American Psychiatric Association, *Diagnostic and Statistical Manual of Mental Disorders*, 3rd ed. (Washington, D.C.: American Psychiatric Association, 1980), 6.

4. American Psychiatric Association, *Diagnostic and Statistical Manual of Mental Disorders*, 4th ed. (Washington, D.C.: American Psychiatric Association, 1994), xxi.

5. Darrel A. Regier et al., "Limitations of Diagnostic Criteria and Assessment Instruments for Mental Disorders: Implications for Research and Policy," *Archives of General Psychiatry* 55, no. 2 (1998): 109–15.

6. W. E. Narrow et al., "Revised Prevalence Estimates of Mental Disorders in the United States: Using a Clinical Significance Criterion to Reconcile 2 Surveys' Estimates," *Archives of General Psychiatry* 59, no. 2 (2002): 115–23.

7. Darrel A. Regier, William E. Narrow, and Donald S. Rae, "For DSM-V, It's the 'Disorder Threshold,' Stupid," *Archives of General Psychiatry* 61, no. 10 (2004): 1051–51.

8. H. A. Pincus, W. W. Davis, and L. E. McQueen, "'Subthreshold' Mental Disorders. A Review and Synthesis of Studies on Minor Depression and Other 'Brand Names,'" *British Journal of Psychiatry* 174, no. 4 (1999): 288–96.

9. R. L. Spitzer, "Diagnosis and Need for Treatment Are Not the Same," *Archives of General Psychiatry* 55, no. 2 (1998): 120.

10. Ibid.

11. Kenneth F. Schaffner, "Comment: A Tail of a Tiger," in *Philosophical Issues in Psychiatry: Explanation, Phenomenology, and Nosology*, ed. Kenneth S. Kendler and Josef Parnas (Baltimore, Md.: Johns Hopkins University Press, 2008).

12. John Mirowsky and Catherine E. Ross, "Measurement for a Human Science," *Journal of Health and Social Behavior* 43 (2002): 152–70.

13. Steven E. Hyman, "The Diagnosis of Mental Disorders: The Problem of Reification," *Annual Review of Clinical Psychology* 6 (2010): 155–79.

14. R. C. Kessler et al., "Short Screening Scales to Monitor Population Prevalences and Trends in Non-Specific Psychological Distress," *Psychological Medicine* 32, no. 6 (2002): 959–76.

15. Blair Wheaton, "Personal Resources and Mental Health," in *Research in Community and Mental Health*, ed. James R. Greenley (Greenwich, Conn.: JAI, 1985), 139–84.

16. Mirowsky and Ross, "Measurement for a Human Science."

17. Denny Borsboom and Angélique O. J. Cramer, "Network Analysis: An Integrative Approach to the Structure of Psychopathology," *Annual Review of Clinical Psychology* 9, no. 1 (2013): 91–121.

18. Denny Borsboom et al., "The Small World of Psychopathology," *PLoS ONE* 6, no. 11 (2011): e27407.

19. Jerome C. Wakefield, "The Concept of Mental Disorder: On the Boundary Between Biological Facts and Social Values," *American Psychologist* 47 (1992): 373–88.

20. R. M. Nesse, "Is Depression an Adaptation?," *Archives of General Psychiatry* 57, no. 1 (2000): 14–20.

21. Allan V. Horwitz and Jerome C. Wakefield, *The Loss of Sadness: How Psychiatry Transformed Normal Sorrow Into Depressive Disorder* (New York: Oxford University Press, 2007).

22. J. C. Wakefield et al., "Extending the Bereavement Exclusion for Major Depression to Other Losses: Evidence from the National Comorbidity Survey," *Archives of General Psychiatry* 64, no. 4 (2007): 433–40.

23. Jerome C. Wakefield and Mark F. Schmitz, "When Does Depression Become a Disorder? Using Recurrence Rates to Evaluate the Validity of Proposed Changes in Major Depression Diagnostic Thresholds," *World Psychiatry* 12, no. 1 (2013): 44–52.

24. See, for a review, Joseph Zohar, "Is There Room for a New Diagnostic Subtype—the Schizo-Obsessive Subtype?," *CNS Spectrums* 2, no. 3 (1997): 49–50.

25. Steven E. Hyman, "Can Neuroscience Be Integrated Into the DSM-V?," *National Review of Neuroscience* 8, no. 9 (2007): 725–32.

26. Paul R. McHugh, "Striving for Coherence: Psychiatry's Efforts Over Classification," *Journal of the American Medical Association* 293, no. 20 (2005): 2526–28.

27. Nick Craddock and Michael J. Owen, "The Kraepelinian Dichotomy—Going, Going . . . but Still Not Gone," *British Journal of Psychiatry* 196, no. 2 (2010): 92–95.

5. HOW PROFESSIONALS USE DIAGNOSES

1. Nancy S. Kim and Woo-kyoung Ahn, "Clinical Psychologists' Theory-Based Representations of Mental Disorders Predict Their Diagnostic Reasoning and Memory," *Journal of Experimental Psychology: General* 131, no. 4 (2002): 451–76.

2. Jennelle E. Yopchick and Nancy S. Kim, "The Influence of Causal Information on Judgments of Treatment Efficacy," *Memory and Cognition* 37, no. 1 (2009): 29–41.

3. Woo-Kyoung Ahn, Laura R. Novick, and Nancy S. Kim, "Understanding Behavior Makes It More Normal," *Psychonomic Bulletin and Review* 10, no. 3 (2003): 746–52.

4. Nancy S. Kim et al., "Proportionate Responses to Life Events Influence Clinicians' Judgments of Psychological Abnormality," *Psychological Assessment* 24, no. 3 (2012): 581–91.

5. Woo-kyoung Ahn et al., "Beliefs About Essences and the Reality of Mental Disorders," *Psychological Science* 17, no. 9 (2006): 759–66.

6. Howard N. Garb, *Studying the Clinician: Judgment Research and Psychological Assessment* (Washington, D.C.: American Psychological Association, 1998); M. Katherine Shear et al., "Diagnosis of Nonpsychotic Patients in Community Clinics," *American Journal of Psychiatry* 157, no. 4 (2000): 581–87.

7. Shear et al., "Diagnosis of Nonpsychotic Patients in Community Clinics," 584.

8. Paul R. Miller et al., "Inpatient Diagnostic Assessments: 1. Accuracy of Structured Vs. Unstructured Interviews," *Psychiatry Research* 105, no. 3 (2001): 255–64.

9. Reuben J. Silver, "Practicing Professional Psychology," *American Psychologist* 56, no. 11 (2001): 1008–14.

10. Monica Ramirez Basco et al., "Methods to Improve Diagnostic Accuracy in a Community Mental Health Setting," *American Journal of Psychiatry* 157, no. 10 (2000): 1599–605.

11. Mark Zimmerman and Jill I. Mattia, "Psychiatric Diagnosis in Clinical Practice: Is Comorbidity Being Missed?," *Comprehensive Psychiatry* 40, no. 3 (1999): 182–91.

12. Steven Reiss, Grant W. Levitan, and Joseph Szyszko, "Emotional Disturbance and Mental Retardation: Diagnostic Overshadowing," *American Journal of Mental Deficiency* 86, no. 6 (1982): 567–74.

13. Jared W. Keeley, Chafen S. DeLao, and Claire L. Kirk, "The Commutative Property in Comorbid Diagnosis: Does A + B = B + A?," *Clinical Psychological Science* 1, no. 1 (2013): 16–29.

14. Carlos E. Climent et al., "A Comparison of Traditional and Symptom-Checklist-Based Histories," *American Journal of Psychiatry* 132, no. 4 (1975): 450–53.

15. Eliot Freidson, *Profession of Medicine: A Study of the Sociology of Applied Knowledge* (Chicago: University of Chicago, 1988), 347.

16. Stefan Timmermans and Emily S. Kolker, "Evidence-Based Medicine and the Reconfiguration of Medical Knowledge," *Journal of Health and Social Behavior* 45 (2004): 177–93; Stefan Timmermans and Alison Angell, "Evidence-Based Medicine, Clinical Uncertainty, and Learning to Doctor," *Journal of Health and Social Behavior* 42, no. 4 (2001): 342–59.

17. See especially Timmermans and Angell, "Evidence-Based Medicine, Clinical Uncertainty, and Learning to Doctor."

18. David Armstrong, "Clinical Autonomy, Individual and Collective: The Problem of Changing Doctors' Behaviour," *Social Science and Medicine* 55, no. 10 (2002): 1771–77.

19. Owen Whooley, "Diagnostic Ambivalence: Psychiatric Workarounds and the Diagnostic and Statistical Manual of Mental Disorders," *Sociology of Health and Illness* 32, no. 3 (2010): 452–69.

20. T. M. Luhrmann, *Of Two Minds: An Anthropologist Looks at American Psychiatry* (New York: Vintage, 2000), 302.

21. Ibid., 48.

22. Ibid., 49.

23. H. G. Pope Jr. and J. F. Lipinski, "Diagnosis in Schizophrenia and Manic-Depressive Illness: A Reassessment of the Specificity of Schizophrenic Symptoms in the Light of Current Research," *Archives of General Psychiatry* 35, no. 7 (1978): 811–28.

24. Carlo Perris, "A Study of Cycloid Psychoses," *Acta Psychiatrica Scandinavica* s253 (1974): 7–79.

25. Edward Shorter, "The History of Lithium Therapy," *Bipolar Disorders* 11, no. 2 (2009): 4–9.

26. Whooley, "Diagnostic Ambivalence."

27. Lorence S. Miller et al., "Opinions and Use of the DSM System by Practicing Psychologists," *Professional Psychology* 12, no. 3 (1981): 385–90.

28. Roel Verheul and Thomas A. Widiger, "A Meta-Analysis of the Prevalence and Usage of the Personality Disorder Not Otherwise Specified (PDNOS) Diagnosis," *Journal of Personality Disorders* 18, no. 4 (2004): 309–19.

29. Christopher G. Fairburn and Kristin Bohn, "Eating Disorder NOS (EDNOS): An Example of the Troublesome 'Not Otherwise Specified' (NOS) Category in DSM-IV," *Behaviour Research and Therapy* 43, no. 6 (2005): 691–701, 693.

30. Harold W. Neighbors et al., "Racial Differences in DSM Diagnosis Using a Semi-Structured Instrument: The Importance of Clinical Judgment in the Diagnosis of African

Americans," *Journal of Health and Social Behavior* 44, no. 3 (2003): 237–56; Marti Loring and Brian Powell, "Gender, Race, and DSM-III: A Study of the Objectivity of Psychiatric Diagnostic Behavior," *Journal of Health and Social Behavior* 29, no. 1 (1988): 1–22.

31. Howard N. Garb, "Race Bias, Social Class Bias, and Gender Bias in Clinical Judgment," *Clinical Psychology: Science and Practice* 4, no. 2 (1997): 99–120.

32. Nicholas A. Christakis, *Death Foretold: Prophecy and Prognosis in Medical Care* (Chicago: University of Chicago, 1999).

33. Luhrmann, *Of Two Minds*, 42.

34. Adrian Angold, quoted in Eliot Marshall, "Duke Study Faults Overuse of Stimulants for Children," *Science* 289, no. 5480 (2000): 721.

35. Susanna N. Visser et al., "Trends in the Parent-Report of Health Care Provider–Diagnosed and Medicated Attention-Deficit/Hyperactivity Disorder: United States, 2003–2011," *Journal of the American Academy of Child and Adolescent Psychiatry* 53, no. 1 (2014): 34–46.e2.

36. Marissa D. King, Jennifer Jennings, and Jason M. Fletcher, "Medical Adaptation to Academic Pressure: Schooling, Stimulant Use, and Socioeconomic Status," *American Sociological Review* 79, no. 6 (2014): 1039–66.

37. Ilina Singh, "Will the 'Real Boy' Please Behave: Dosing Dilemmas for Parents of Boys with ADHD," *American Journal of Bioethics* 5, no. 3 (2005): 34–47.

38. David H. Autor and Mark G. Duggan, "The Growth in the Social Security Disability Rolls: A Fiscal Crisis Unfolding," *Journal of Economic Perspectives* 20, no. 3 (2006): 71–96.

39. Ibid., 79.

40. John Bound, "The Health and Earnings of Rejected Disability Insurance Applicants," *American Economic Review* 79, no. 3 (1989): 482–503; Susan Chen and Wilbert van der Klaauw, "The Work Disincentive Effects of the Disability Insurance Program in the 1990s," *Journal of Econometrics* 142, no. 2 (2008): 757–84.

41. Autor and Duggan, "The Growth in the Social Security Disability Rolls," 93.

42. David H. Autor and Mark G. Duggan, "The Rise in the Disability Rolls and the Decline in Unemployment," *Quarterly Journal of Economics* 118, no. 1 (2003): 157–206.

43. Ibid.

44. Jeannette Rogowski et al., "Final Report for Policy Evaluation of the Effect of the 1996 Welfare Reform Legislation on SSI Benefits for Disabled Children," (Santa Monica, Calif.: RAND Corporation, 2002).

45. Ronald C. Kessler and Richard G. Frank, "The Impact of Psychiatric Disorders on Work Loss Days," *Psychological Medicine* 27, no. 4 (1997): 861–73.

46. Ibid., 870.

47. David Mechanic, Scott Bilder, and Donna D. McAlpine, "Employing Persons with Serious Mental Illness," *Health Affairs* 21, no. 5 (2002): 242–53.

48. David H. Autor, Mark G. Duggan, and David S. Lyle, "Battle Scars? The Puzzling Decline in Employment and Rise in Disability Receipt Among Vietnam Era Veterans," *American Economic Review* 101, no. 3 (2011): 339–44.

49. Eric T. Dean Jr., *Shook Over Hell: Post-Traumatic Stress, Vietnam, and the Civil War* (Cambridge, Mass.: Harvard University Press, 1997).

50. American Psychiatric Association, *Diagnostic and Statistical Manual of Mental Disorders*, 3rd. ed. (Washington, D.C.: American Psychiatric Association, 1980), 238.

51. American Psychiatric Association, *Diagnostic and Statistical Manual of Mental Disorders*, 4th ed. (Washington, D.C.: American Psychiatric Association, 1994), 427.

52. Marilyn Laura Bowman, "Individual Differences in Posttraumatic Distress: Problems with the DSM-IV Model," *Canadian Journal of Psychiatry* 44 (1999): 21–33.

53. Patricia B. Sutker et al., "War Zone Stress, Personal Resources, and PTSD in Persian Gulf War Returnees," *Journal of Abnormal Psychology* 104, no. 3 (1995): 444–52.

54. Metin Basoglu et al., "Psychological Effects of Torture: A Comparison of Tortured with Nontortured Political Activists in Turkey," *American Journal of Psychiatry* 151, no. 1 (1994): 76–81.

55. Bowman, "Individual Differences in Posttraumatic Distress."

56. Lee Hyer et al., "Relationship of Neo-Pi to Personality Styles and Severity of Trauma in Chronic PTSD Victims," *Journal of Clinical Psychology* 50, no. 5 (1994): 699–707.

57. Lauraine Casella and Robert W. Motta, "Comparison of Characteristics of Vietnam Veterans with and Without Posttraumatic Stress Disorder," *Psychological Reports* 67, no. 2 (1990): 595–605.

58. Bowman, "Individual Differences in Posttraumatic Distress."

59. Alex J. Mitchell, Amol Vaze, and Sanjay Rao, "Clinical Diagnosis of Depression in Primary Care: A Meta-Analysis," *The Lancet* 374, no. 9690 (2009): 609–19.

60. H.-U. Wittchen, M. Höfler, and W. Meister, "Prevalence and Recognition of Depressive Syndromes in German Primary Care Settings: Poorly Recognized and Treated?," *International Clinical Psychopharmacology* 16, no. 3 (2001): 121–35.

61. Maria Vuorilehto et al., "Depressive Disorders in Primary Care: Recurrent, Chronic, and Co-Morbid," *Psychological Medicine* 35, no. 5 (2005): 673–82.

62. Nancy S. Kim et al., "The Influence of Framing on Clinicians' Judgments of the Biological Basis of Behaviors," *Journal of Experimental Psychology: Applied* 22, no. 1 (2016): 39–47.

63. Ibid., 4.

64. For example, a good deal of Peter Conrad's review of medicalization as an instrument of social control focuses on the formal diagnostic criteria for assorted psychiatric disorders. Peter Conrad, "Medicalization and Social Control," *Annual Review of Sociology* 18 (1992): 209–32.

65. Mechanic, Bilder, and McAlpine, "Employing Persons with Serious Mental Illness."

6. HOW THE PUBLIC USES DIAGNOSES

1. Allen J. Frances, *Saving Normal: An Insider's Revolt Against Out-of-Control Psychiatric Diagnosis, DSM-5, Big Pharma, and the Medicalization of Ordinary Life* (New York: William Morrow, 2014).

2. Edward Shorter, *From Paralysis to Fatigue: A History of Psychosomatic Illness in the Modern Era* (New York: The Free Press, 1992).

3. Thomas J. Scheff, "The Labelling Theory of Mental Illness," *American Sociological Review* 39, no. 3 (1974): 444–52.

4. See, for example, Danny C. K. Lam, Paul M. Salkovskis, and Lorna I. Hogg, "'Judging a Book by Its Cover': An Experimental Study of the Negative Impact of a Diagnosis of Borderline Personality Disorder on Clinicians' Judgements of Uncomplicated Panic Disorder," *British Journal of Clinical Psychology* (2015), doi:10.1111/bjc.12093.

5. The data are drawn from Bernice A. Pescosolido et al., "'A Disease Like Any Other'? A Decade of Change in Public Reactions to Schizophrenia, Depression, and Alcohol Dependence," *American Journal of Psychiatry* 167, no. 11 (2010): 1321–30.

6. Andrew R. Payton and Peggy A. Thoits, "Medicalization, Direct-to-Consumer Advertising, and Mental Illness Stigma," *Society and Mental Health* 1, no. 1 (2011): 55–70.
7. Paul Meehl, *Psychodiagnosis: Selected Papers* (Minneapolis: University of Minnesota, 1973).
8. Woo-Kyoung Ahn, Laura R. Novick, and Nancy S. Kim, "Understanding Behavior Makes It More Normal," *Psychonomic Bulletin and Review* 10, no. 3 (2003): 746–52.
9. Nancy S. Kim and Stefanie T. LoSavio, "Causal Explanations Affect Judgments of the Need for Psychological Treatment," *Judgment and Decision Making* 4, no. 1 (2009): 82–91.
10. Nancy S. Kim and Woo-kyoung Ahn, "Clinical Psychologists' Theory-Based Representations of Mental Disorders Predict Their Diagnostic Reasoning and Memory," *Journal of Experimental Psychology: General* 131, no. 4 (2002): 451–76.
11. Kristian Pollock, "Maintaining Face in the Presentation of Depression: Constraining the Therapeutic Potential of the Consultation," *Health* 11, no. 2 (2007): 163–80.
12. Richard L. Kravitz et al., "Influence of Patients' Requests for Direct-to-Consumer Advertised Antidepressants," *Journal of the American Medical Association* 293, no. 16 (2005): 1995–2002.
13. R. A. Bell, M. S. Wikes, and R. L. Kravitz, "Advertisement-Induced Prescription Drug Requests: Patients' Anticipated Reactions to a Physician Who Refuses," *Journal of Family Practice* 48(1999): 446–52.
14. Talcott Parsons, *The Social System* (Glencoe, Ill.: The Free Press, 1951).
15. Bernice A. Pescosolido, Steven A. Tuch, and Jack K. Martin, "The Profession of Medicine and the Public: Examining Americans' Changing Confidence in Physician Authority from the Beginning of the 'Health Care Crisis' to the Era of Health Care Reform," *Journal of Health and Social Behavior* 42, no. 1 (2001): 1–16.
16. Scheff, "The Labelling Theory of Mental Illness."
17. Walter R. Gove, "Societal Reaction as an Explanation of Mental Illness: An Evaluation," *American Sociological Review* 35, no. 5 (1970): 873–84.
18. Bruce G. Link et al., "A Modified Labeling Theory Approach to Mental Disorders: An Empirical Assessment," *American Sociological Review* 54, no. 3 (1989): 400–23.
19. Bruce G. Link et al., "On Stigma and Its Consequences: Evidence from a Longitudinal Study of Men with Dual Diagnoses of Mental Illness and Substance Abuse," *Journal of Health and Social Behavior* 38, no. 2 (1997): 177–90; Link et al., "A Modified Labeling Theory Approach to Mental Disorders"; Bruce G. Link et al., "The Social Rejection of Former Mental Patients: Understanding Why Labels Matter," *American Journal of Sociology* 92, no. 6 (1987): 1461–500.
20. Jo C. Phelan et al., "Public Conceptions of Mental Illness in 1950 and 1996: What Is Mental Illness and Is It to Be Feared?," *Journal of Health and Social Behavior* 41 (2000): 188–207.
21. The data are drawn again from, Pescosolido et al., "'A Disease Like Any Other'?"
22. Dorothy Nelkin and M. Susan Lindee, *The DNA Mystique: The Gene as a Cultural Icon* (New York: W. H. Freeman, 1995).
23. Nikolas Rose, *The Politics of Life Itself: Biomedicine, Power, and Subjectivity in the Twenty-First Century* (Princeton, N.J.: Princeton University, 2007).
24. Ibid., 125.
25. Jason Schnittker, "An Uncertain Revolution: Why the Rise of a Genetic Model of Mental Illness Has Not Increased Tolerance," *Social Science and Medicine* 67, no. 9 (2008): 1370–81.
26. Matthew S. Lebowitz and Woo-kyoung Ahn, "Emphasizing Malleability in the Biology of Depression: Durable Effects on Perceived Agency and Prognostic Pessimism," *Behaviour Research and Therapy* 71 (2015): 125–30.

27. Ilan Dar-Nimrod, Miron Zuckerman, and Paul R. Duberstein, "The Effects of Learning About One's Own Genetic Susceptibility to Alcoholism: A Randomized Experiment," *Genetics in Medicine* 15, no. 2 (2013): 132–38.

28. Link et al., "The Social Rejection of Former Mental Patients."

29. Bruce G. Link et al., "On Describing and Seeking to Change the Experience of Stigma," *Psychiatric Rehabilitation Skills* 6, no. 2 (2002): 201–31.

30. Peggy A. Thoits, "Resisting the Stigma of Mental Illness," *Social Psychology Quarterly* 74, no. 1 (2011): 6–28.

31. Sue E. Estroff et al., "Everybody's Got a Little Mental Illness: Accounts of Illness and Self Among People with Severe, Persistent Mental Illnesses," *Medical Anthropology Quarterly* 5, no. 4 (1991): 331–69.

32. Ibid., 363.

33. Ibid., 337.

34. Ibid., 344.

35. Ibid., 349.

36. Adrian Furnham, "Explaining Health and Illness: Lay Perceptions on Current and Future Health, the Causes of Illness, and the Nature of Recovery," *Social Science and Medicine* 39, no. 5 (1994): 715–25; Furnham, "Explaining Health and Illness: Lay Beliefs on the Nature of Health," *Personality and Individual Differences* 17, no. 4 (1994): 455–66; Bernice A. Pescosolido, "The Public Stigma of Mental Illness: What Do We Think; What Do We Know; What Can We Prove?," *Journal of Health and Social Behavior* 54, no. 1 (2013): 1–21.

37. John A. Clausen and Marian Radke Yarrow, "Introduction: Mental Illness and the Family," *Journal of Social Issues* 11, no. 4 (1955): 3–5.

7. HOW SCIENTISTS USE THE *DSM*

1. Steven E. Hyman, "The Diagnosis of Mental Disorders: The Problem of Reification," *Annual Review of Clinical Psychology* 6 (2010): 157, 173.

2. Professional Staff of the U.S.-UK Cross-National Project, "The Diagnosis and Psychopathology of Schizophrenia in New York and London," *Schizophrenia Bulletin* 1, no. 11 (1974): 80–102.

3. Robert Kendell and Assen Jablensky, "Distinguishing Between the Validity and Utility of Psychiatric Diagnoses," *American Journal of Psychiatry* 160, no. 1 (2003): 4–12.

4. Christopher G. Fairburn and Kristin Bohn, "Eating Disorder NOS (EDNOS): An Example of the Troublesome 'Not Otherwise Specified' (NOS) Category in DSM-IV," *Behaviour Research and Therapy* 43, no. 6 (2005): 691–701.

5. David B. Herzog, Julie D. Hopkins, and Craig D. Burns, "A Follow-up Study of Thirty-Three Subdiagnostic Eating Disordered Women," *International Journal of Eating Disorders* 14, no. 3 (1993): 261–67.

6. Christopher G. Fairburn and Paul J. Harrison, "Eating Disorders," *The Lancet* 361, no. 9355 (2003): 407–16.

7. H. A. Pincus, W. W. Davis, and L. E. McQueen, "'Subthreshold' Mental Disorders: A Review and Synthesis of Studies on Minor Depression and Other 'Brand Names,'" *British Journal of Psychiatry* 174, no. 4 (1999): 289.

8. Jay C. Fournier et al., "Antidepressant Drug Effects and Depression Severity," *Journal of the American Medical Association* 303, no. 1 (2010): 47–53.

9. Pincus, Davis, and McQueen, "'Subthreshold' Mental Disorders."

10. Ibid., 294.
11. Scott O. Lilienfeld, Irwin D. Waldman, and Allen C. Israel, "A Critical Examination of the Use of the Term and Concept of Comorbidity in Psychopathology Research," *Clinical Psychology: Science and Practice* 1, no. 1 (1994): 71–83.
12. Timothy A. Brown et al., "Current and Lifetime Comorbidity of the DSM-IV Anxiety and Mood Disorders in a Large Clinical Sample," *Journal of Abnormal Psychology* 110, no. 4 (2001): 585–99.
13. Robert H. Howland et al., "Concurrent Anxiety and Substance Use Disorders Among Outpatients with Major Depression: Clinical Features and Effect on Treatment Outcome," *Drug and Alcohol Dependence* 99, no. 1–3 (2009): 248–60; A. John Rush et al., "Acute and Longer-Term Outcomes in Depressed Outpatients Requiring One or Several Treatment Steps: A Star*D Report," *FOCUS* 6, no. 1 (2008): 128–42.
14. S. Kapur, A. G. Phillips, and T. R. Insel, "Why Has It Taken So Long for Biological Psychiatry to Develop Clinical Tests and What to Do About It?," *Molecular Psychiatry* 17, no. 12 (2012): 1174–79.
15. Ian Smith et al., "Two-Year Follow-up of Trastuzumab After Adjuvant Chemotherapy in HER2-Positive Breast Cancer: A Randomised Controlled Trial," *The Lancet* 369, no. 9555 (2007): 29–36.
16. For a discussion of this broader issue, including this example, see Hyman, "The Diagnosis of Mental Disorders."
17. Stefan Leucht et al., "Second-Generation Versus First-Generation Antipsychotic Drugs for Schizophrenia: A Meta-Analysis," *The Lancet* 373, no. 9657 (2009): 31–41.
18. Richard S. E. Keefe, "Neurocognitive Effects of Antipsychotic Medications in Patients with Chronic Schizophrenia in the CATIE Trial," *Archives of General Psychiatry* 64, no. 6 (2007): 633.
19. Michael Foster Green, "What Are the Functional Consequences of Neurocognitive Deficits in Schizophrenia?," *American Journal of Psychiatry* 153, no. 3 (1996): 321–30.
20. Thomas A. Ban, "The Role of Serendipity in Drug Discovery," *Dialogues in Clinical Neuroscience* 8, no. 3 (2006): 335–44.
21. Steven E. Hyman, "Depression Needs Large Human-Genetics Studies," *Nature* 515 (2014): 189–91.
22. Steven E. Hyman and Wayne S. Fenton, "What Are the Right Targets for Psychopharmacology?," *Science* 299, no. 5605 (2003): 350–51.
23. Steven E. Hyman, "Revolution Stalled," *Science Translational Medicine* 4, no. 155 (2012): 155cm11.
24. Greg Miller, "Is Pharma Running out of Brainy Ideas?," *Science* 329, no. 5991 (2010): 502–4.
25. Hyman, "Revolution Stalled."
26. Kapur, Phillips, and Insel, "Why Has It Taken So Long for Biological Psychiatry to Develop Clinical Tests?"
27. Miller, "Is Pharma Running out of Brainy Ideas?"
28. Ibid.
29. David J. Kupfer, Michael B. First, and Darrel A. Regier, *A Research Agenda for DSM-V* (Washington, D.C.: American Psychiatric Association, 2002).
30. Ibid., xix.
31. Ibid.

32. Jeffrey H. Boyd et al., "Exclusion Criteria of DSM-III: A Study of Co-Occurrence of Hierarchy-Free Syndromes," *Archives of General Psychiatry* 41, no. 10 (1984): 983–89.

33. T. Slade and G. Andrews, "DSM-IV and ICD-10 Generalized Anxiety Disorder: Discrepant Diagnoses and Associated Disability," *Social Psychiatry and Psychiatric Epidemiology* 36, no. 1 (2001): 45–51.

8. HOW CULTURES USE DIAGNOSES

1. Jean-Baptiste Michel et al., "Quantitative Analysis of Culture Using Millions of Digitized Books," *Science* 331, no. 6014 (2011): 176–82.

2. For this history, see Robert L. Spitzer, "The Diagnostic Status of Homosexuality in DSM-III: A Reformulation of the Issues," *American Journal of Psychiatry* 138, no. 2 (1981): 210–15.

3. American Psychiatric Association, *Diagnostic and Statistical Manual of Mental Disorders*, 3rd ed. rev. (Washington, D.C.: American Psychiatric Association, 1987), 296.

4. Ibid., 371.

5. American Psychiatric Association, *Diagnostic and Statistical Manual of Mental Disorders*, 3rd ed. (Washington, D.C.: American Psychiatric Association, 1980), 314.

6. Jonas F. Bakkevig and Sigmund Karterud, "Is the Diagnostic and Statistical Manual of Mental Disorders, Fourth Edition, Histrionic Personality Disorder Category a Valid Construct?," *Comprehensive Psychiatry* 51, no. 5 (2010): 462–70.

7. James W. Pennebaker, Matthias R. Mehl, and Kate G. Niederhoffer, "Psychological Aspects of Natural Language Use: Our Words, Our Selves," *Annual Review of Psychology* 54, no. 1 (2003): 570.

8. James W. Pennebaker, *The Secret Life of Pronouns: What Our Words Say About Us* (New York: Bloomsbury, 2011).

9. THE CONTEMPORARY SCIENCE OF PSYCHIATRIC NOSOLOGY

1. Roger K. Blashfield et al., "The Cycle of Classification: DSM-I through DSM-5," *Annual Review of Clinical Psychology* 10, no. 1 (2014): 25–51.

2. E. Kraepelin and A. R. Diefendorf, *Clinical Psychiatry: A Textbook for Students and Physicians*, 7th ed. (New York: MacMillan, 1907).

3. Patrick F. Sullivan, Mark J. Daly, and Michael O'Donovan, "Genetic Architectures of Psychiatric Disorders: The Emerging Picture and Its Implications," *Nature Reviews Genetics* 13, no. 8 (2012): 537–51.

4. Steven E. Hyman, "Can Neuroscience Be Integrated Into the DSM-V?," *Nature Reviews Neuroscience* 8, no. 9 (2007): 725–32.

5. Irving I. Gottesman, *Schizophrenia Genesis: The Origins of Madness* (New York: Freeman, 1991).

6. Peter Conrad, "Genetic Optimism: Framing Genes and Mental Illness in the News," *Culture, Medicine, and Psychiatry* 25 (2001): 225–47.

7. Kenneth S. Kendler, "'A Gene for . . .': The Nature of Gene Action in Psychiatric Disorders," *American Journal of Psychiatry* 162 (2005): 1243–52.

8. Ibid., 1246.

9. Consortium Schizophrenia Working Group of the Psychiatric Genomics, "Biological Insights from 108 Schizophrenia-Associated Genetic Loci," *Nature* 511, no. 7510 (2014): 421–27.

10. Gwas Consortium Major Depressive Disorder Working Group of the Psychiatric Genomics, "A Mega-Analysis of Genome-Wide Association Studies for Major Depressive Disorder," *Molecular Psychiatry* 18, no. 4 (2013): 497–511.

11. Sadik A. Khuder, "Effect of Cigarette Smoking on Major Histological Types of Lung Cancer: A Meta-Analysis," *Lung Cancer* 31, no. 2–3 (2001): 139–48, 143.

12. Avshalom Caspi et al., "Influence of Life Stress on Depression: Moderation by a Polymorphism in the 5-HTT Gene," *Science* 301 (2003): 386–89.

13. Tyrone D. Cannon and Matthew C. Keller, "Endophenotypes in the Genetic Analyses of Mental Disorders," *Annual Review of Clinical Psychology* 2, no. 1 (2006): 267–90; Irving I. Gottesman and Todd D. Gould, "The Endophenotype Concept in Psychiatry: Etymology and Strategic Intentions," *American Journal of Psychiatry* 160, no. 4 (2003): 636–45.

14. Gregor Hasler et al., "Discovering Endophenotypes for Major Depression," *Neuropsychopharmacology* 29, no. 10 (2004): 1765–81.

15. Gottesman and Gould, "The Endophenotype Concept in Psychiatry."

16. K. S. Kendler et al., "The Structure of Genetic and Environmental Risk Factors for Common Psychiatric and Substance Use Disorders in Men and Women," *Archives of General Psychiatry* 60, no. 9 (2003): 929–37.

17. Francesca Happe, Angelica Ronald, and Robert Plomin, "Time to Give up on a Single Explanation for Autism," *Nature Neuroscience* 9, no. 10 (2006): 1218–20.

18. K. S. Kendler et al., "Major Depression and Generalized Anxiety Disorder: Same Genes, (Partly) Different Environments?," *Archives of General Psychiatry* 49, no. 9 (1992): 716–22.

19. Nick Craddock and Michael J. Owen, "The Kraepelinian Dichotomy—Going, Going . . . but Still Not Gone," *British Journal of Psychiatry* 196, no. 2 (2010): 92–95.

20. Wade Berrettini, "Bipolar Disorder and Schizophrenia," *NeuroMolecular Medicine* 5, no. 1 (2004): 109–17; Craddock and Owen, "The Kraepelinian Dichotomy."

21. Cross-Disorder Group of the Psychiatric Genomics Consortium, "Identification of Risk Loci with Shared Effects on Five Major Psychiatric Disorders: A Genome-Wide Analysis," *The Lancet* 381, no. 9875 (2013): 1371–79.

22. G. S. Malhi and J. Lagopoulos, "Making Sense of Neuroimaging in Psychiatry," *Acta Psychiatrica Scandinavica* 117, no. 2 (2008): 100–17.

23. Tyrone D. Cannon et al., "Cortex Mapping Reveals Regionally Specific Patterns of Genetic and Disease-Specific Gray-Matter Deficits in Twins Discordant for Schizophrenia," *Proceedings of the National Academy of Sciences* 99, no. 5 (2002): 3228–33.

24. Wayne C. Drevets, "Functional Neuroimaging Studies of Depression: The Anatomy of Melancholia," *Annual Review of Medicine* 49, no. 1 (1998): 341–61.

25. Malhi and Lagopoulos, "Making Sense of Neuroimaging in Psychiatry."

26. P. Videbech, "MRI Findings in Patients with Affective Disorder: A Meta-Analysis," *Acta Psychiatrica Scandinavica* 96, no. 3 (1997): 157–68.

27. Tatjana Aue, Leah A. Lavelle, and John T. Cacioppo, "Great Expectations: What Can fMRI Research Tell Us About Psychological Phenomena?," *International Journal of Psychophysiology* 73, no. 1 (2009): 10–16.

28. Malhi and Lagopoulos, "Making Sense of Neuroimaging in Psychiatry."

29. Max Coltheart, "What Has Functional Neuroimaging Told Us About the Mind (So Far)? (Position Paper Presented to the European Cognitive Neuropsychology Workshop, Bressanone, 2005)," *Cortex* 42, no. 3 (2006): 323–31.

30. S. Nassir Ghaemi, *The Concepts of Psychiatry: A Pluralistic Approach to the Mind and Mental Illness* (Baltimore, Md.: Johns Hopkins University Press, 2003).

31. Daniel Dennett, *Consciousness Explained* (Boston: Little, Brown, 1991).

32. Rachel V. Cooper, "Avoiding False Positives: Zones of Rarity, the Threshold Problem, and the DSM Clinical Significance Criterion," *Canadian Journal of Psychiatry* 58, no. 11 (2013): 606–11.

33. Paul E. Meehl, "What's in a Taxon?," *Journal of Abnormal Psychology* 113, no. 1 (2004): 39–43; Paul E. Meehl, "Bootstraps Taxometrics: Solving the Classification Problem in Psychopathology," *American Psychologist* 50, no. 4 (1995): 266–75.

34. Nick Haslam, "Categories Versus Dimensions in Personality and Psychopathology: A Quantitative Review of Taxometric Research," *Psychological Medicine* 42, no. 5 (2012): 903–20.

35. Jean-Pierre Guay, "A Taxometric Analysis of the Latent Structure of Psychopathy: Evidence for Dimensionality," *Journal of Abnormal Psychology* 116, no. 4 (2007): 701–16.

36. Kenneth S. Kendler and Charles O. Gardner Jr., "Twin Studies of Adult Psychiatric and Substance Dependence Disorders: Are They Biased by Differences in the Environmental Experiences of Monozygotic and Dizygotic Twins in Childhood and Adolescence?," *Psychological Medicine* 28 (1998): 625–33.

37. Jason Schnittker, "The Proximity of Common Unhappiness and Misery," *Society and Mental Health* 2, no. 3 (2012): 135–53.

38. Kenneth S. Kendler, Laura M. Thornton, and Charles O. Gardner, "Genetic Risk, Number of Previous Depressive Episodes, and Stressful Life Events in Predicting Onset of Major Depression," *American Journal of Psychiatry* 158 (2001): 582–86.

39. David T. Lykken, *Happiness: What Studies on Twins Show Us About Nature, Nurture, and the Happiness Set Point* (New York: Golden Books, 1999).

40. K. S. Kendler, J. Myers, and L. J. Halberstadt, "Should the Diagnosis of Major Depression Be Made Independent of or Dependent Upon the Psychosocial Context?," *Psychological Medicine* 40, no. 5 (2010): 771–80.

41. Sidney Zisook and Kenneth S. Kendler, "Is Bereavement-Related Depression Different Than Non-Bereavement-Related Depression?," *Psychological Medicine* 37, no. 6 (2007): 779–94; Sidney Zisook, Katherine Shear, and Kenneth S. Kendler, "Validity of the Bereavement Exclusion Criterion for the Diagnosis of Major Depressive Episode," *World Psychiatry* 6, no. 2 (2007): 102–7.

42. Kenneth S. Kendler, John Myers, and Sidney Zisook, "Does Bereavement-Related Major Depression Differ from Major Depression Associated with Other Stressful Life Events?," *American Journal of Psychiatry* 165, no. 11 (2008): 1449–55.

43. Ramin Mojtabai, "Bereavement-Related Depressive Episodes Characteristics, Three-Year Course, and Implications for the DSM-5," *Archives of General Psychiatry* 68, no. 9 (2011): 920.

44. Stephen E. Gilman et al., "Bereavement and the Diagnosis of Major Depressive Episode in the National Epidemiologic Survey on Alcohol and Related Conditions," *Journal of Clinical Psychiatry* 73, no. 2 (2012): 208–15.

45. Stephen E. Gilman et al., "Epidemiologic Evidence Concerning the Bereavement Exclusion in Major Depression," *Archives of General Psychiatry* 69, no. 11 (2012): 1179–81.

46. Ibid., 1179.

47. Jerome C. Wakefield, "The DSM-5 Debate Over the Bereavement Exclusion: Psychiatric Diagnosis and the Future of Empirically Supported Treatment," *Clinical Psychology Review* 33, no. 7 (2013): 825–45.

48. Ibid., 837.

49. Kenneth S. Kendler and Sidney Zisook, "Drs. Kendler and Zisook Reply," *American Journal of Psychiatry* 166, no. 4 (2009): 492–93.

50. J. C. Wakefield et al., "Extending the Bereavement Exclusion for Major Depression to Other Losses: Evidence from the National Comorbidity Survey," *Archives of General Psychiatry* 64, no. 4 (2007): 433–40.

51. This percentage is presented in Wakefield and colleagues' sample-selection flowchart; ibid., 435.

52. Ibid.

53. Sidney Zisook et al., "The Bereavement Exclusion and DSM-5," *Depression and Anxiety* 29, no. 5 (2012): 425–43.

54. American Psychiatric Association, *Diagnostic and Statistical Manual of Mental Disorders*, 5th ed. (Arlington, Va.: American Psychiatric Association, 2013).

55. Ibid., 5.

56. Ibid., 6–10.

57. American Psychiatric Association, "From Planning to Publication: Developing DSM-5" (Washington, D.C., 2013).

58. Ibid., 8.

59. Ibid., 5.

60. Ibid., 9.

61. Ibid., 12.

62. Ibid., 5–6.

63. APA, *DSM-5*, 811.

64. Ibid., 812.

65. Ibid., 813.

66. Ibid., 814.

67. Ibid.

68. Ibid., 155.

69. Ibid., 161.

70. Ibid.

71. Ibid., 5.

72. Ibid.

73. David J. Kupfer and Darrel A. Regier, "Neuroscience, Clinical Evidence, and the Future of Psychiatric Classification in DSM-5," *American Journal of Psychiatry* 168, no. 7 (2011): 672.

74. Kenneth Kendler et al., "Guidelines for Making Changes to DSM-V" (Washington, D.C.: American Psychiatric Association, 2009).

75. APA, *DSM-5*, 20.

76. Ibid., 12.

77. Ibid., 21.

78. Ibid., 13.
79. Helena Chmura Kraemer, "DSM Categories and Dimensions in Clinical and Research Contexts," *International Journal of Methods in Psychiatric Research* 16, no. S1 (2007): S8–S15, 264.

10. THE ENDLESS SEARCH FOR VALIDITY

1. Rachel V. Cooper, "Avoiding False Positives: Zones of Rarity, the Threshold Problem, and the DSM Clinical Significance Criterion," *Canadian Journal of Psychiatry* 58, no. 11 (2013): 606–11, 162.
2. For an example of this, see evidence linking advanced parental age and de novo mutations in the case of autism among children. Ka-Yuet Liu, Marissa King, and Peter S. Bearman, "Social Influence and the Autism Epidemic," *American Journal of Sociology* 115, no. 5 (2010): 1387–434.
3. Robert Kendell and Assen Jablensky, "Distinguishing Between the Validity and Utility of Psychiatric Diagnoses," *American Journal of Psychiatry* 160, no. 1 (2003): 4–12.
4. E. G. Boring, "Intelligence as the Tests Test It," *New Republic* 35 (1923): 35–37, 35.
5. Allan V. Horwitz and Jerome C. Wakefield, *The Loss of Sadness: How Psychiatry Transformed Normal Sorrow Into Depressive Disorder* (New York: Oxford University Press, 2007).
6. Ibid., 216, 111, 12, 213, and 9 and 117 for "obvious."
7. Ibid., 14, 90.
8. Robert L. Spitzer, "Values and Assumptions in the Development of DSM-III and DSM-III-R: An Insider's Perspective and a Belated Response to Sadler, Hulgus, and Agich's 'On Values in Recent American Psychiatric Classification,'" *Journal of Nervous and Mental Disease* 189 (2001): 351–59, 353.
9. Kendell and Jablensky, "Distinguishing Between the Validity and Utility of Psychiatric Diagnoses."
10. Ibid., 4.
11. Kenneth S. Kendler, "Toward a Scientific Psychiatric Nosology: Strengths and Limitations," *Archives of General Psychiatry* 47, no. 10 (1990): 969.
12. Eli Robins and Samuel B. Guze, "Establishment of Diagnostic Validity in Psychiatric Illness: Its Application to Schizophrenia," *American Journal of Psychiatry* 126, no. 7 (1970): 983–87.
13. Kenneth S. Kendler, "A History of the DSM-5 Scientific Review Committee," *Psychological Medicine* 43, no. 9 (2013): 1793–800.
14. Nancy C. Andreasen, "The Validation of Psychiatric Diagnosis: New Models and Approaches," *American Journal of Psychiatry* 152, no. 2 (1995): 161–62.
15. Ibid., 162.
16. Ibid.
17. Ibid.
18. For this distinction, see Scott O. Lilienfeld and Lori Marino, "Essentialism Revisited: Evolutionary Theory and the Concept of Mental Disorder," *Journal of Abnormal Psychology* 108, no. 3 (1999): 400–11.
19. Jeremy Freese, "Genetics and the Social Science Explanation of Individual Outcomes," *American Journal of Sociology* 114 (2008): S1–S35.

20. Kenneth S. Kendler, "Reflections on the Relationship Between Psychiatric Genetics and Psychiatric Nosology," *American Journal of Psychiatry* 163, no. 7 (2006): 1138–46.

21. Paul W. Andrews and J. Anderson Thomson Jr., "The Bright Side of Being Blue: Depression as an Adaptation for Analyzing Complex Problems," *Psychological Review* 116, no. 3 (2009): 620–54.

22. Scott O. Lilienfeld and Lori Marino, "Mental Disorder as a Roschian Concept: A Critique of Wakefield's 'Harmful Dysfunction' Analysis," *Journal of Abnormal Psychology* 104, no. 3 (1995): 411–20.

23. Stephen Jay Gould and Elisabeth S. Vrba, "Exaptation—A Missing Term in the Science of Form," *Paleobiology* 8, no. 1 (1982): 4–15.

24. Stephen Jay Gould, "Exaptation: A Crucial Tool for an Evolutionary Psychology," *Journal of Social Issues* 47, no. 3 (1991): 43–65.

25. Horwitz and Wakefield, *The Loss of Sadness*, esp. 51, 123, 33.

26. Michael D. Sockol, David A. Raichlen, and Herman Pontzer, "Chimpanzee Locomotor Energetics and the Origin of Human Bipedalism," *Proceedings of the National Academy of Sciences* 104, no. 30 (2007): 12265–69.

27. Daniel Nettle, "The Evolution of Personality Variation in Humans and Other Animals," *American Psychologist* 61, no. 6 (2006): 622–31.

28. Lawrence H. Cohen, Lynn C. Towbes, and Regina Flocco, "Effects of Induced Mood on Self-Reported Life Events and Perceived and Received Social Support," *Journal of Personality and Social Psychology* 55, no. 4 (1988): 669–74.

29. Kendler, "Toward a Scientific Psychiatric Nosology."

30. Michael S. McCabe et al., "Symptom Differences in Schizophrenia with Good and Poor Prognosis," *American Journal of Psychiatry* 128, no. 10 (1972): 1239–43.

31. Patrick F. Sullivan, Mark J. Daly, and Michael O'Donovan, "Genetic Architectures of Psychiatric Disorders: The Emerging Picture and Its Implications," *Nature Reviews Genetics* 13, no. 8 (2012): 537–51.

32. Ibid.

33. Norman Sartorius, "Disability and Mental Illness Are Different Entities and Should Be Assessed Separately," *World Psychiatry* 8, no. 2 (2009): 86–86.

34. Freud appears not to have said this directlly, although the statement is often attributed to him, and the idea is implied in some of his work, especially Sigmund Freud, *Civilization and Its Discontents* (New York: Norton, 1961).

35. Jürgen Rehm et al., "On the Development and Psychometric Testing of the WHO Screening Instrument to Assess Disablement in the General Population," *International Journal of Methods in Psychiatric Research* 8, no. 2 (1999): 110–22.

36. J. Ormel et al., "Common Mental Disorders and Disability Across Cultures: Results from the WHO Collaborative Study on Psychological Problems in General Health Care," *Journal of the American Medical Association* 272, no. 22 (1994): 1741–48.

37. Ronald C. Kessler and Richard G. Frank, "The Impact of Psychiatric Disorders on Work Loss Days," *Psychological Medicine* 27, no. 4 (1997): 861–73.

38. Dominic P. Murphy, "Levels of Explanation in Psychiatry," in *Philosophical Issues in Psychiatry I: Explanation, Phenomenology, and Nosology*, ed. Kenneth S. Kendler and Josef Parnas (Baltimore, Md.: Johns Hopkins University Press, 2008).

39. Gregor Hasler et al., "Discovering Endophenotypes for Major Depression," *Neuropsychopharmacology* 29, no. 10 (2004): 1765–81.

40. S. R. Chamberlain et al., "The Neuropsychology of Obsessive Compulsive Disorder: The Importance of Failures in Cognitive and Behavioural Inhibition as Candidate Endophenotypic Markers," *Neuroscience and Biobehavioral Reviews* 29, no. 3 (2005): 399–419.

41. Jonathan Flint and Marcus R. Munafò, "The Endophenotype Concept in Psychiatric Genetics," *Psychological Medicine* 37, no. 2 (2007): 163–80.

42. Ibid.

43. Kenneth S. Kendler and Peter Zachar, "The Incredible Insecurity of Psychiatric Nosology," in *Philosophical Issues in Psychiatry*, ed. Kenneth S. Kendler and Josef Parnas (Baltimore, Md.: Johns Hopkins University Press, 2008).

44. Kendler and Zachar attribute this idea to S. D. Mitchell, *Biological Complexity and Integrative Pluralism* (Cambridge: Cambridge University Press, 2003).

45. William E. Schlenger et al., "Psychological Reactions to Terrorist Attacks: Findings from the National Study of Americans' Reactions to September 11," *Journal of the American Medical Association* 288, no. 5 (2002): 581–88.

46. Roxane Cohen Silver et al., "Mental- and Physical-Health Effects of Acute Exposure to Media Images of the September 11, 2001, Attacks and the Iraq War," *Psychological Science* 24, no. 9 (2013): 1623–34.

47. Edgar Jones and Simon Wessely, *Shell Shock to PTSD: Military Psychiatry from 1900 to the Gulf War* (Hove: Psychology Press, 2006); Edgar Jones et al., "Flashbacks and Post-Traumatic Stress Disorder: The Genesis of a Twentieth-Century Diagnosis," *British Journal of Psychiatry* 182, no. 2 (2003): 158–63.

48. Jones et al., "Flashbacks and Post-Traumatic Stress Disorder," 163.

49. Richard J. McNally, "Progress and Controversy in the Study of Posttraumatic Stress Disorder," *Annual Review of Psychology* 54, no. 1 (2003): 229–52.

50. American Psychiatric Association, *Diagnostic and Statistical Manual of Mental Disorders*, 3rd ed. (Washington, D.C.: American Psychiatric Association, 1980), 236.

51. American Psychiatric Association, *Diagnostic and Statistical Manual of Mental Disorders*, 4th ed. (Washington, D.C.: American Psychiatric Association, 1994).

52. Naomi Breslau and Ronald C. Kessler, "The Stressor Criterion in DSM-IV Posttraumatic Stress Disorder: An Empirical Investigation," *Biological Psychiatry* 50, no. 9 (2001): 699–704, 701.

53. Ibid., 702.

54. Pamela K. Keel and Kelly L. Klump, "Are Eating Disorders Culture-Bound Syndromes? Implications for Conceptualizing Their Etiology," *Psychological Bulletin* 129, no. 5 (2003): 747–69.

55. Ethan Watters, *Crazy Like Us: The Globalization of the American Psyche* (New York: Simon and Schuster, 2011).

56. Shan Guisinger, "Adapted to Flee Famine: Adding an Evolutionary Perspective on Anorexia Nervosa," *Psychological Review* 110, no. 4 (2003): 745–61.

57. Joel Gold and Ian Gold, "The 'Truman Show' Delusion: Psychosis in the Global Village," *Cognitive Neuropsychiatry* 17, no. 6 (2012): 455–72.

58. Ian Hacking, *Mad Travelers: Reflections on the Reality of Transient Mental Illnesses* (Cambridge, Mass.: Harvard University, 1998).

59. Ma-Li Wong and Julio Licinio, "Research and Treatment Approaches to Depression," *Nature Reviews Neuroscience* 2, no. 5 (2001): 343–51.

60. Jan M. Deussing, "Animal Models of Depression," *Drug Discovery Today: Disease Models* 3, no. 4 (2006): 375–83.

61. M. R. Delgado, A. Olsson, and E. A. Phelps, "Extending Animal Models of Fear Conditioning to Humans," *Biological Psychology* 73, no. 1 (2006): 39–48.

62. Paul M. Plotsky and Michael J. Meaney, "Early, Postnatal Experience Alters Hypothalamic Corticotropin-Releasing Factor (CRF) mRNA, Median Eminence CRF Content and Stress-Induced Release in Adult Rats," *Molecular Brain Research* 18, no. 3 (1993): 195–200.

63. Josef Parnas, Louis A. Sass, and Dan Zahavi, "Rediscovering Psychopathology: The Epistemology and Phenomenology of the Psychiatric Object," *Schizophrenia Bulletin* 39, no. 2 (2013): 270–77.

64. M. Cermolacce, L. Sass, and J. Parnas, "What Is Bizarre in Bizarre Delusions? A Critical Review," *Schizophrenia Bulletin* 36, no. 4 (2010): 667–79.

65. Adrian M. Owen, "Detecting Consciousness: A Unique Role for Neuroimaging," *Annual Review of Psychology* 64, no. 1 (2013): 109–33.

66. Parnas, Sass, and Zahavi, "Rediscovering Psychopathology," 274.

67. Josef Parnas and Pierre Bovet, "Psychiatry Made Easy: Operationalism and Some of Its Consequences," in *Philosophical Issues in Psychiatry III*, ed. Kenneth S. Kendler and Josef Parnas (New York: Oxford University Press, 2014).

68. D. J. Chalmers, "Facing up to the Problem of Consciousness," *Journal of Consciousness Studies* 2, no. 3 (1995): 200–19.

69. John Searle remains optimistic about the scientific study of consciousness, although he catalogues the complexities of the endeavor. John R. Searle, "How to Study Consciousness Scientifically," *Philosophical Transactions: Biological Sciences* 353, no. 1377 (1998): 1935–42.

70. Ibid., 1941.

71. Alva Noë, *Out of Our Heads: Why You Are Not Your Brain, and Other Lessons from the Biology of Consciousness* (New York: Farrar, Straus and Giroux, 2009).

72. J. Levine, "Materialism and Qualia: The Explanatory Gap," *Pacific Philosophical Quarterly* 64 (1983): 354–61.

73. Eric A. Storch, Jonathan Abramowitz, and Wayne K. Goodman, "Where Does Obsessive-Compulsive Disorder Belong in DSM-V?," *Depression and Anxiety* 25, no. 4 (2008): 336–47.

74. John Dupré, "Scientific Classification," *Theory, Culture, and Society* 23, no. 2–3 (2006): 30–32; John Dupré, "On the Impossibility of a Monistic Account of Species," in *Species: New Interdisciplinary Essays*, ed. R. A. Wilson (Cambridge, Mass.: MIT Press, 1999).

75. D. L. Hull, "The Ontological Status of Species as Evolutionary Units," in *Philosophy of Biology*, ed. M. Ruse (New York: Macmillan, 1989), 174.

76. Dupré, "Scientific Classification," 206.

77. Ernst Mayr, *Systematics and the Origin of Species from the Viewpoint of a Zoologist* (New York: Columbia University Press, 1942).

78. Dupré, "Scientific Classification."

79. Dupré, "On the Impossibility of a Monistic Account of Species," 18.

80. Allen J. Frances, "DSM in Philosophyland: Curiouser and Curiouser," in *Making the DSM-5*, ed. Joel Paris and James Phillips (New York: Springer, 2013), 100.

81. Leda Cosmides and John Tooby, "Toward an Evolutionary Taxonomy of Treatable Conditions," *Journal of Abnormal Psychology* 108, no. 3 (1999): 453–64.

82. Samuel Cartwright, "Diseases and Peculiarities of the Negro Race," *DeBow's Review* 11 (1851).

83. Jerome C. Wakefield, "The DSM-5 Debate Over the Bereavement Exclusion: Psychiatric Diagnosis and the Future of Empirically Supported Treatment," *Clinical Psychology Review* 33, no. 7 (2013): 825–45, 840.

84. B. Timothy Walsh et al., "Placebo Response in Studies of Major Depression: Variable, Substantial, and Growing," *Journal of the American Medical Association* 287, no. 14 (2002): 1840–47.

85. S. Leucht et al., "How Effective Are Second-Generation Antipsychotic Drugs? A Meta-Analysis of Placebo-Controlled Trials," *Molecular Psychiatry* 14, no. 4 (2008): 429–47.

86. Alexander H. A. Tuttle et al., "Increasing Placebo Responses Over Time in U.S. Clinical Trials of Neuropathic Pain," *Pain* 156, no. 12 (2015): 2616–26.

87. Raúl de la Fuente-Fernández et al., "Expectation and Dopamine Release: Mechanism of the Placebo Effect in Parkinson's Disease," *Science* 293, no. 5532 (2001): 1164–66.

88. A. Pollo et al., "Placebo Analgesia and the Heart," *Pain* 102, no. 1–2 (2003): 125–33.

89. F. Benedetti et al., "Conscious Expectation and Unconscious Conditioning in Analgesic, Motor, and Hormonal Placebo/Nocebo Responses," *Journal of Neuroscience* 23, no. 10 (2003): 4315–23.

90. Damien G. Finniss et al., "Biological, Clinical, and Ethical Advances of Placebo Effects," *The Lancet* 375, no. 9715: 686–695.

91. Richard J. McNally, *What Is Mental Illness?* (Cambridge, Mass.: Harvard University Press, 2011), 69.

92. Barbara L. Andersen, "Primary Orgasmic Dysfunction: Diagnostic Considerations and Review of Treatment," *Psychological Bulletin* 93, no. 1 (1983): 105–36; W. H. Masters and V. E. Johnson, *Human Sexual Inadequacy* (Boston: Little Brown, 1970).

93. Barbara L. Andersen, "A Comparison of Systematic Desensitization and Directed Masturbation in the Treatment of Primary Orgasmic Dysfunction in Females," *Journal of Consulting and Clinical Psychology* 49, no. 4 (1981): 568–70.

94. Joseph LoPiccolo and W. Charles Lobitz, "The Role of Masturbation in the Treatment of Orgasmic Dysfunction," *Archives of Sexual Behavior* 2, no. 2 (1972): 163–71.

95. Jerome Wakefield, "Female Primary Orgasmic Dysfunction: Masters and Johnson Versus DSM-III-R on Diagnosis and Incidence," *Journal of Sex Research* 24(1988): 363–77.

96. Ibid., 363.

97. APA, *DSM-III*, 279.

98. Kenneth S. Kendler et al., "Issues for DSM-V: DSM-V Should Include a Conceptual Issues Work Group," *American Journal of Psychiatry* 165, no. 2 (2008): 174–75.

99. Ibid., 174.

100. John Dupré, "In Defence of Classification," *Studies in History and Philosophy of Science Part C: Studies in History and Philosophy of Biological and Biomedical Sciences* 32, no. 2 (2001): 203–19. For a discussion of this issue as it is applied to psychiatric disorders, see Peter Zachar and Kenneth S. Kendler, "Psychiatric Disorders: A Conceptual Taxonomy," *American Journal of Psychiatry* 164, no. 4 (2007): 557–65.

11. THE ENDURANCE OF THE DIAGNOSTIC SYSTEM

1. Robert L. Spitzer, "Psychiatric Diagnosis: Are Clinicians Still Necessary?," *Comprehensive Psychiatry* 24 (1983): 399–411, 312.

2. Mark Nichter, "Idioms of Distress Revisited," *Culture, Medicine, and Psychiatry* 34, no. 2 (2010): 401–16.

3. David Mechanic, "The Concept of Illness Behavior," *Journal of Chronic Diseases* 15, no. 2 (1962): 189–94.

4. Laurence J. Kirmayer, "Cultural Variations in the Response to Psychiatric Disorders and Emotional Distress," *Social Science and Medicine* 29, no. 3 (1989): 327–39.

5. Robert A. Aronowitz, "The Converged Experience of Risk and Disease," *Milbank Quarterly* 87, no. 2 (2009): 417–42.

6. Lisa M. Schwartz et al., "Enthusiasm for Cancer Screening in the United States," *Journal of the American Medical Association* 291, no. 1 (2004): 71–78.

7. Aronowitz, "The Converged Experience of Risk and Disease."

8. Ronald C. Kessler, "The Effects of Stressful Life Events on Depression," *Annual Review of Psychology* 48 (1997): 191–214.

9. A. Banerjee, S. L. Jadhav, and J. S. Bhawalkar, "Probability, Clinical Decision Making, and Hypothesis Testing," *Industrial Psychiatry Journal* 18, no. 1 (2009): 64–69.

10. S. Nassir Ghaemi, *The Concepts of Psychiatry: A Pluralistic Approach to the Mind and Mental Illness* (Baltimore, Md.: Johns Hopkins University Press, 2003).

11. Jerome C. Wakefield, "High Mental Disorder Rates Are Based on Invalid Measures: Questions About the Claimed Ubiquity of Mutation-Induced Dysfunction," *Behavioral and Brain Sciences* 29, no. 4 (2006): 424–26.

12. Douglas Porter, "Establishing Normative Validity for Scientific Psychiatric Nosology: The Significance of Integrating Patient Perspectives," in *Making the DSM-5: Concepts and Controversies*, ed. Joel Paris and James Philips (New York: Springer, 2013).

13. Elizabeth H. Flanagan, Larry Davidson, and John S. Strauss, "The Need for Patient-Subjective Data in the DSM and the ICD," *Psychiatry: Interpersonal and Biological Processes* 73, no. 4 (2010): 297–307.

14. Larry Davidson and David Stayner, "Loss, Loneliness, and the Desire for Love: Perspectives on the Social Lives of People with Schizophrenia," *Psychiatric Rehabilitation Journal* 20, no. 3 (1997): 3–12.

15. Larry Davidson, *Living Outside Mental Illness: Qualitative Studies of Recovery in Schizophrenia* (New York: New York University, 2003).

16. Bruce Cuthbert and Thomas Insel, "The Data of Diagnosis: New Approaches to Psychiatric Classification," *Psychiatry: Interpersonal and Biological Processes* 73, no. 4 (2010): 311–14.

17. Ibid., 312.

18. Ibid.

19. Ibid.

20. American Psychiatric Association, *Diagnostic and Statistical Manual of Mental Disorders*, 5th ed. (Arlington, Va.: American Psychiatric Association, 2013), 20.

21. Peter Conrad, "Medicalization and Social Control," *Annual Review of Sociology* 18 (1992): 209–32.

22. Edward Shorter, *From Paralysis to Fatigue: A History of Psychosomatic Illness in the Modern Era* (New York: The Free Press, 1992).

23. Ibid., 295.

24. Gerald L. Klerman and Myrna M. Weissman, "Increasing Rates of Depression," *Journal of the American Medical Association* 261, no. 15 (1989): 2229–35.

25. Jean M. Twenge, "The Age of Anxiety? The Birth Cohort Change in Anxiety and Neuroticism, 1952–1993," *Journal of Personality and Social Psychology* 79, no. 6 (2000): 1007–21.

26. Joel Lexchin et al., "Pharmaceutical Industry Sponsorship and Research Outcome and Quality: Systematic Review," *British Medical Journal* 326 (2003): 1167–70.

27. Shorter, *From Paralysis to Fatigue.*

28. Ibid., x.

29. E. J. M. Campbell, J. G. Scadding, and R. S. Roberts, "The Concept of Disease," *British Medical Journal* 2, no. 6193 (1979): 757–62.

30. For an endorsement of RDoC see, David J. Kupfer and Darrel A. Regier, "Neuroscience, Clinical Evidence, and the Future of Psychiatric Classification in DSM-5," *American Journal of Psychiatry* 168, no. 7 (2011): 672–74.

31. APA, *DSM-5*, xii.

32. This distinction was emphasized by Claire Pouncey and elaborated by James Phillips. See Claire Pouncey, "The Six Most Essential Questions in Psychiatric Diagnosis: A Pluralogue, Mental Disorders, Like Diseases, Are Constructs, So What?," *Philosophy, Ethics, and Humanities in Medicine* 7, no. 3 (2012): 6–7; James Phillips, "The Conceptual Status of DSM-5 Diagnoses," in *Making the DSM-5: Concepts and Controversies*, ed. Joel Paris and James Phillips (New York: Springer, 2013).

INDEX

addiction, and diagnostic criteria, 6

adjustment disorders, prescribing rates for, 151

adjustment-related problems, in children, 45–46

advertising, pharmaceutical, direct-to-consumer, 147, 276. *See also* pharmaceuticals

affective disorders, in *DSM-II*, 21

African Americans, 127

aging, and onset of psychiatric disorders, 70

Ahn, Woo-kyoung, 113, 114

alcohol abuse, 10, 158–159

alcohol dependence: in GSS, 145, 146 table; and social distance, 157 table, 158

alcoholism: endophenotype associated with, 258; and psychiatric disorders, 42

Alzheimer's disease, 106

American culture, antiauthoritarian streak in, 27

American Psychiatric Association (APA), 291; and *DSM* limitations, 176; on homosexuality, 29, 35, 184, 186

Andreasen, Nancy, 244–245

Andrews, G., 177

Andrews, Paul, 249

anger, and use of labels, 161

animals, study of depression in, 265–266

anorexia, 113, 114, 126, 170; and cultural considerations, 261

antidepressants: and comorbidity, 172; responses to, 274; use of, 14

antidepressants, name-brand, in treatment-seeking behavior, 150

antisocial personality, in male patients, 127

anxiety: in early *DSM* editions, 46; endophenotype associated with, 258; normal, 224; symptoms of, 97 fig., 99; use of term, 201

"anxiety attack," in *DSM* lexicon, 192 fig., 193

anxiety disorders: age of onset for, 69–70; comorbidity with, 64; and conditionalities, 258; in *DSM* lexicon, 189–190, 189f, 191, 192 fig., 193; global prevalence of, 72–74, 73 table; increase in, 297–298; medication for, 124; misclassification of, 233; prevalence of, 61 table, 62; public's view of, 294; severity of, 66 table. *See also* generalized anxiety disorder

"anxiety symptoms," in *DSM* lexicon, 191, 192 fig., 193

Aronowitz, Robert, 286

articles (of speech), in *DSM* lexicon, 194, 195

association studies, genome-wide, 214

AstraZeneca, 174

attention deficit/hyperactivity disorder (ADHD): *DSM-IV* criteria for, 91–92; in *DSM* lexicon, 185 fig., 187–188; endophenotype associated with, 258; filling prescriptions for, 129–130; institutional pressures on diagnosis of, 128–134; parents of children diagnosed with, 131; prevalence of, 298; seeking